The Science of Climbing and Mountaineering

This is the first book to explore in-depth the science of climbing and mountaineering. Written by a team of leading international sport scientists, clinicians and climbing practitioners, it covers the full span of technical disciplines, including rock climbing, ice climbing, indoor climbing and mountaineering, across all scientific fields from physiology and biomechanics to history, psychology, medicine, motor control, skill acquisition and engineering.

Striking a balance between theory and practice, this unique interdisciplinary study provides practical examples and illustrative data to demonstrate the strategies that can be adopted to promote safety, injury prevention, recovery and mental preparation. Divided into six parts, the book covers all essential aspects of the culture and science of climbing and mountaineering, including:

- physiology and medicine
- biomechanics
- motor control and learning
- psychology
- equipment, technology and safety devices.

Showcasing the latest cutting-edge research and demonstrating how science translates into practice, *The Science of Climbing and Mountaineering* is essential reading for all advanced students and researchers of sport science, biomechanics and skill acquisition, as well as all active climbers and adventure sport coaches.

Ludovic Seifert is Professor at the Faculty of Sport Sciences at the University of Rouen in France. He gained a PhD in expertise and coordination dynamics in swimming at the University of Rouen in 2003, then a certification to supervise research in 2010. He conducts his research in the field of motor learning and motor control. He is a mountain guide certified by IFMGA.

Peter Wolf studied sports engineering at the Chemnitz University of Technology, Germany, and carried out his PhD thesis on foot biomechanics at the Institute for Biomechanics, ETH Zurich, Switzerland. For the last few years, he has been the Scientific Coordinator of the SMS-Lab, ETH Zurich. His research interests include (i) the design of sport simulators in virtual environments, (ii) the development of devices measuring performance in sports and motor learning and (iii) the establishment of augmented, real-time feedback displays facilitating motor learning of complex tasks.

Andreas Schweizer is Deputy Head of Hand Surgery at the Balgrist University Hospital, Zurich, Switzerland. He is adept in wrist surgery, surgery on peripheral nerves, surgical treatment of hand fractures, ultrasound on the hand, and 3D computer aided analysis of malunions. Currently, he is also the medical advisor for the technical committee of the Swiss Alpine Club.

Routledge Research in Sport and Exercise Science

The *Routledge Research in Sport and Exercise Science* series is a showcase for cutting-edge research from across the sport and exercise sciences, including physiology, psychology, biomechanics, motor control, physical activity and health, and every core sub-discipline. Featuring the work of established and emerging scientists and practitioners from around the world, and covering the theoretical, investigative and applied dimensions of sport and exercise, this series is an important channel for new and ground-breaking research in the human movement sciences.

Available in this series:

Complex Systems in Sport
Edited by Keith Davids, Robert Hristovski, Duarte Araújo, Natalia Balague Serre, Chris Button and Pedro Passos

Mixed Methods Research in the Movement Sciences
Case Studies in Sport, Physical Education and Dance
Edited by Oleguer Camerino, Marta Castaner and Teresa M Anguera

Eccentric Exercise
Physiology and Application in Sport and Rehabilitation
Hans Hoppeler

Computer Science in Sport
Research and Practice
Edited by Arnold Baca

Life Story Research in Sport
Understanding the Experiences of Elite and Professional Athletes through Narrative
Kitrina Douglas and David Carless

The Psychology of Doping in Sport
Edited by Vassilis Barkoukis, Lambros Lazuras and Haralambos Tsorbatzoudis

Detecting Doping in Sport
Stephen Moston and Terry Engelberg

The Science of Climbing and Mountaineering

Edited by Ludovic Seifert, Peter Wolf and Andreas Schweizer

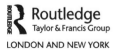
Routledge
Taylor & Francis Group

LONDON AND NEW YORK

First published 2017
by Routledge
2 Park Square, Milton Park, Abingdon, Oxon OX14 4RN

and by Routledge
711 Third Avenue, New York, NY 10017

First issued in paperback 2018

Routledge is an imprint of the Taylor & Francis Group, an informa business

British Library Cataloguing-in-Publication Data
A catalogue record for this book is available from the British Library

Library of Congress Cataloging in Publication Data
A catalog record for this book has been requested

ISBN 13: 978-1-138-59523-1 (pbk)
ISBN 13: 978-1-138-92758-2 (hbk)

Typeset in Times New Roman
by HWA Text and Data Management, London

Contents

List of figures   viii
List of tables   xii
List of contributors   xiii
Preface   xvii
LUDOVIC SEIFERT, PETER WOLF AND ANDREAS SCHWEIZER

1 A cultural history of mountaineering and climbing   1
OLIVIER HOIBIAN

PART I
Physiology   17

2 Physiology of climbing   19
LUISA GILES AND JASON BRANDENBURG

3 Economy in difficult rock climbing   48
PHILLIP (PHIL) B. WATTS

PART II
Medicine   57

4 Sport climbing related injuries and overuse syndromes   59
VOLKER RAINER SCHÖFFL AND ANDREAS SCHWEIZER

5 High altitude medicine and cold effects in mountaineering   76
JEAN PAUL RICHALET AND EMMANUEL CAUCHY

6 Hypoxic training   91
GRÉGOIRE MILLET AND OLIVIER GIRARD

PART III
Biomechanics   **109**

7   Postural regulation and motion simulation in rock climbing   111
    FRANCK QUAINE, LIONEL REVERET, SIMON COURTEMANCHE
    AND PAUL G. KRY

8   Grip capabilities of climbers' hands and fingers   129
    LAURENT VIGOUROUX

9   Muscular strength and endurance in climbers   147
    JIŘÍ BALÁŠ

10 Biomechanics of ice tool swinging movement   164
    ANNIE ROUARD, THOMAS ROBERT AND LUDOVIC SEIFERT

PART IV
Motor control and learning   **179**

11 How expert climbers use perception and action during
    successful climbing performance   181
    LUDOVIC SEIFERT, DOMINIC ORTH, CHRIS BUTTON
    AND KEITH DAVIDS

12 What current research tells us about skill acquisition
    in climbing   196
    DOMINIC ORTH, CHRIS BUTTON, KEITH DAVIDS
    AND LUDOVIC SEIFERT

13 Visual-motor skill in climbing   210
    CHRIS BUTTON, DOMINIC ORTH, KEITH DAVIDS
    AND LUDOVIC SEIFERT

PART V
Psychology   **225**

14 Climbing grades: Systems and subjectivity   227
    NICK DRAPER

15 Psychological processes in the sport of climbing 244
   GARETH JONES AND XAVIER SANCHEZ

16 Exposure and engagement in mountaineering 257
   ERIC BRYMER AND ERIK MONASTERIO

PART VI
Equipment, technology and safety devices in climbing **267**

17 The engineering of climbing equipment 269
   FRANZ KONSTANTIN FUSS AND PETER WOLF

18 Simul-climbing progression and falls analysis 282
   PHILIPPE BATOUX

   Index 301

Figures

1.1 Social field of outdoor activities   14

3.1 Line of Motion and Geometric Entropy (GE) for the same climber during an on-sight ascent (A1) and the ninth ascent (A9) of the same route   54

4.1 Typical full crimp grip position (a) to hold a small ledge   61

4.2 Finger flexor tendon sheath   62

4.3 Lumbrical tears happen most often between the middle/ring and the ring/small fingers where the two heads of the common lumbrical muscle belly   64

4.4 High load to finger bones leading to impressive increase of cortical thickness of the middle and distal phalanx   65

4.5 Epiphyseal fractures at the base of the middle phalanx due to crimp grip position in a 14-year-old climber   66

4.6 Proximal biceps femoris tendon/muscle avulsion injury during a foot-hook pull   69

4.7 The shoe size reduction forces the foot to conform to the shoe and changes the biomechanical position of the foot within the shoe   71

5.1 Grading severity of frostbite and bone amputation risk after rewarming   84

5.2 First-degree frostbite: no lesion after rapid rewarming   85

5.3 Third-degree frostbite: lesions with hemorrhagic blisters on intermediate and distal phalanges   85

5.4 Fourth-degree with extended lesions up to carpus   86

5.5 Late stage necrosis of the thumb   86

6.1 Panorama of the different hypoxic/altitude training methods used by athletes in the late 2000s   93

6.2 Panorama of the different hypoxic/altitude training methods used by athletes in 2015   94

6.3 Nightly pattern of A) breathing frequency, and B) O2 saturation (SpO_2) in 'real altitude' (HH) versus 'simulated altitude' (NH) at 2250 m during 18 days of LHTL training   96

6.4 Effect of pre-acclimatization on performance   97

6.5   Change in 3 km running time trial performance and in maximal
      oxygen consumption (ΔVO_{2max})   99
7.1   Typical force variations following a right-foot release in the
      imposed position   116
7.2   Schematic representation of the moments at work in a vertical and
      an overhanging posture   118
7.3   The instrumented bouldering wall used for the data capture   121
7.4   Results for average prediction of contact forces along each
      sequence of 15 performers as percentage of body mass with 95 per
      cent confidence interval   122
7.5   Contact force prediction with no constraint on ankle joint torques   123
7.6   Sensibility analysis for timing prediction   125
7.7   Timing optimization for a large climbing wall, and the given
      input poses   126
8.1   Illustration of the slope (a), half crimp (b) and full crimp (c) grip
      techniques used in rock climbing   131
8.2   Experimental devices used in Vigouroux et al. (2005) and
      Philippe et al. (2012)   132
8.3   A: Mean maximum vertical force (N) and standard deviation
      according to the hold depth with the slope, half crimp and full
      crimp grips reported by Amca et al. (2012)   135
8.4   Evolution of fingertip forces according to fatigue   137
8.5   Mean estimations of tendon and pulley force computed for the
      crimp and slope grips in a one-finger grip in six expert climbers   139
8.6   Examples of experimental design used to estimate tendon tension
      in a one-finger crimp grip (Vigouroux et al., 2006b) and the muscle
      maximal strength of the five main hand muscle groups   140
8.7   Estimated maximal muscle moment potential at wrist joint level
      and MCP joint level according to Vigouroux et al. (2015)   142
9.1   a) Handgrip dynamometry; b) finger flexor strength testing
      proposed by Grant et al. (1996, 2001) and lately used by
      MacLeod et al. (2007), Philippe et al. (2012) and Fryer et al. (2015)   149
9.2   Finger position on the gauge (a, b), handgrip - grip strength
      measurement with shoulder at 0°; and elbow fully extended
      (c) (Baláš, Mrskoč, Panáčková, & Draper, 2014).   152
9.3   The four different grips and the position on the scale: a) open grip;
      b) crimp grip; c) middle and ring fingers; d) index and middle
      fingers; e) the basic position on the scale   153
9.4   The starting and finishing position for the narrow and wide grip
      power tests of shoulder girdle muscles   159
10.1 Example of the ice tool striking task (left panel) and of the
      exhaustion task   168
10.2 The three ice tools used in this study   168
10.3 Angle (average ± SD across trials) between the horizontal
      and the line joining the axe's tip and axe's head for the 11 subjects   169

10.4   Example of joint angles for a typical subject
       (average ± SD across trials) related to the time (in percentage of the
       total time of the swing)   170
10.5   Normalized IEMG (%) for the two phases (cocking/strike) for
       upper limb muscles: digitorum (flexor and extensor), carpi (flexor
       and extensor), elbow (biceps and triceps brachii) and shoulder
       (deltoidus anterior and teres major)   171
10.6   Joint angles amplitude (average ± SD across subjects and trials) for
       the different arm's degrees of freedom in four different conditions   172
10.7   Burst mean power frequency during strike phase for muscles   174
11.1   Framework to intertwine the outcome variables (climbing
       performance outcome) and process variables (key components of
       skill)   183
11.2   Inter-limb coordination in ice climbing   190
12.1   Data adapted from Cordier et al. (1993, p. 373) showing practice
       and skill effects as indexed by entropy of the hip trajectory when
       climbing the same route over ten trials   198
12.2   Recall performance and verbal reports during a route recall task
       reported in Boschker et al. (2002)   200
12.3   Affordance perception and skill in climbing   203
12.4   Geometric index of entropy for each trial (A), for each condition
       (B) and for the interaction between trial and condition (C).
       Hor. = horizontal edge condition, Ver.=vertical edge condition,
       Both = double-edged condition, TR= transfer test   204
13.1   The optical flow presented to a climber as he examines holds on
       an indoor climbing route   212
13.2   Mean visual search data of five skilled climbers   216
13.3   Summary of visual search variables collected during six climbs   219
13.4   Perceived maximum reaching height and actual maximum r
       eaching height before climbing, after climbing 2, 4, 6 and 8 trials,
       and after climbing to exhaustion   220
14.1   IRCRA Reporting Scale against existing difficulty scales   233
15.1   Basic processes of capturing and processing information in sport
       climbing   246
15.2   Motivational aspects in sport climbing   247
15.3   Emotional aspects in sport climbing   248
15.4   The Climbing Self-Efficacy Scale (CSES).   253
17.1   Instrumented hold mounted on wall   270
17.2   Fully instrumented climbing wall (with eight smart holds)   271
17.3   Two degrees of freedom instrumentation of an arbitrary hold   272
17.4   Development of the contact force over time   273
17.5   Climber in static position on a wall   275
17.6   ATC Guide (with Magic plate function)   278

17.7   (a) Logarithmic spiral (b) and camming device; (c) camming
       device inserted in a crack with two different widths; θ = pitch angle;
       COP = centre of pressure; the downward arrow in (c) indicates the
       load direction   279
18.1   Fall factors during normal and simul-climbing falls   286
18.2   Configuration of the simul-climb tests   287
18.3   Simultaneous release of two 80 kg dummies to simulate the fall
       of two climbers on the north face of Pointe Lachenal   288
18.4   Forces measured on the anchor point (in N) versus time (in
       seconds) for the following types of rope – single, double and twin   289
18.5   Screenshots from the high-speed film: movements of the Ice twin
       rope with both ropes running through the carabiner   290
18.6   Screenshots from the high-speed film: movements of the Ice Line
       rope during a simul-climb fall; the rope opened the screw   290
18.7   Leader fall with the second climber held by a Tibloc™   292
18.8   Repeatable protocol of a crevasse fall   293
18.9   The braking system   294
18.10 Comparison of the force transmitted to the rescuer during a
       crevasse fall with a double rope (Beal, Ice Line and Ice Twin)
       and a single rope (Beal Joker and Diablo) with and without
       friction knots   295
18.11 Force generated on the rope depending on the rope distance
       between the climbers   296

Tables

2.1 VO_{2max} of climbers during different modes of exercise   21

2.2 VO_2 and heart rate during climbing   25

2.3   Lactate reponses to climbing   33

5.1   Definition of altitude ranges   78

5.2   Wind-chill index chart   88

6.1   Historical perspectives on the implementation of altitude/hypoxic training methods   94

6.2   Main hypoxic methods and associated mechanisms   103

6.3   Practical recommendations for the different hypoxic methods   104

8.1   Examples of results (mean ±SD) reported in the literature (Quaine et al., 2003a and 2004; Schweizer, 2001; Vigouroux et al., 2008; Quaine et al., 2011; Cutts & Bollen, 1993 for each line respectively) for maximum grip exertion in different population during different grip tests   134

9.1   Bivariate and partial correlations among climbing abilities and finger strength in four different grip positions   154

9.2   Maximal voluntary contraction (MVC), continual and intermittent tests on "climbing specific" devices in males (M) and females (F) of different climbing abilities   156

9.3   Normative values for simple strength and endurance tests related to climbing ability RP in lead climbing   160

12.1   Specific forms of exploration directed toward qualitatively distinct affordance   205

13.1   Summary of gaze behaviour from unskilled climbers contrasting between traverses associated with low and high anxiety   217

14.1   Climbing grades comparison   229

14.2   The British adjectival system   230

14.3   Summary of self-report methods and reported grades in rock climbing studies post 2000   234

18.1   Maximal force generated on the protection point by the s imultaneous falls of the second and the leader, depending on the type of rope   288

18.2   Maximum force measured on the climbing protection during the fall of the second on the self-blocking pulley   291

Contributors

Jiří Baláš is a lecturer at outdoor sports department and an exercise physiology researcher at Charles University in Prague. He has published more than 20 scientific papers on climbing related topics with a focus on performance diagnostics, recovery and effect of climbing programmes on physical fitness. He is a member of a commission for competitive climbing under the Czech Mountaineering Federation where he is responsible for the performance diagnostics of the national climbing team. Jiří is passionate climber and mountaineer.

Philippe Batoux gained a PhD in mathematics and is a mountain guide certified by the International Federation of Mountain Guides Association (IFMGA). He is a teacher and researcher at the National School of Skiing and Mountaineering.

Jason Brandenburg is an associate professor in the kinesiology department at the University of the Fraser Valley located in Chilliwack, British Columbia. His research and teaching interests fall in the area of exercise physiology. Jason enjoys sport and trad climbing as well as bouldering.

Eric Brymer is a reader at Leeds Beckett University in the UK, and also holds an adjunct associate professor position at Queensland University of Technology, Australia, and a research fellow position at the University of Cumbria, UK. He specialises in extreme sport research.

Chris Button is associate professor in motor control at the School of Physical Education at the University of Otago, New Zealand.

Emmanuel Cauchy is emergency medical doctor in the rescue team in the Mont-Blanc Massif (Chamonix), founder and chief executive of IFREMMONT (Mountain Medicine Institute for Training and Research), teacher and researcher in mountain medicine, and master in environment physiology, specialized in cold injuries. He is also a mountain guide certified by the IFMGA and himalayist.

Simon Courtemanche recently defended his PhD at INRIA Rhone-Alpes, France. He received his MSc from Grenoble Institute of Technology and his PhD in mathematics and computer science from Grenoble University. His primary research interests are physically based computer animation and rock climbing.

Keith Davids is professor of motor control at the Centre for Sports Engineering Research, Sheffield Hallam University and Finnish Distinguished Professor at the University of Jyväskylä in Finland.

Nick Draper has been involved in rock climbing for nearly 30 years and has taught outdoor education in the UK and New Zealand. His research interests in rock climbing relate to the psychophysiology of the sport and the development of new sport-specific methods for testing climbers. He is a professor of sport science at the University of Canterbury, New Zealand.

Franz Konstantin Fuss is the professor of sports engineering at RMIT University, the editor-in-chief of sports technology, and the editor of the *Routledge Handbook of Sports Technology and Engineering*. He specializes in smart equipment and wearable technology, non-linear engineering and sports aerodynamics.

Luisa Giles is a faculty member in the department of Sport Science at Douglas College in New Westminster, British Columbia. Her training/research focuses on environmental exercise physiology and she formerly worked as a sport scientist with the Canadian BMX team. In her spare time Luisa enjoys all kinds of climbing especially climbing on alpine granite.

Olivier Girard is currently working at Lausanne University. His research (more than 65 articles in peer-reviewed journals) is focused on identifying, quantifying and explaining mechanisms responsible for fatigue and associated neuro-mechanical adjustments during high-intensity intermittent exercises performed under challenging environmental conditions (i.e. heat stress or hypoxia).

Olivier Hoibian is an associate professor at the Faculty of Sport Sciences (University Paul Sabatier of Toulouse 3, France). His research focuses on the cultural history and sociology of sport, outdoor leisure activities, and physical education from the end of the eighteenth century to the present. He is also a mountain guide certified by the IFMGA.

Gareth Jones is a senior lecturer in physiotherapy, and sport and exercise medicine at Leeds Beckett University. Gareth possesses an MSc in physiotherapy and a BSc in sports and exercise science. Clinically Gareth has experience of the treatment and management of climbing related injuries.

Paul G. Kry is an associate professor at McGill University. He received his B.Math at the University of Waterloo, and his MSc and PhD in computer science from the University of British Columbia. His primary research interest is physically based computer animation.

Grégoire Millet is a professor and the author of books on endurance and altitude training, 40 book chapters and more than 200 indexed scientific articles. Grégoire is the chief editor of *Frontiers in Exercise Physiology*. His research area is on the therapeutic use of altitude/hypoxia in patients (obesity, hypertension etc.) and for performance enhancement (endurance athletes, team-sport players). He has co-authored two books on altitude training: Millet

(*Entrainement en altitude dans les sports collectifs*, deBoeck Supérieur, 2015 and *S'entraîner en altitude,* deBoeck Supérieur, 2011)

Erik Monasterio is a consultant in forensic psychiatry, clinical director and senior lecturer in the Department of Psychological Medicine, University of Otago, Christchurch, New Zealand. He has 20 years mountaineering experience.

Dominic Orth gained a joined-tutorage PhD in sport sciences at the Faculty of Sport Sciences, University of Rouen, France and at the School of Exercise & Nutrition Science, Queensland University of Technology, Brisbane, Australia. He now has a post-doctoral position at the CETAPS laboratory at the University of Rouen, France.

Franck Quaine is an associate professor in Grenoble University. His PhD was on the biomechanics of balance in rock climbing. His current work aims to develop new methods for modelling the human hand. Major applications concern the evaluation of human movement biomechanics for health and care, muscle–computer interfaces and human movement performance.

Lionel Reveret is a research scientist at INRIA Rhone-Alpes, France. He received his MSc and PhD in computer science from Grenoble Institute of Technology (INPG, France). His primary research interests are computer animation, motion capture and anatomical motion analysis.

Jean Paul Richalet is professor of physiology at University Paris 13, a medical doctor and PhD. He dedicated his career to the mechanisms of adaptation to altitude hypoxia. He has led three scientific expeditions to high altitude (Numbur, Annapurna IV, Sajama) and organized a great number of studies at the Observatoire Vallot.

Thomas Robert has a MSc degree in mechanical engineering and a PhD in biomechanics. He is a researcher in the Biomechanics and Impact Mechanics Laboratory (LBMC) in Lyon and his main research interests are the analysis of human movement dynamics.

Annie Rouard is full professor of biomechanics at the University of Savoy Mont Blanc (France) and with Inter-university Laboratory on Biology of Motor skills (LIBM). She works on the biomechanical evaluation of fatigue and coordination in sports.

Xavier Sanchez is associate professor in sport and performance psychology at the department of medical and sport sciences, University of Cumbria, Lancaster, UK. Xavier possesses psychology and sport psychology degrees, and has international and multidisciplinary experience in both higher education and the sporting arena.

Volker Rainer Schöffl is a professor and medical specialist in sports medicine, general surgery, trauma surgery and orthopaedics at the Klinikum Bamberg, Germany. He received a Master of Health Business Administration from the University of Erlangen-Nuremberg where he also gives lectures in orthopaedic and trauma surgery. He is the physician of the German competition climbing team and member of the medical commissions of the International Climbing and Mountaineering Federation (UIAA) and International Federation of Sport Climbing (IFSC).

Andreas Schweizer is deputy head of hand surgery at the Balgrist University Hospital, Zurich, Switzerland. He is adept in wrist surgery, surgery on peripheral nerves, surgical treatment of hand fractures, ultrasound on the hand, and 3D computer aided analysis of malunions. Currently, he is also the medical advisor for the technical committee of the Swiss Alpine Club.

Ludovic Seifert is professor at the Faculty of Sport Sciences at the University of Rouen in France. He gained a PhD in expertise and coordination dynamics in swimming at the University of Rouen in 2003, then a certification to supervise research in 2010. He conducts his research in the field of motor learning and motor control. He is mountain guide certified by IFMGA.

Laurent Vigouroux started his research in sport-climbing by analysing the different physiological states of forearm fatigue in rock climbers. His PhD thesis addressed the development of biomechanical models of the hand and fingers to quantify the muscle forces and the pulley forces while using slope and crimp grip techniques. This work brought new information for the understanding of pulley rupture pathomechanism which has been used by surgeons to improve surgical reconstruction techniques. More recently as assistant professor, he has focused on the hand and forearm muscle capacity adaptations in climbers and on finger coordination while gripping different type of holds.

Phillip (Phil) B. Watts is a professor and exercise physiologist at Northern Michigan University and a Fellow of the American College of Sports Medicine. His primary research interests include the physiology of cross-country ski racing and physiological aspects of rock climbing and mountaineering. Dr. Watts is the author of *Rock Climbing* (1996, Human Kinetics). He has also written for *Summit*, *Rock & Ice*, and *The Master Skier* magazines.

Peter Wolf studied sports engineering at the Chemnitz University of Technology, Germany, and carried out his PhD thesis on foot biomechanics at the Institute for Biomechanics, ETH Zurich. For the last few years, he has been the scientific coordinator of the SMS-Lab, ETH Zurich. His research interests include (i) the design of sport simulators in virtual environments, (ii) the development of devices measuring performance in sports and motor learning and (iii) the establishment of augmented, real-time feedback displays facilitating motor learning of complex tasks.

List of reviewers

Most of the authors of the book have reviewed chapters of this book, and additional external reviewers have also contributed: Peter Bärtsch, Thomas Bayer, Hermann Brugger, Lars Donath, Davids Giles, Peter Gilliver, Charly Machemelh, Ferran Rodriguez, Urs Stoecker.

Preface

Ludovic Seifert, Peter Wolf and
Andreas Schweizer

As you all certainly know, the book you are holding in your hands is not the first book ever published on climbing. Numerous books on climbing have already seen the public light. Why then another book on climbing? The answer is 'because of climbing science'. The scientific knowledge on all the different aspects of climbing has increased so that high performance climbing on various surfaces (artificial climbing wall, rock, ice and mixed route), with hands or various tools, at various altitudes, in various conditions (competitive, traditional, sport climbing, soloing) is no longer just the result of a natural gift or ability, it is also a science.

This statement is supported by the following events: the International Rock Climbing Research Association (IRCRA; http://www.ircra.rocks) was funded during the first International Rock Climbing congress in 2011 at the University of Canterbury, New Zealand. Three years later, the second congress occurred in Pontresina, Switzerland, organized by the University Hospital Balgrist and ETH Zurich welcoming 50 attendees from 12 different countries (http://www.climbing.ethz.ch). Actually, the IRCRA has around 70 researchers and the third International Rock Climbing congress will take place in Colorado, USA in 2016.

In January 2016, the most widely used internet database for biological and medical sciences (PubMed) displayed 3332 human studies when the search word 'climbing' was entered. However, as climbing is a primary quadruped mode of locomotion used when biped mode is not suitable, this search includes many studies about stair-climbing, tree-climbing, and so on. Therefore, when the search phrase 'rock climbing' is entered, only 191 human studies were found. The first publication about 'rock climbing' dates from 1962. Twelve papers about rock climbing were published between 1962 and 1990 versus 38 papers between 1991 and 2000, and 91 papers between 2001 and 2010. Within the last six years, 51 papers have been published, thus, climbing is getting more and more attention in the scientific community. As climbing can be practised in many ways, we extended our book scope and our search to 'mountaineering' and 2365 human studies were found, and 21 human studies appeared when the search phrase was 'ice climbing'. Therefore, a huge body of scientific data seems to be available to improve the coaches', the instructors', the teachers', the students' and the climbers' knowledge of their own sport.

Unfortunately, most of these studies are hardly ever available to potentially interested people, and even when they are, it is extremely difficult for them to translate the reported results into day-to-day training practice. With this book, we intend to translate the latest body of scientific knowledge consistent with on-deck coaches', instructors' and their climbers' language. It is our goal to make the most significant results from some of the world's leading climbing researchers available to them, so that their coaching and teaching strategies can be improved and the climbers' qualities and performance potential can be optimized.

There is little doubt that climbing is becoming an international sport, notably because it became easy to practise on indoor climbing walls, which appeared in the 1960s in England and in the 1980s in Europe and the USA, then going on to increase all around the world (for instance, the surrounding suburbs of Paris had 342 indoor climbing walls as of 2012: http://www.irds-idf.fr/fileadmin/Etudes/etude_479/irds_01.pdf). Similarly, the use of artificial ice climbing walls has emerged recently, opening up the possibility to practice with ice year round (e.g. http://winter.champagny.com/resort-guide/unmissable/ice-tower.html). Accordingly, the selection of 'state-of-the-art' chapters that compose this book have been written by 30 experts from nine different countries in Europe, Australasia and America. All the authors have a PhD, are on the editorial board of a journal and/or are a director of a research laboratory, and have significant experience of research in climbing. They are also currently actively involved in climbing research, all having recently published papers on the research topics represented in this book. In each review, the authors present the 'state-of-the-art' and the new knowledge (mostly published in indexed journals) in their area of research that is destined for researchers, graduate students, climbers, instructors and coaches. In addition, most of the authors practice climbing or mountaineering, and some are involved in the practice of teaching and coaching climbing.

A large body of the pioneering studies relate to climbing injuries, risk and mountain sickness, and more broadly concern physiology and medicine (i.e. when the search words are 'rock climbing' AND 'physiology', 101 studies were found among the 191 rock climbing studies). Our goal is to enlarge the scope of the scientific knowledge by introducing humanities and technology sciences, in order to provide a pluri-disciplinary approach to climbing science. The book is divided into an introduction and six distinct parts (Physiology, Medicine, Biomechanics, Motor Control and Learning, Psychology, and Equipment, Technology and Safety Devices).

In the introductory chapter, Olivier Hoibian shows how the most relevant *historical* and *sociological aspects* of mountaineering and climbing became practiced on various surfaces and in various conditions year to year. In fact, mountaineering and climbing have been closely related since their respective origins at the dawn of the nineteenth century. In some respects, they are unique in the world of sport as both are practised without formal regulations or refereeing. The introduction of new technical equipment, however, has regularly sparked conflict and tensions around how these two sports should be defined. Yet despite all the protestations from various corners, these traditional activities have recently split off into highly specific sporting categories like via ferrata, ice climbing and indoor wall climbing. Competitions are now held alongside traditional mountain climbing and rock climbing in natural settings. The diversification in activities has in many ways been a positive development for the climbing community, as there is now something for everyone. Thus, by starting this book with a historical perspective on climbing and mountaineering and explaining the dynamics that have characterized the changes in these sports, Olivier Hoibian provides an important rationale for a pluri-disciplinary approach to climbing and mountaineering in this book.

The first part about *physiology* comprises two chapters. Chapter 2, 'Physiology of climbing' by Luisa Giles and Jason Brandenburg, presents the acute physiological demands of climbing. Metabolic and physiological responses, and recovery interventions are discussed. Chapter 3 by Phil Watts, entitled 'Economy in difficult rock climbing', reviews concepts and related research to estimate energy expenditure during climbing.

The second part is about *medicine* and contains three chapters. Chapter 4, 'Sport climbing related injuries and overuse syndromes' is by Volker Schöffl and Andreas Schweizer. After an overview of the most common climbing related injuries, the authors outline that new pathologies like closed finger flexor tendon pulley injuries and epiphyseal fractures of the fingers in young climbers have emerged as significant risks. The authors also present diagnosis and treatment options on sport-specific overstrain syndromes. In Chapter 5, entitled 'High altitude medicine and cold effects in mountaineering', Jean Paul Richalet and Emmanuel Cauchy review the mechanisms of acclimatization that help the organism to cope with altitude hypoxia and cold. Then, the authors explain the symptoms of acute mountain sickness and high altitude pulmonary or cerebral oedema when incomplete acclimatization occurs. They also present ways of preventing altitude diseases. The second section of the chapter deals with the physiological mechanisms when the body is exposed to cold and the several degrees of frostbite severity. Practical applications about rewarming are provided. The next chapter (Chapter 6), written by Grégoire Millet and Olivier Girard, logically presents how mountaineers can take advantage of 'hypoxic training'. Hypoxic training emerged in 1960s and was limited to the 'Live High Train High' method for endurance athletes looking to increase their haemoglobin mass and oxygen transport. This 'classical' method was complemented in the 1990s by the 'Live High Train Low' method where athletes benefit from long hypoxic exposure and from the higher intensity of training at low altitude. The authors also present more recent methods and discuss the potential physiological differences between 'real altitude' and 'simulated altitude'.

The third part of the book is about *biomechanics* and includes four chapters. Chapter 7 is 'Postural regulation and motion simulation in rock climbing' and is written by Franck Quaine, Lionel Reveret, Simon Courtemanche and Paul Kry. The first section of this chapter describes the load distribution of the different limbs. The second section of the chapter focuses on the kinematics of rock climbing and introduces a modelling technique to estimate contact forces without force sensors. Chapter 8 is entitled 'Grip capabilities of climbers' hands and fingers' and is written by Laurent Vigouroux. This chapter summarizes the studies investigating the maximum grip capacity and the forearm muscle fatigue of rock climbers compared to non-climbers and/or according to the grip technique used. In addition, Laurent Vigouroux presents biomechanical models that allow the estimation of forces withstood by tendons and ligaments while gripping a hold. As the strong forces exerted on the musculoskeletal systems of the hand and fingers are an important risk factor of pulley rupture, the author outlines the need for developing new training tools and programmes. Chapter 9, written by Jiří Baláš, continues in this field and is entitled 'Muscular strength and endurance in climbers'. This chapter discusses climbing-specific tests which consider the loading, movement and body positions typically found in climbing. The last chapter of this part (Chapter 10) focuses on the 'Biomechanics of ice tool swinging movement' and is written by Annie Rouard, Thomas Robert and Ludovic Seifert. This chapter describes the kinematics, kinetics and electromyography activation of upper limbs during ice tool swinging. The effect of using different parts of the ice tool and the effect of fatigue are presented and practical applications for greater effectiveness are proposed.

The fourth part concerns *motor control and learning* and includes four chapters. Chapter 11 explores 'How expert climbers use perception and action during successful climbing performance'. In particular, Ludovic Seifert, Dominic Orth, Chris Button and Keith Davids highlight how climbers use perception and action to enhance their expertise in climbing, through the continuous and active exploration of environmental properties. From this perspective, the authors emphasize that adaptability is the foundation of expertise because it underpins the ongoing co-adaptation of each climber's behaviours to a set of dynamically changing, interacting constraints, which are individually perceived and acted upon. Chapter 12, written by Dominic Orth, Chris Button, Keith Davids and Ludovic Seifert, is entitled 'What current research tells us about skill acquisition in climbing'. This chapter reviews the effects of practice constraints on skilled behaviour in climbing. A theoretical framework is developed to guide perceptual-motor learning in route climbing through learning design. Chapter 13 deals with 'Visual-motor skill in climbing' and is by Chris Button, Dominic Orth, Keith Davids and Ludovic Seifert. This chapter presents an overview on the visual-motor behaviours used by climbers and how to acquire them. The authors also discuss how influential factors such as anxiety and fatigue affect visual-motor behaviour.

The fifth part is related to *psychology* and includes three chapters. Chapter 14, entitled 'Climbing grades – systems and subjectivity', by Nick Draper, presents the debate around the different grading systems in climbing, and the implication and challenges with its usability for research, but also the ability of climbers to self-assess their skills. Chapter 15 is about the psychological processes which influence climbing and is written by Gareth Jones and Xavier Sanchez. The chapter outlines the impact of visual inspection on successful completion of the route. In addtion, self-efficacy and anxiety are reviewed with respect to climbing performance and motivation, e.g. in terms of risk taking. Chapter 16 deals with 'Exposure and engagement in mountaineering' and is written by Eric Brymer and Erik Monasterio. This chapter questions the traditional risk-focused approach that has dominated mountaineering literature and presents an alternative perspective. This alternative perspective emphasizes that mountaineering involves a considerable range of experiences that includes a search for mastery in challenging and unstable environments, unique camaraderie found in situations of mutual reliance in isolated, stressful and dangerous situations and the search for freedom and transcendence. From there, the chapter provides practical advice for mental preparation and coaching.

The sixth part of this book is about *equipment, technology and safety devices* and includes two chapters. Chapter 17 looks at 'The engineering of climbing equipment'. This chapter is written by Tino Fuss and Peter Wolf, who present current means to measure contact forces between hand/foot and hold. Performance metrics extracted from contact force–time curves, the benefit of chalk, and the advantages and disadvantages of various rope breaks and the functionality of rock protection devices are also discussed. Last, Chapter 18 by Philippe Batoux relates to 'Simul-climbing progression and falls analysis'. This chapter presents an analysis of the different types of falls occurring during simul-climbing progression. The author also presents an analysis of forces during a crevasse fall on horizontal glacial terrain.

1 A cultural history of mountaineering and climbing

Olivier Hoibian

Mountaineering and climbing have been closely related since their respective origins at the dawn of the nineteenth century. In some respects, they are unique in the world of sport as both are practised without formal regulations or refereeing. The introduction of new technical equipment, however, has regularly sparked conflict and tensions around how these two sports should be defined. Moreover, between the two world wars, attempts to streamline the processes of ascension provoked heated controversy over the status of mountaineering and rock climbing as elite activities, with some practitioners fearing that they would become mere 'sports like any other'. Similar concerns were voiced in the 1960s over the advent of 'artificial rock climbing', which was denounced by many as a form of 'technological drift' that threatened the very objective of engaging in these two activities. Yet despite all the protestations from various corners, these traditional activities have recently split off into highly specific sporting categories like via ferrata, ice climbing and indoor wall climbing, and competitions are now held alongside traditional mountain climbing and rock climbing in natural settings. The diversification in activities has in many ways been a positive development for the climbing community, as there is now something for everyone: climbing appeals as much to those who want to push themselves to their limits as to those who find climbing an opportunity for contemplation, and international competitions are a magnet for those who want to measure their performance against the best. A historical perspective on climbing and mountaineering will provide insight into the dynamics that have characterised the changes in these sports and will help to understand the social challenges they have posed.

Introduction

Mountaineering and rock climbing have been closely related since their respective origins at the dawn of the nineteenth century. Rock climbing, which in 1840 was given its first name, 'varappe' (Le Comte, 2008), in the Salève foothills of the French Alps, has often been thought of as a kind of preparation for mountaineering, although in certain geographic locations rock climbing in its earliest forms was practised in and of itself. Both activities have always been based on ethical principles, yet these principles have never been formally articulated. Instead they have been passed down through the generations as a guide to climbers everywhere, which gives these activities a unique standing in the sporting world. And in recent times, both have been confronted by radical changes and challenges.

The introduction of various technical advances in climbing has often caused dissension among climbers around the essential question of what constitutes legitimate practice. Between the two world wars, steps to streamline climbing practices provoked considerable controversy about whether such advances would turn climbing into 'a sport like any other', forever stripped of its elite status. Controversy surged again in the 1960s with the creation of artificial climbing walls, which were soundly denounced by many as either a technological deformation of the sport or a crass attempt at opening it up to all and any, thereby threatening its core values and the symbolic benefits that practitioners derived from it. Although today's conflicts have taken on a different form, they nevertheless persist, with the controversial project to have climbing declared an Olympic sport being a good example.

The two climbing activities have recently split off into several categories: via ferrata, icefall climbing, dry-tooling, indoor wall climbing, and practices on bouldering and multi-pitches, and today competitions have become common. Yet, despite these innovations, traditional high-altitude mountaineering and rock climbing in natural settings continue to thrive. The diversification of climbing practices has broadened the range of motivations driving climbers, with some finding a means to exceed personal limits and others finding a meditative, contemplative practice. And situated somewhere in between is the desire to achieve elite performance at international competitions. A historical perspective on the successive phases that have marked mountaineering and rock climbing might help to better understand the dynamics in play and the social issues at stake.

A cultural approach

Mountaineers have always had at least one thing in common with those who are passionate about deep-water and desert sports: a penchant for writing about their impressions. The number of works on mountaineering and climbing far exceeds the number of works on any other land-based sport or leisure activity. The authors have often brought a historical perspective to their writing, with some looking far back in time to find clues as to why certain people have always been driven to conquer the highest mountain peaks. Somewhat opposed to this abundant historiography, historians have tended to conduct more methodical investigations within well-defined conceptual frameworks. In the 1970s, epistemological debates about the discipline of history led to a certain relativism (Veyne, 1971). The ambition of a 'total history' promoted by the French 'Annales' school of Lucien Febvre and Marc Bloch was much discussed in the interwar period, to the ultimate benefit of more circumscribed approaches (Poirrier, 2004). Although today historians will readily acknowledge that their work can be challenged, they nevertheless stand firm in their claim that history is a scientific discipline. A historical accounting is, to their eyes, quite different from a fictional narrative because it is truth-based and the facts can be verified by historical methods (Ricoeur, 2000).

In the midst of these debates about the nature of historical research, cultural history emerged as a distinct field of investigation. Defined as 'the social history of representations', it is based on a broad interpretation of 'culture' as defined by anthropologists, and this therefore encompasses physical leisure and sport practices (Chartier, 1998). Cultural history, however, pays particular attention to the significations or meanings associated with such activities by incorporating the corporeal know-how and the specific techniques of the social universe being studied (Ory, 2011). According to Roger Chartier, this essentially means incorporating clear thoughts and personal intentions and desires into a system of collective constraints that both makes them possible and standardises them (Chartier, 1993).

Mountaineering and rock climbing have a unique position in the world of leisure sport. These activities arouse scientific curiosity; attract those with aesthetic and contemplative sensibilities, a spirit of adventure or a desire to attain high levels of performance; and offer an unusual form of tourism. In this sense, they can be said to be characterised by a certain ambivalence. Up until quite recently, they were practised without regard to regulations or referees, yet conformed to an unwritten code of ethics transmitted by the practitioners themselves, thereby lending themselves to multiple appropriations over time, notably between the different parts of the social elite. For this reason, writing the cultural history of mountaineering and rock climbing is far more than retracing the major steps in their development and dissemination throughout the world: close examination of the evolution in the collective representations associated with them is called for. One such examination concerns the debates and conflicts around the legitimate definition of these sports and how these debates developed and became structured. By necessity, this field of investigation also includes a historical accounting of elitism, especially with regard to the educated faction in societies that are organised hierarchically according to a logic of social distinction (Hoibian, 2008).

The cultural conditions for the invention of mountaineering

Since the dawn of time, mountains have been a part of the landscape: permanent landmarks on the horizon. Palaeontologists have shown that the valleys and the most accessible mountain passes have been inhabited since the earliest traces of humankind. These areas have always been important for travel and trade routes, even in the dead of winter. The remains of Otzi, the Neolithic hunter whose mummified corpse was found in a crevasse of one of the Tyrolean glaciers, provides evidence that this was so even in very early times.

On the highest mountains peaks, however, the situation has always been quite different. Summits are sterile and inhospitable places, long associated in the popular mind with supernatural powers (fairies, dragons, evil beings) that were believed to be at the root of a good number of the catastrophes that have regularly befallen the valleys (torrential flooding, avalanches, mudslides, etc.).

In the eighteenth century, the expansion of urban lifestyles began to transform the representations of the educated elite. These new sensibilities, promulgated by the Enlightenment philosophers and the pre-Romantic writers, marked a new era in the relationship between humankind and the mountains. The works of Jean-Jacques Rousseau and Albrecht von Haller helped spread this new appreciation for the summits and glaciers of the Alps and Pyrenees as objects of contemplation throughout Europe (Engel, 1930). The inhabited valleys and the pasture lands began to pique the curiosity of the European elite, and they started to frequent these rustic areas with some regularity, embarking on excursions and admiring the picturesque settings. This set the stage for a new type of aristocratic and worldly tourism.

Ascending Mont Blanc

The process of legitimising this fascination with high altitudes was supported by a growing scientific curiosity about the unexplored parts of the world. The great voyages of explorers like Cook, Bougainville and La Pérouse were part of a vast movement to explore and inventory the planet, and the snow-covered mountain peaks were terra incognita. However, to overcome prejudices and break through the natural and symbolic barriers to a world of eternal snow, the authority of science based on reason and faith in progress were needed. In 1762, the Geneva scientist Horace Bénédicte de Saussure provided the decisive incentive by promising a large reward to anyone who would set out to find a viable route to the top of the mountain considered at that time to be the highest in Europe: Mont Blanc. In the popular mind, the imperative of scientific discovery legitimised and justified the ambition to conquer this emblematic summit, even at the risk of the lives of local guides (De Bellefon, 2003).

In 1786, the summit of Mount Blanc was conquered and the response to this success was confirmation that these intrepid exploits were fully in line with the sensibilities of the social elite of the period. A cultural barrier had been breached. In contrast to the worries previously evoked at the thought of the 'accursed mountains' came the overwhelming desire to contemplate and even ascend these 'sublime mountains', forevermore perceived as worthy of interest. 'Mountaineering, with its technical imperatives, its need for extreme caution, a thirst to conquer, and a feeling for the summit, was born right here and still promises many more mutations' (Vigarello, 2008).

The mountain, stripped of any spiritual connotation by rational science, could thus now be surveyed. Some weeks after the ascent of Mont Blanc by De Saussure himself in August 1787, Marc Beaufroy, a young British subject staying in Berne, repeated the exploit. Setting foot on the highest mountain peaks of the European continent soon became a challenge for the most enterprising members of the ruling class. Momentum built to conquer the main summits of the Alps and Pyrenees and this was accomplished within a few years: Little Matterhorn in 1792, Grossglockner in 1800, the Girardin pass of Monte Rosa in 1801, Mont Perdu in 1802, Jungfrau in 1810, Breithorn in 1813, the Vincent Pyramid of Monte Rosa in 1819, Finsteraarhorn in 1829, Eiger in 1859, the Ecrins in 1864, the Grandes Jorasses and the Matterhorn in 1865, and so on.

In this crucial period for mountaineering, the British set themselves apart as fervent 'collectors of firsts' (Ring, 2000). Between 1786 and 1853, they made twenty-six of the forty initial ascents of Mont Blanc and before 1880 they made half of the first ascents of summits in Europe.

The era of clubs

For 'tourists' and mountaineering adepts in the early nineteenth century, the living conditions in the villages nestled into the valleys of the Alps and Pyrenees appeared rather crude. Comfortable hotels and inns were rare, transport was irregular despite progress in railways, the guides from local companies were not always reliable, and trails and shelters were cruelly lacking. The mountaineers of Europe began to see a strong need to organise into specialised clubs. The English were the first, with the 'Alpine Club' created on 22 December 1857, in London during a 'gentlemen's' meeting of public school graduates. These members quickly adopted statutes that clearly spelled out the aim of this very elite group: 'Fostering opportunities for climbers to meet and plan for the most difficult climbs, exchange information, and publish the narratives of these exploits' (Tailland, 1997).

On 19 November 1862, the Viennese followed in their steps and founded the Austrian Alpine Club, and this was soon followed by their colleagues in Berne with the creation of the Swiss Alpine Club on 16 August 1863, in Olten (Haver, 2008). A few weeks later, their transalpine neighbours in Italy created the Italian Alpine Club on 23 October 1863, in Turin (Zuanon, 2008). In 1866, the German Alpine Club was established in Munich and in 1873 it merged with the Austrian club to become the biggest club in Europe in terms of membership. The Austrian-German Club had more than 100,000 members on the eve of the Great War (Mestre, 2000).

Amidst this vast movement, France seemed to be lagging behind. The Ramon Company had been founded in 1865 by the friends of the illustrious explorer of the Pyrenees, Ramond de Carbonnières, but it had no national ambitions. On the eve of the Prussian War of 1870, a group of Parisian mountaineers established the bases for a French Alpine Club but the defeat at Sedan and the events of the Paris Commune hindered this initiative. The founders of the French Alpine Club thus had to wait until 2 April 1874, to adopt the slogan 'Excelsior' and fix their aim as 'Fostering and propagating exact knowledge of the mountains of France and the surrounding countries.' The club founders were completely favourable to the participation of women and organised caravans for young school girls (Ottogali-Mazzacavallo, 2006).

Although the members of the alpine clubs were oriented towards the conquest of mountains by engaging the services of the best guides of the moment, the national clubs of the continent were more interested in acting as interlocutors with government representatives. The educated elite who had control of their destiny were able to define what constituted legitimate practices in planning for moderate climbs, following the most accessible routes, and being led by experienced local guides. They preferred a kind of 'cultivated excursionism' that made room for contemplative, scientific, literary or artistic practices, which were in keeping with their ethical and aesthetic values. Along the way, this enlightened bourgeoisie arranged the mountain, organised the guide business, created trails and shelters, wrote up scientific notices and invented a literature around tourism. They thus helped their fellow citizens to learn about an alpine type of tourism, contemplative and yet worldly.

As part of the same movement, alpine clubs were formed on other continents, especially in the United States with the Appalachian Alpine Club in 1876 and the American Alpine Club in 1902, and in Canada with the Alpine Club of Canada in 1906.

From 1865 onward, the most active members of the British Alpine Club began to think that the challenges of the Alps had been exhausted and turned to the conquest of mountains outside Europe. E. Whymper covered Greenland in 1867, the Andes in 1880 and the Canadian Rockies in 1900; A. F. Mummery organised an expedition in the Caucasus in 1888 and to Nanga Parbat in the Himalayas, where he disappeared in 1895. The routes traced out by these two legendary British explorers would then be followed by a growing number of mountaineers in the following decades, beginning with the Duke of Abruzzi and his expeditions to Ruwenzori in Africa in 1906 and to K2 in the Himalayas in 1909 (Bonnington, 1992).

The first debates on the legitimate practice of mountaineering and rock climbing: the emergence of 'technical elitism'

At the end of the nineteenth century, the classic way of ascending mountains with the aid of local guides began to be contested and the reason was that new types of climbing became more and more present with the development of competition. New methods began to be practised, such as winter climbing, seeking out the technically most difficult routes, climbing without guides, mountain skiing and rock climbing. At the end of the 1880s, first in Austria, then in Berlin and soon in Switzerland, 'Academic Clubs' were created to bring together students who were passionate about climbing. They promoted 'acrobatic climbing' using solo ropes, despite the reservations expressed by the heads of the national clubs. In 1904, the Italian Academic Alpine Club was founded on the initiative of A. Hess. These clubs were soon to become associations for a new type of climbing elite.

The notion of technical training in winter began to take hold, encouraging the regular frequentation of a new kind of training site: climbing schools. The Salève, already popular before 1870, the small limestone mountains of the eastern Alps and the sandstone rocks of the Elbe and Fontainebleau were all located near good-sized cities and gradually became overrun by climbers (Le Comte, 2008). In England, a similar phenomenon was observed in 1886, with the beginnings of rock wall climbing in the Lake District (Jones, 1984).

During this time, climbing techniques and procedures were steadily improving with the introduction of new materials like carabiners and pitons and new belay methods. All these innovations aroused heated debate over what should be permissible for the climbing community and what should be rejected.

One of the most famous feuds was between P. Preuss and T. Piaz about the use of modern belay techniques. Pitons and carabiners were condemned by the former as 'contrary to the honour of mountaineers'. These 'artificial means' were also treated with hostility in England, from such climbers as W. P. Hasket Smith, who climbed the Napes Needle 'without using illegitimate means' in 1886, and O. G. Jones, author of 'Pinnacles' a few years later (Clark and Pyatt, 1957). In the massive Elbe Sandstone Mountains near Dresden, O. Schuster and R. Freshman recommended free climbing as early as 1890–1910. These climbers had strict rules limiting the number of protection points that could be permanently installed, while accepting their use as resting points, and their conception was close to the principles adopted by the English. In the United States, climbers familiar with the principles of European free climbing started to open climbing sites in Colorado, California and the Schawagunk Mountains of New York.

The process of streamlining the training techniques and methods in the climbing schools during the winter continued in the period between the two world wars. Notable progress was made in the design of crampons and ice axes, and in the different techniques used for rappelling in Europe. Much of this progress was oriented towards improving performances, led by the British-inspired spread of competition climbing and the initial media success in covering major international meetings. In France, the High Mountain Group was created in 1919 on the model of technical excellence promoted by the academic clubs of neighbouring countries. This initiative aroused virulent criticism from the proponents of traditional 'cultivated excursionism', who dominated the French Alpine Club. Another intense debate in this period concerned the projects to rank the climbing routes according to difficulty. The Austrian W. Welzenbach proposed a set of objective criteria for ranking the difficulty with grades up to VIth degree (traditional cotation), and this completely divided the world of mountaineers between promoters of sport climbing and individuals who would like to keep mountaineering away from competition climbing system (see Chapter 14 for further discussion about grading system). The controversies of this epoch indicate that defining the correct way to climb had become a control issue for practitioners.

Mountaineering also became a propaganda tool at the hands of authoritarian regimes in this period. The rising nationalism in certain European countries led to the exaltation of a virile type of heroism that was at times pushed to the point of self-sacrifice for the glory of one's country. This ideology was echoed somewhat in the mountaineering world of those nations, where alpine clubs were subject to strict state control. In Fascist Italy, youth were indoctrinated around extreme values of commitment (i.e. supreme sacrifice for national glory) that sometimes had the whiff of morbidity (Pastore, 2003). A similar phenomenon was observed in Nazi Germany (Müller, 1979). The conquest of the last 'big problems' in the Alps, including the north face of the Eiger, which was finally climbed in 1938 by the Austro-German team of A. Heckmair, L. Worg, H. Harrer, and F. Kasparek, was achieved against a background of heightened international rivalries that soon infected the great expeditions to conquer the highest peaks on the planet. The equipment and knowledge available at the time did not meet the extreme conditions of such high altitudes. Many of the attempts to conquer the Himalayan peaks were disastrous, both for the English on the slopes of Everest with the disappearance of G. Mallory and A. Irvine in 1924, and for the Germans in their multiple attempts to climb Nanga Parbat that resulted in the tragedies of 1934 and 1937 and many deaths (Raspaud, 2003).

Not until the end of World War II would a modern conception of mountaineering emerge, founded on technical excellence but avoiding excessive competition. The formula according to which 'mountaineering is of course a sport, but a sport like no other' underlined its uniqueness and the resolve of its practitioners to resist its trivialisation by refusing to allow it to conform to the model of classic athletic competition. This vision of climbing began to gain consensus in 1945 to the point of it becoming the 'classic' mode for this practice. Mountaineers who had achieved levels of high popularity presented themselves as individuals capable of associating high physical and technical performances with the expression of an artistic or literary sensibility. The icons of this time like W. Bonatti, M. Herzog, L. Terray and G. Rebuffat undoubtedly owe their fame to their talents in these two areas of competence (Hoibian, 2001).

The development of 'aid climbing'

In the 1950s, the climbing community throughout the world began to be introduced to new materials like ropes and clothing in synthetic fibres, light-alloy carabiners, and expanding pitons, and the use of new techniques like chocks and fixed ropes, which gave rise to a new way of climbing: 'aid climbing'. Thanks to these innovations, climbers were able to tackle rock walls that were completely smooth and compact. They were able to grab on to holds bolted into the rock with the help of drilling tools (tamponoirs) and climb from one point to another with occasional help from small ladders. The most impressive ascents were direct: straight up to the top on the vertical, and winter routes in the mountains of Europe using the Himalayan techniques of fixed ropes. The climbing schools were quick to accommodate climbers wanting to practise these techniques.

In the United States, aid climbing also enjoyed great success with the rise of 'big wall' climbing in Yosemite Valley, with W. Harding, T. Frost and Y. Chouinard (Roper, 1979).

To conquer the highest peaks in the world, the developed nations entered into fierce competition and tended towards cumbersome expeditions. The prevailing view at the time was that a veritable siege was called for, with camps successively set up at each new altitude and continually refuelled by an endless stream of high-altitude porters. This design was adopted for the French expedition of 1950, which ended with the conquest of Annapurna by the team of M. Herzog and L. Lachenal, the first time a peak over 8000 m had been reached. It was the same for the ascent of Everest by the British expedition in 1953, conquered by E. Hillary, a New Zealander, and the Sherpa Tenzing Norgay. In 1965, on an expedition in Patagonia, an Italian climber used a compressor drill to facilitate placing expansion pitons into the rock wall, which caused a scandal in the alpine club journals of the epoch.

Challenging 'technological drift': a social issue?

From 1960, these developments began to raise questions and concerns among certain climbers. By publishing articles in the mountaineering journals of several countries, these climbers sought to sound the alert about the adverse effects of the 'abuse of artificial means'. They denounced the risks of this technological orientation to the sport itself: the risk of an 'imbalance between the physical and the moral, the body and the mind, to the benefit of only the athletic dimension'. From their viewpoint, the logic of using artificial means would lead to only one conclusion: 'the one with the biggest muscles wins' (Le Prince Ringuet, 1964).

At the same time, the youngest climbers were also starting to reject the use of aids. While continuing to be interested in high-altitude mountaineering, they adopted other principles in the way they climbed rock walls. This movement burgeoned almost simultaneously in different parts of Europe and the United States.

The 1960s were, of course, a time of mounting anti-authoritarianism and anti-technological sensibilities that exploded in the spring of 1968 in France and in many developed countries around the world. The youth of that time, coming of age in the midst of economic expansion, affluence and mass consumption, shared not only a 'culture of hedonism', but also growing environmental concerns and demands for sexual liberation, greater parity between men and women and greater equality in children's education (Hamon & Rotman, 1987).

As a generation, they distanced themselves from the adult world and its faith in science and technology, and its beliefs in the good of centralised power and the benefits of a 'consumer society' as opposed to the 'ascetic culture' that grew out of the hardships experienced during World War II (Baudrillard, 1970).

In the South of France, small groups of climbers began to limit the number of pitons that could be driven into the walls along ascension routes. At this time, every protection point was removed after each climber had passed. These climbers above all sought to 'hang free' between two pitons, placing them as far apart as possible and then resting on a protection point once it was driven into the wall. The level of difficulty reached in these conditions, notably by F. Guillot, was graded around 6c–7a (modern cotation), which required a very high skill level given the height from which they could fall. The argument advanced by these innovators to justify their taste for 'free climbing' was essentially based on a rejection of 'artificial climbing'. This last was described as a 'tedious' activity, for 'amateurs', 'handymen', 'porters', the 'indigent'. Conversely, they described themselves as 'intellectuals', looking for leisure time activities less dependent on 'predominantly muscle'. Instead, they emphasised free climbing as a sport by which to express one's 'capacities for taking decisions, committing to a decision, and sensing the right route to follow'. They also touted the hedonistic pleasure they derived, closely related to their cultivation and fashionable sensibilities. Implicitly, the distinction they drew was social, and it dealt more than anything with the desire to maintain control over the definition of climbing. It was as if these young climbers feared more than anything the appropriation of their sport by the lower classes with their emphasis on athletic as opposed to intellectual values. Their commitment to free climbing was a way to conserve their dominant position in this space. Perhaps unconsciously, they sought to continue giving the tone to the sport and to impose practices in harmony with their own ethical and aesthetic inclinations: that is, with their own 'ethos' as the representatives of the educated faction (Hoibian, 1995).

The same developments could be observed in the climbing schools in the Paris region (Saussois, Surgy, Fontainebleau, etc.), as well as in the east of France. Claudio Barbier painted all the pitons he did not use in yellow while climbing the Rochers de Freyr in Belgium, giving birth to the expression 'jaunir un passage', meaning to paint a climbing route in yellow. This expression spread quickly through this climbing community. In Elbsandstein, which became part of the German Democratic Republic in 1945, the rules in force were essentially the same and favoured free climbing between two protection points (i.e. climbers can have a rest at the level of a protection point, but climb between them). Similar practices were developing in England and the United States, though in these countries there was greater concern to preserve the rock walls from degradation due to intensive climbing, with pitons driven into the walls with each new passage of a rope. In the Anglo-American countries, 'clean climbing' encouraged practitioners to replace pitons by other means that were more respectful of the rock, such as cord knots or stones stuck in fissures, soon to be replaced by mechanical bolts with the rope running through, innovations that later gave rise to the first mass-produced chocks (Godfrey & Dudley, 1977).

Expedition style versus alpine style

For expeditions, disputes erupted around the excessive means that were often deployed. The most critical mountaineers argued that overly equipped expeditions were limited in their ability to adapt quickly enough to the changing situations of very high altitude. Various articles defended the principle of lightly equipped expeditions, more mobile and flexible in extreme conditions. The difference in budget between the two types of expedition was also mentioned as an argument in favour of simpler logistics to increase the number of expeditions that could be funded. These debates led to a renewal in design in the following years, with the first alpine-style expeditions without oxygen, which made the reputation of mountaineers like Reinhold Messner in subsequent decades.

From free climbing to climbing competition: the 'sportivisation' process

The inspiration for the free climbing movement, which touted the merits of climbing without protection points for rest or aid, appears to have been significantly different than 'hang free' between two pitons as was done in the South of France at the same time. Free climbing took hold in the Anglo-American countries, with some variation in the rules from one climbing group to another. The main difference concerned climbing 'on sight', with no prior identification or testing of routes, as opposed to climbing 'after preparation', sometimes with rehearsals of key passages assured from the top of the route (Aubel, 2005).

Beyond these distinctions, which indicated more or less radical positions on ethics in climbing, it is important to recall that for this new generation of climbers, streamlining the practice of climbing was part of a 'comparative' logic. The stricter codification of ascent conditions served primarily to ensure the high ranking of the best climbers. This development should be seen within the context of the new journals from the marketing sector, which were then competing with the traditional publications from the climbing clubs. Magazines like *Mountain* in Britain (1969), *Climbing* in the United States (1970), *Mountaineering and Hiking* and *Mountain Magazine* in France (1977) became the new vectors for spreading information on these practices. For the publishing companies, backed by private investors and manufacturers' advertising, it became important to rank the best climbers of the moment based on relatively objective criteria (see Chapter 14). The emblematic figures of this evolution seem to have been J. Stannard, H. Barber and J. Collins in the United States, P. Livesey and R. Fawcett in England, and J. P. Droyer and J. C. Bouvier in France. Despite minor variations in the practices, often linked to the context of each country, their vision of climbing created a process of the universalisation of climbing as a 'sport' that was set to affect the worldwide climbing community. All the while claiming to challenge aid climbing, the free climbers imported a kind of 'sport normalisation' into the world of mountaineering and climbing, which had been kept at bay until that point!

Reported on by the press and supported by sponsors, these climbers were often from the middle classes and they soon sought to trade their 'sporting excellence' for financial remuneration and media coverage. The rise in communication, travel and international meetings among the key representatives of free climbing clearly reflected their ambitions and their intention to impose this form of sport codification, despite the reluctance of a large portion of the practitioners.

With hindsight, the free climbing proponents actually appear to have been a vanguard of what would become the mainstream in the 1980s and 1990s in the world of outdoor leisure sports: the 'fun culture' (Loret, 1995). This culture effectively replaced the anti-institutional culture of the post-1968 years, which were characterised by the drive to establish an alternative to the idealised consumer society of the 1960s.

Contrary to the view expressed by Alain Loret, however, the growth of this 'fun culture' reflected the remarkable penetration of commerce into the world of leisure sport, which was fast becoming a booming economic sector. The anti-authoritarian slogans of the 1960s were re-purposed for mass marketing, as exemplified by the advertising slogan of Reebok's brand campaign: 'Break the rules' (Bouchet & Hilliairet, 2009). After some debate and controversy, the 'sporting standardisation' would lead to the first climbing competitions in 1985.

The paradoxical evolution in climbing under the influence of an anti-capitalist alternative culture from the 1960s and a later consumer-driven 'fun culture' provide insight into the divisions and tensions that erupted in France between the rock climbers in the South, who supported free climbing and remained close to the alternative culture, and the proponents of free climbing like J. C. Droyer and J. P. Bouvier, who supported the sport standardisation process.

In the 1990s, the level of difficulty that could be reached rose significantly with the rationalisation of training thanks to scientific input. P. Edlinger was a pioneer in this field and gained an international reputation with the release of J. P. Jansen's films *Vertical Opera* in 1982 and *Life at your Fingertips* in 1983. With W. Güllich and B. Moon, Edlinger opened the first eight-level routes, only to be followed by a new generation of very young climbers, both men and women, who attempted to go beyond the ninth level. In this period, women's achievements in high-level climbing were led by C. Destivelle and Lynn Hill. Since that time, the performance gap between the sexes has become smaller, underlining the critical importance of the power to weight ratio in this discipline (Tribout & Chambre, 1987).

Simultaneously, climbing was following the classic model for sporting federations with the creation of national and international competition circuits. In the former USSR, speed contests reserved for Soviet athletes had been held since 1947. In the early 1980s, exchanges with Western climbers became more frequent and the first international competition was held in Bardonecchia in 1985. Trials in artificial wall climbing were then organised in Vaulx-en-Velin the following year despite the protests of some practitioners.

The International Climbing and Mountaineering Federation (UIAA) began to recognise 'world series' like the 'Masters of Bercy' in 1988. The first World Cup was held in 1989 with difficulty tests and was won by the British climber S. Nadin and the French climber N. Raybaud. The World Cup Tour included competitions in speed in 1998 and multi-pitch climbing in 1999, with participants qualifying by accumulating points throughout the year among the top thirty routes with a minimum of five stages each.

A World Championship now takes place every two years since being established in Frankfurt in 1991. The Championship comprises three disciplines: speed, lead and bouldering. Notably, one can observe a form of professionalisation of these competition climbers. Initially, the organisation of these official events resided with the UIAA. The UIAA instituted the International Council for Competition Climbing (ICC) in 1997 and supported the foundation of the International Federation of Sport Climbing (IFCS) in 2007 (Chambre, 2015). The federation is now actively trying to have sport climbing recognised as an Olympic discipline. First, it was able to have climbing included among the events of the World Games in 2005 and in the following two seasons. It had high hopes for the Tokyo Olympics in 2020 but this has ultimately failed, and it is now trying to win the case for 2024. This initiative has been received with criticism from those climbers hostile to what they see as the trivialisation of climbing and its assimilation into the model of classic sports.

The current segmentation of practices in mountaineering and climbing

The cultural environment of 1990–2000 was marked by a remarkable increase in physical forms of recreation, undoubtedly related to trends towards a focus on personal well-being and health. During this period, mountaineering and climbing activities again underwent a process of differentiation and segmentation.

First, climbing began to be urbanised with the development of artificial structures. This phenomenon started in England in the early 1960s, that is, at Leeds University in 1964, and in the early 1980s had spread to Europe and the United States. It has since undergone explosive growth. In addition to the artificial equipment installed in schools to promote climbing for pupils, investors have backed the creation of private climbing gyms, on the model of commercial gyms dedicated to health maintenance and physical culture. These facilities are designed according to a sporting logic that also promotes indoor wall climbing competitions among younger generations.

In the mountains also, new forms of climbing emerged in the 1990s, including frozen waterfall climbing and dry-tooling (climbing rock walls using ice axes). Since 1996, these practices have gained a reputation for festive gatherings, especially among dry-toolers, such as in Pont-Rouge, Quebec, and international competitions have been organised with an Ice Climbing World Cup in 2000.

Other outdoor leisure activities have been just as much in demand in mountain areas, surely one of the repercussions of the success of the 'fun culture'. New sites have mushroomed in the valleys, where strong sensations are guaranteed in relative safety. Canyoning, the via ferrata and acrobranching have all seen remarkable growth in popularity. They ensure passive safety through the systematic design of safe environments (with lifelines, safety nets, etc.) rather than requiring that participants learn to manage their own safety.

Simultaneously, high altitude remains a space of accomplishment for 'advanced climbers' with extreme ascents to the highest peaks in the world. With funding from sponsors, the most recent achievements seem to be part of a movement towards increasingly technical ascents in alpine style and even solo winter ascents on walls at very high altitude.

Conclusion

The social space of mountaineering and climbing activities is today structured into different clusters (Hoibian, 2014) (Figure 1.1). A hedonistic cluster attracts families and youthful populations around safe, recreational and fun culture. The standardisation of sporting equipment in natural climbing environments tends to bring these environments closer to the practice conditions of artificial structures. The same hedonist and fun culture is true for many winter activities that promise a broad range of sensations and ease of use, ensuring the success of snowshoeing, ice-hiking or off-trail skiing with improved parabolic skis.

A competitive cluster has also gained ground in natural areas with the proliferation of participatory events, bringing together an elite and all other practitioners on the model of urban racing. Adventure, trail and ultra-trail races have flourished, with the offer of a wide range of race intensities held in grandiose sites and timely logistical assistance to keep the races safe. The races of the 'Tour du Mont-Blanc', organised every year at the end of August and starting in Chamonix, are a good illustration, with climbing competitions slowly becoming a part of this movement.

A third cluster, more in line with traditional representations of the ever-looming mountains, responds more directly to the need for 'authenticity' in a natural environment. Although the degree of physical engagement can vary substantially, from a contemplative approach to extreme performance, confronting uncertainty in the environment and managing one's own safety are important aspects.

In this updated configuration, the practices and representations in the field of leisure, mountain and climbing activities nevertheless continue to reflect the

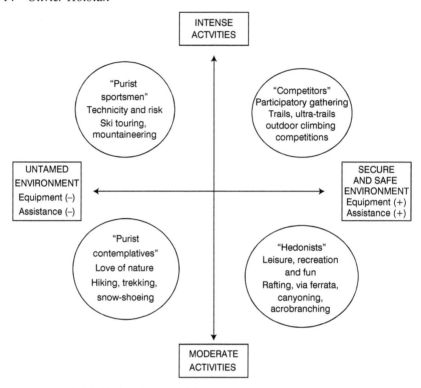

Figure 1.1 Social field of outdoor activities

logic of social distinction. This space appears crisscrossed by tensions between the various types of practitioners and their differing needs. The structuring of this space into several clusters against a backdrop of sometimes antagonistic trends and the recent intensification of conflicts seems to reveal the main lines of division. Undoubtedly, the best interpretation is that these conflicts express a transition between two states in the field of mountaineering climbing and activities.

The cultural history of mountaineering and climbing is an attempt to understand the processes at work in this cultural universe by observing the debates and tensions around defining legitimate practice, in order to better identify the relevant social issues. How these activities are practised and their modes of sociability have been defined by the dominant groups in these social worlds and then have tended to spread to all practitioners. Based on the logic of 'distinction', the conceptions that were imposed in different periods were intended to ensure that certain forms of practice would prevail, in harmony with the ethical and aesthetic inclinations of the educated classes. Traditionally, climbers have sought to protect their sport from becoming 'like other sports'; they have fought against the danger of having their sport trivialised by being opened up to the masses in order to continue deriving the 'symbolic benefits' of being members of a 'rare' community. This has essentially meant that they have struggled to reserve these activities for an elite.

The analysis of the cultural conditions that allowed for the emergence of and successive transformations in these two activities provides insight into how collective identities are constructed in developed and hierarchical societies and how social relations are structured among national elites. Therefore, can we not imagine, in the words of Norbert Elias, that 'knowledge of sport is the key to knowledge of society' (Elias and Dunning, 1994)?

Summary

- The history of mountaineering and climbing has regularly sparked conflict and tensions around how these two activities would become mere 'sports like any other'.
- During the 1930s, a process of streamlining the training techniques began to contest 'cultivated excursionism' and gave rise to classic mountaineering.
- 'Aid climbing' appeared in the 1950s before being denounced by certain climbers for the 'abuse of artificial means'.
- The emergence of 'free climbing' took hold at the end of the 1960s by climbers who also had growing environmental concerns.
- With the 'sportivisation process' and the development of competitions and participatory gathering, this space appears crisscrossed by tensions between the various types of practitioners.

References

Aubel, O. (2005). *L'escalade libre en France, sociologie d'une prophétie sportive*. Paris, France: L'Harmattan.

Baudrillard, J. (1970). *La société de consommation*. Paris, France: Denoël.

Bonnington, C. (1992). *The Climbers: A History of Mountaineering*. London, England: BBC Books.

Bouchet, P., & Hilliairet, D. (2009). *Marques de sport: Approches marketing et stratégiques*. Bruxelles, Belgium: De Boeck.

Chambre, D. (2015). *Le 9e degree, 150 ans d'escalade*. Chamonix, France: Edition du Mont Blanc.

Chartier, R. (1993). Le temps des doutes, *Le Monde*, 18.3.1993.

Chartier, R. (1998). *Au bord de la falaise, l'histoire entre certitude et inquiétude*. Paris, France: Albin Michel.

Clark, R. W., & Pyatt, E. C. (1957). *Mountaineering in Britain*. London, England: Phoenix House.

De Bellefon, R. (2003). *Histoire des guides de montagne, 1760-1980*. Paris, France: Milan.

Elias, N. & Dunning, E. (1994). *Sport et civilisation, la violence maitrisée*. Paris, France: Fayard.

Engel, C. E. (1930). *La litterature alpestre en France et en Angleterre au XVIIIe et XIXe siècles*. Paris, France: Victor Attinger.

Godfrey, B., & Dudley, C. (1977). *Climb! Rock Climbing in Colorado*. Boulder, CO: Alpine House Publishing, Westview Press.

Hamon, H., & Rotman, P. (1987). *Génération*. Paris, France: Le seuil.

Haver, G. (2008). Le club alpin suisse. In O. Hoibian (Ed.), *L'invention de l'alpinisme.* Paris, France: Belin.

Hoibian, O. (1995). De l'Alpinisme à l'escalade libre: l'invention d'un style? *Revue STAPS*, 36, 7–15.

Hoibian, O. (2001). *Les alpinistes en France, une histoire culturelle.* Paris, France: L'Harmattan.

Hoibian, O. (2008). *L'invention de l'alpinisme. La montagne et l'affirmation de la bourgeoisie cultivée, 1786-1914.* Paris, France: Belin.

Hoibian, O. (2014). Les professionnels du tourisme sportif de montagne sont-ils préservés du risque de burn out? *Juristourisme*, 163, 24–29.

Jones, D. (1984). *Rock Climbing in Britain.* Glasgow, Scotland: Collins.

Le Comte, E. (2008). *Citadins au sommet.* Genève, Switzerland: Slatkine.

Le Prince Ringuet, D. (1964). Les moyens de l'alpinisme. *La Montagne*, 307–314.

Loret, A. (1995). *Génération glisse.* Paris, France: Autrement.

Mestre, M. (2000). Le alpi contese alpinismo e nazionalismi. Torino, Italy: CDA.

Müller A. M. (1979). *Geschichte des Deutschen und Österreichischen Alpenvereins. Ein Beitrag zur Sozialgeschichte des Vereinswesens.* Münster, Germany: Westfälische Wilhelms-Universität Münster.

Ory, P. (2011). *L'histoire culturelle.* Paris, France: PUF.

Ottogali-Mazzacavallo, C. (2006). *Femmes et alpinisme, un genre de compromis, 1874-1919,* Paris, France: L'Harmattan.

Pastore, A. (2003). *Alpinismo e storia d'Italia. Dall'Unità alla Resistenza.* Bologna, Italy: Mulino.

Poirrier, P. (2004). *Les enjeux de l'histoire culturelle.* Paris, France: Seuil.

Raspaud, M. (2003). *L'aventure himalayenne.* Grenoble, France: PUG.

Ricoeur, P. (2000). *La mémoire, l'histoire, l'oubli.* Paris, France: Le Seuil.

Ring, J. (2000). *How the Englishmen Made the Alps.* London, England: John Murray.

Roper, S. (1979). *Camp 4, Chroniques du Yosémite,* Chamonix, Switzerland: Editions Guérin.

Tailland, M. (1997). *Les alpinistes victoriens.* Villeneuve d'Ascq, France: PUS.

Tribout, J. B., & Chambre, D. (1987). *Le huitième degré, dix ans d'escalade libre en France.* Paris, France: Editions Denoël.

Veyne, P. (1971). *Comment on écrit l'histoire: essai d'épistémologie.* Paris, France: Le seuil.

Vigarello, G. (2008). Préface. In O. Hoibian (Ed.), *L'invention de l'alpinisme.* Paris, France: Belin.

Zuanon, J. P. (2008). Le club alpin italien (1863-1914). In O. Hoibian (Ed.), *L'invention de l'alpinisme.* Paris, France: Belin.

Part I
Physiology

2   Physiology of climbing

Luisa Giles and Jason Brandenburg

Rock climbing relies heavily on the relatively small musculature of the upper body, specifically the finger and elbow flexors. Consequently, upper body rowing or cycling, rather than treadmill or bicycling modes of exercise testing, are more closely related to climbing ability. The acute physiological demands of climbing increase as the climb difficulty increases. However, when route difficulty increases by reducing hold size and increasing the distance between holds, the physiological responses are more pronounced than when route grade is increased by simply increasing steepness but maintaining hold configuration. Forearm vasculature adaptations that result from climbing allow for faster re-oxygenation of the forearm muscles during short recovery periods and improved muscular endurance. Activation of the forearm muscles is altered by grip styles and, practically, climbers should incorporate a variety of grip styles during their training. Climbers may also want to include active and/or cold-water immersion recovery strategies as both have been shown expedite muscle recovery.

Introduction

Climbing encompasses a broad spectrum of difficulties and within each level of difficulty there are a variety of route styles; all of which can place different physiological demands on the body. Furthermore, as climbers become more competent the physiological demands of climbing may change. To this end, the purpose of this chapter is to summarise the metabolic and physiological responses to climbing.

Metabolic responses

Maximal oxygen consumption of climbers

Peak oxygen consumption (VO_{2peak}), which refers to the peak oxygen consumption during an incremental test to maximum, is an indicator of aerobic fitness and cardiovascular function. As climbing increases the demand on aerobic energy production, aerobic fitness may be an important characteristic for climbers (Bertuzzi, Franchini, Kokubun, & Kiss, 2007). Furthermore, good general aerobic fitness could be beneficial when climbers are faced with short recovery periods between climbs, such as during competition climbing (Pires et al., 2011).

When performing a graded exercise test on a treadmill or cycling ergometer, the VO_{2peak} of climbers is generally considered to be excellent to superior (American College of Sports Medicine, 2014) and ranges between 50.5 and 60.2 mL•kg^{-1}•min^{-1} (see Table 2.1). As expected, the VO_{2peak} of climbers is lower than endurance athletes (>60 mL•kg^{-1}•min^{-1}); however, these values are consistent with team sport athletes (50–64 mL•kg^{-1}•min^{-1}) (Kenney, Wilmore, Costill, & Wilmore, 2012). Although the VO_{2peak} of climbers represents excellent to superior aerobic fitness, there is no clear relationship between a high VO_{2peak} (on a treadmill/ bicycle) and rock climbing performance/ability. For example, Fryer et al. (2012) observed no significant difference in treadmill VO_{2peak} between intermediate (56.5 ± 12.2 mL•kg^{-1}•min^{-1}; mean ± SD) and elite level climbers (59.7 ± 8.2 mL•kg^{-1}•min^{-1}). The absence of a positive relationship between climbing ability and VO_{2peak} may be due to the mode of exercise used for assessing aerobic fitness. Running on a treadmill or cycling on an ergometer are not specific to the muscles used during climbing or those that limit climbing performance (Pires et al., 2011; Sheel, Seddon, Knight, McKenzie, & Warburton, 2003).

The VO_{2peak} during upper body tests, such as arm ergometry and rowing, is lower than that achieved on a treadmill (Table 2.1: 22.3–36.8 vs. 50.5–60.2 mL•kg^{-1}•min^{-1}). However, because upper body tests use the muscles involved during climbing, they may be better related to climbing ability. In fact, there was a significant positive relationship between self-reported climbing ability (redpoint and on-sight) and VO_{2peak} during upper body rowing but not treadmill running (Michailov, Morrison, Ketenliev, & Pentcheva, 2014). Furthermore, VO_{2peak} during upper body cycling was significantly lower in non-climbers than climbers, highlighting the potential for upper body tests to discriminate between climbers of different abilities (Pires et al., 2011). However, as some studies have shown no differences between intermediate and elite climbers (Bertuzzi et al., 2007; Pires et al., 2011) future research should continue to explore the relationship between climbing performance and upper body VO_{2peak}.

To further increase test specificity, several studies have measured VO_{2peak} during climbing-specific tests. During such tests, climbers are challenged until exhaustion by either increasing the angle of the climbing wall or by increasing the speed of climbing using a climbing treadmill. During tests of increasing speed, VO_{2peak} (43.8–51.9 mL•kg^{-1}•min^{-1}, on-sight range 6b–8b) tends to be less than that achieved on a running treadmill using similar ability climbers (on-sight range 6b–7b+) (see Table 2.1) (Booth, Marino, Hill, & Gwinn, 1999; Espana-Romero et al., 2009). During tests of increasing steepness, VO_{2peak} (40.3–43.8 mL•kg^{-1}•min^{-1}) is also less than that achieved on a running treadmill (Balas et al., 2014; Booth et al., 1999), and represented 68 per cent of treadmill VO_{2peak} within the same subjects (Balas et al., 2014).

Although VO_{2peak} during climbing is different from that obtained from non-specific modes of exercise, it does not appear to be better at predicting climbing ability. Specifically, one study found no correlation between climbing VO_{2peak} and

Table 2.1 VO$_{2max}$ of climbers during different modes of exercise

Author	Participants	Climbing ability	VO$_{2max}$/VO$_{2peak}$ (mL•kg^{-1}•min^{-1})	HRmax (bpm)
Treadmill running				
Balas et al., 2014	26 M	Redpoint 3–8b	59.7 (5.1)	193 (8)
Billat, Palleja, Charlaix, Rizzardo, and Janel, 1995	4	> 7b	54.8 (5.9)	205 (12)
de Geus, Villanueva O'Driscoll, and Meeusen, 2006	15 M	Indoor: on-sight 7b–7c, redpoint 7c–8a. Outdoor: on-sight 7b+, redpoint 8a	52.2 (5.1)	192 (13)
Dickson et al., 2012	9 (8 M, 1 F)	6b+–6c	57.7 (5.9)	192 (8)
Draper et al., 2012	19 (13 M, 6 F)	Redpoint 5+–6b On-sight 5+–6a	51.8 (8.7)	
Draper, Jones, Fryer, Hodgson, and Blackwell, 2010	9 M	LC 6a–6c	58.7 (6)	195 (8)
Draper, Jones, Fryer, Hodgson, and Blackwell, 2008	10 M	LC 4+–5 (traditional climb)	58.0 (6.0)	195 (8)
Fryer, Dickson, Draper, Blackwell, and Hillier, 2013	21 (18 M, 3 F)	On-sight 6b+–6c Redpoint 6c+–7b Participants were split into LC and TR groups	LC: 60.2 (8.5) TR: 52.0 (9.5)	LC: 189 (10) TR: 193 (11)
Fryer et al., 2012	22 (17 M, 5 F)	Intermediate: On-sight 6a Advanced: On-sight 6c+	56.5 (12.2) 59.7 (8.2)	
Magalhaes et al., 2007	14 M	'indoor climbers' climbing grade ability unclear	54.5 (2.1)	197.5 (6)
Michailov, Morrison, Ketenliev, and Pentcheva, 2014	11 M	Redpoint: 8a+ (range: 7b+–8c+) On-sight: 7b (range: 6c+–8a)	58.3 (2.6)	197.1 (8)

continued…

Table 2.1 continued…

Author	Participants	Climbing ability	VO_{2max}/VO_{2peak} $(mL{\cdot}kg^{-1}{\cdot}min^{-1})$	HRmax (bpm)
Watts and Drobish, 1998	16 (9 M, 7 F)	Completed a 1 credit climbing course and 10 days of climbing over the last year. Climbing grade ability unclear.	50.5 (7.0)	
Upper body rowing/pulling using a vertical rowing machine				
Billat et al., 1995	4	> 7b	22.3 (2.6)[a]	190 (10)[a]
Michailov et al., 2014	11 M	Redpoint: 8a+ (range: 7b+–8c+) On-sight: 7b (range: 6c+–8a)	34.1 (4.1)[b]	184 (8)
Upper body cycling				
Bertuzzi, Franchini, Kokubun, and Kiss, 2007	13	Elite (n=6): > 7c Recreational (n=7): > 6c+	36.5 (6.2) 35.5 (5.2)	
Pires et al., 2011	21	Elite (n=7): > 7a+ Intermediate (n=7): > 6c+ Control (n=7): n/a	36.8 (5,7) 35.5 (5.2) 28.8 (5.0)[c]	184 (7) 175 (9) 159 (22)[d]
Cycling				
Rosponi, Schena, Leonardi, and Tosi, 2012	6 M	On-sight 7b+–8a	56.3 (4.9)	178 (6)
Sheel, Seddon, Knight, McKenzie, and Warburton, 2003	9 (6 M, 3 F)	7a+–8c+	45.5 (6.6)	192 (11)
Climbing test to exhaustion. Incremental increase in climbing angle or speed of climbing				
Balas et al., 2014	26 M	Redpoint: 3–8b	40.3 (3.5)	178 (11)
Bertuzzi et al., 2012	11	Elite (n=6): 7c–8b Recreational (n=7): 6a+–6c+	51.8 (7.3) 47.7 (8.9)	188 (6) 183 (6)
Booth, Marino, Hill, and Gwinn, 1999	7 (6 M, 1 F)	On-sight 6b–7a	43.8 (2.2)	190 (4)

| Espana-Romero et al., 2009 | 16 (8 M, 8 F) Also split into Expert and Elite | Men: On-sight 8a Women: On-sight 7a Expert (n=12): On-sight 7b Elite (n=4): On-sight 8b | 53.6 (3.7) 49.2 (3.5)[e] 51.3 (4.5) 51.9 (3.4) |

Of the 16 participants data is displayed as a male and female split, as well as an elite and expert split.

Notes:

a p<0.05, significantly less than treadmill values
b Upper body vertical rowing related to self-reported climbing ability
c p<0.05, significantly less than other groups;
d p<0.05, significantly less than elite
e p<0.05, significantly different from men

Unless otherwise stated the climbing ability of participants was determined using self-reported sport climbing ability. All grades have been converted to the French sport grading system. Data represents mean (sd). Abbreviations: HR: heart rate, LC: lead climb, TR: Top rope self-reported on-sight climbing ability, nor were there differences in climbing VO_{2peak} between expert (on-sight: 7b) and elite (on-sight: 8b) climbers (Espana-Romero et al., 2009). Although surprising, these findings imply that climbing-specific VO_{2peak} is not predictive of climbing performance and/or ability (Espana-Romero et al., 2009). Based on current research, upper body cycling and rowing, because they are related to climbing performance/ability, appear to be the preferred modes of exercise when assessing the aerobic fitness of climbers.

Oxygen consumption during climbing

At the onset of climbing, oxygen consumption sharply increases and typically plateaus during the remainder of the climb (Dickson, Fryer, Blackwell, Draper, & Stoner, 2012; Fryer, Dickson, Draper, Blackwell, & Hillier, 2013; Watts, Daggett, Gallagher, & Wilkins, 2000). Average oxygen consumption during climbing ranges between 20 and 37 mL•kg^{-1}•min^{-1} (Table 2.2), corresponding to 40–70 per cent of treadmill VO_{2peak} and 75 per cent of climbing VO_{2peak} (Booth et al., 1999), and may be influenced by route difficulty, climbing ability, ascent style, that is, top rope versus lead climb, and the speed of ascent.

Route difficulty

It is generally assumed if hold size and placement are maintained but steepness increases, or if the steepness of the climb is maintained but the climbing holds are smaller or placed further apart, the climbing grade increases; both of which may affect climbing VO_2. In some instances increasing steepness did not affect climbing VO_2 (Watts & Drobish, 1998), which could be related to the fact that as the steepness increased climbing distance (and thus ascent speed) progressively decreased. An increase in steepness combined with a progressive decrease in speed of ascent may result in a similar workload, thus explaining the similar VO_2 responses between the different climbing angles. To support this, when the speed of ascent was controlled VO_2 was higher during a steeper climb (105° vs. 90° ; 32.4 vs. 28.5 mL•kg^{-1}•min^{-1}; significance unreported) (Balas et al., 2014), suggesting VO_2 during climbing is a product of steepness and speed of ascent.

The lack of difference in VO_2 between the different angles found by Watts and Drobish (1998) may also be attributed to the small differences in steepness between the climbs (80°, 86°, 91°, 96°). Likewise, Mermier et al. (1997) found no differences in VO_2 when climbers completed routes that only differed by 16° (90°: 20.7 mL•kg^{-1}•min^{-1} vs. 106°: 21.9 mL•kg^{-1}•min^{-1}). However, when route steepness increased to 151° a significant increase in oxygen consumption was observed (24.9 mL•kg^{-1}•min^{-1}). These findings indicate that the oxygen demand of climbing is only influenced by large changes in steepness. This notion was further supported by de Geus et al. (2006), who observed a significant difference in oxygen consumption between two traversing routes (both graded 7c) with a large difference in angle (90°: 32 mL•kg^{-1}•min^{-1} vs. 135–180°: 34.9 mL•kg^{-1}•min^{-1}). Intuitively, a large increase in the steepness of a climb places considerably more

Table 2.2 VO$_2$ and HR responses during climbing

Author	Participants	Experimental design/protocol	Mean VO$_2$ (mL·kg^{-1}·min^{-1})	Mean heart rate (bpm)
Steepness of ascent and climbing difficulty				
Balas et al., 2014	26 M Redpoint: 3–8b	90°, 3+ 105°, 4 Maximal climbing test	28.5 (3.6), 48% 32.4 (4.3), 54% 40.3 (3.5), 68%	130 (17), 67% 146 (19), 76%
		5 circuits × 15 movements over 3 minutes (25 moves/minute) at 90°, followed by the same circuit at 105°. Not a randomised order.	The authors found a significant relationship between climbing ability and submaximal VO$_2$ at 90° and 105°. % represents percentage of treadmill max	
Bertuzzi, Franchini, Kokubun, & Kiss, 2007	13 Elite (n=6): 7c–8b Recreational (n=7): 6a+– 6c+	Easy: 90°, 5+ Moderate: 120°, 6c Hard: 110°, 7b VO$_2$ and HR were only compared in elite climbers as recreational climbers were unable to complete moderate and hard routes. 10 m high wall, ~ 25 movements, self-selected pace, TR	37.2 (7.6), 102% 38.0 (6.3), 106% 38.6 (5.4), 108% % represents percentage of arm cycle max * $p<0.05$, significantly greater than easy	162 (8) 175 (5)* 181 (7)*
de Geus, Villanueva O'Driscoll, & Meeusen, 2006	15 M On-sight 7b–8a	Overhanging route: 120–135° Vertical route: 90° Overhanging traverse 135–180° Vertical traverse: 90° All routes were graded 7c, 13–17 m in length and had between 26 and 33 moves.	35.9 (3.2), 70%** 35.9 (3.6), 68%** 34.9 (3.1), 66%** 32.0 (3.8), 62% % represents percentage of VO$_{2max}$ and HRmax achieved on a treadmill * $p<0.05$, significantly different from overhanging and vertical route ** $p<0.05$, significantly > vertical traverse	169 (8), 88% 168 (10), 88%* 160 (8), 84%* 162 (8), 86%*

continued…

Table 2.2 continued...

Author	Participants	Experimental design/protocol	Mean VO_2 ($mL \cdot kg^{-1} \cdot min^{-1}$)	Mean heart rate (bpm)
Mermier, Robergs, McMinn, & Heyward, 1997	14 (9 M, 5 F) Ability unclear	Easy: 90°, 5.6 Moderate: 106°, 5.9 Difficult: 151°, 5.11+	20.7 (8.1) 21.9 (5.3) 24.9 (4.9)*	142 (19)** 155 (15)** 163 (15)**
		3 × 5 minutes of climbing and lowering with 20 minutes rest. Each climb was performed on the same day in from easiest to hardest (not randomised)	* p<0.05, significantly greater than easy ** p<0.05, each route was significantly different from the others	
Sheel, Seddon, Knight, McKenzie, & Warburton, 2003	9 (6 M, 3 F) 7a+–8c+	Easier: 6a+ Harder: 6c+	20.1 (3.3), 45% 22.7 (3.7)*, 52%	
		Easier: climbers maximum climbing ability minus 3 grades. Harder: climbers maximum climbing ability minus 2 grades, TR	% represents percentage of cycling max * p<0.05, significantly greater than easy	
Watts & Drobish, 1998	16 (9 M, 7 F) Completed a 1 credit climbing course and 10 days of climbing over the last year.	80° 86° 91° 96° 102° Treadmill run matching HR at 86°	31.3 (4.0) 31.7 (4.6) 31.2 (4.6) 29.5 (5.2) 30.9 (3.7) 36.6 (5.5)*	156 (17) 165 (16)* 171 (17)** 173 (15)** 171 (16) 163 (16)
	Climbing grade ability unclear.	5.7 for the least steep angle. 4 minutes at each angle, 6 minutes rest between, order not randomised, performed on a rock climbing treadmill	* p<0.05, significantly > 86° * p<0.05, significantly > preceding angle	

Climber ability

Balas et al., 2014	26 M Redpoint: 3–8b	90°, 3+ 105°, 4 Maximal climbing test 5 circuits × 15 movements over 3 minutes (25 moves/minute) at 90°, followed by the same circuit at 105°. Not a randomised order.		Significant negative correlation between VO_2 at 90° and 105° and climber ability for VO_2 (r = –0.82, p<0.05; r = –0.84, p<0.05) and HR (r = –0.43, p<0.05; r = –0.78, p<0.05)
Bertuzzi et al., 2007	13 Elite (n=6): 7c– 8b Recreational (n=7): 6a+– 6c+	Recreational Elite Easy route at 90°, 5+, 10 m high wall, ~25 movements, self-selected pace, TR	36.0 (5.5), 104% 37.2 (7.6), 102%	171 (6)* 162 (8) % represents percentage of arm cycle max data represents VO_{2peak} and peak HR * p<0.05, significantly greater than elite
Fryer et al., 2012	22 (17 M, 5 F) On-sight > 7b	Intermediate 7 M, 4 F, 6a on-sight Advanced: 10 M, 1 F, 6c+ on-sight 12.15 m, 7 bolts, climbing grade 6a for intermediate climbers and 6c for advanced	38 42	data represents VO_{2peak} and no standard deviations were reported

Ascent style: TR vs. LC; on-sight vs. redpoint

Aras & Akalan, 2014	26 (22 M, 4 F) 4+–5+	LC TR 15 m high wall, climb graded 5+ TR included mimicking LC clipping	25.9 (4.4) 24.4 (5.5)*	145 (20) 140 (16) * p=0.022, significantly different from LC

continued…

Table 2.2 continued…

Author	Participants	Experimental design/protocol	Mean VO_2 ($mL \cdot kg^{-1} \cdot min^{-1}$)	Mean heart rate (bpm)
Dickson, Fryer, Blackwell, Draper, & Stoner, 2012	15 (14 M, 1 F) On-sight > 7b	LC TR 12.13 m, 7b, LC had a significantly greater climbing time (135.7 vs. 167.2)	34.3 (1.2), 58% 36.9 (4.2), 64% % represents percentage of treadmill max	166 (9), 87% 171 (10), 88%
Draper, Jones, Fryer, Hodgson, & Blackwell, 2008	10 M Lead 4+–5 Traditional climbs	Not a within-subjects design On-sight LC Redpoint LC 9.38 m, 5b. On-sight significantly greater climbing time than redpoint (213 vs. 199 s)	 26.5 (2.4), 46% 26.0 (2.5), 45% % represents percentage of treadmill max	 161 (6) 159 (6)
Draper, Jones, Fryer, Hodgson, & Blackwell, 2010	9 M Best sport lead 6a–6c	LC TR 9.38 m, 6a, 6 clips, 5° overhang during the first 2 m then vertical to the top. LC had significantly greater climbing time than redpoint (188 vs. 136 s)	VO_{2peak} for LC and TR: 40.9 (6.6) and 32.3 (5.9), respectively	159 (6) 151 (5)
Fryer, Dickson, Draper, Blackwell, & Hillier, 2013	21 (18 M, 3 F) On-sight: 6b+–6c Redpoint: 6c+–7b	LC TR 6c, not a within-subjects design. Climbing time for lead TC climbs were 109.9 and 163.7 s, respectively.	64% 55% % represents percentage of treadmill max	78% 83%
Climbing route style				
Billat, Palleja, Charlaix, Rizzardo, & Janel, 1995	4 Regular climbers, 6 hours a week for 3 years	Route 1: Smaller holds Route 2: Steeper, larger holds Both graded 7b	24.9 (1.4), 46/114% 20.6 (0.9), 38/98% % represents percentage of treadmill max/arm pulling max	176 (14) 86/93% 159 (15), 78/84%

Climbing speed

Study	Sample	Protocol		
			Trial 1, trial 2	Trial 1, trial 2
Rosponi, Schena, Leonardi, & Tosi, 2012	6 M On-sight: 7b+–8a	Self-selected pace (SS) Low speed (50% slower than SS) High speed (50% faster than SS)	35.9 (6.7), 35.7 (6.1)* 28.3 (7.4), 27.4 (7.5) 43.9 (6.0), 44.8 (4.3)* **	157 (15), 159 (16)* 145 (21), 144 (23) 172 (11), 175 (10)* **
		13 m, 6a+, 10° overhang, TR, 5 minutes per speed including rapid lowering, minimum of 10 minutes in between speeds/ascents. Each speed completed twice, not randomized	* $p<0.05$, significantly greater than low speed ** $p<0.05$, significantly greater than SS	

Descriptive response

Study	Sample	Protocol		
Booth, Marino, Hill, & Gwinn, 1999	7 (6 M, 1 F) On-sight 6b–7a	5c redpoint climb (outdoors) 24.4 m overhanging	32.8 (2.0) 75% of a maximal climbing test data represents VO_{2peak} and peak HR	157 (8) 83% of a maximal climbing test
Rodio, Fattorini, Rosponi, Quattrini, & Marchetti, 2008	13 (8 M, 5 F) M > 7a, F > 5	Men Women 4a, 25 m outdoor climb	28.3 (1.5) 27.5 (3.6) * $p<0.05$, significantly > men	144 (16) 164 (13)*
Watts, Daggett, Gallagher, & Wilkins, 2000	15 M Redpoint: 7b+–8c+	20 m, overhanging, 12b, self-selected pace, LC	24.7 (4.3) Peak: 31.9 (5.3)	148 (16) Peak: 162 (17)

Abbreviations: HR: heart rate, LC: lead climb, TR: Top rope.

stress on the upper body musculature required to support and propel the climber (Mermier, Robergs, McMinn, & Heyward, 1997). Consequently, more muscle may be recruited and the force production requirements of the muscles increase; both of which could account for the increase in climbing VO_2 experienced with large increases in climbing angle. Currently, however, there is no consensus for the physiological mechanisms underlying the increase in climbing VO_2 that appears to accompany large increases in climb steepness.

Rather than manipulating climb steepness, Sheel et al. (2003) altered climb difficulty by changing climbing hold size and the distance between holds; with a harder route having smaller sized holds and more distance in between holds. In this study, the climbing VO_2 of experienced climbers (7a+–8c+) was significantly greater (22.7 vs. 20.1 mL•kg^{-1}•min^{-1}) during the harder climb (two grades below maximum climber ability) than the easier climb (three grades below maximum climber ability). Collectively, these findings suggest that as climbing grade increases, by manipulating hold size, the distance between holds, or through large increases in steepness, oxygen demands also increase.

Climber ability

A limitation when comparing the climbing VO_2 of different studies is the heterogeneity in climber ability, which could influence the VO_2 response. However, there were no differences in climbing VO_2 between recreational (climber ability: ≤6c+, 36.0 mL•kg^{-1}•min^{-1}) and elite (climber ability: >7c, 37.2 mL•kg^{-1}•min^{-1}) climbers when climbing the same route (graded 5+) on top rope (Bertuzzi et al., 2007) or between intermediate (climber ability: 6a, 38 mL•kg^{-1}•min^{-1}) and advanced (climber ability: 6c+, 42 mL•kg^{-1}•min^{-1}) climbers when lead climbing routes relative to their ability (6a for intermediate and 6c for advanced) (Fryer et al., 2012). The similarity in climbing VO_2 could be the result of comparable climbing times, and thus a similar speed of ascent, between groups in both studies. One concern with the above studies is that the difference in climbing ability between the higher and lower level climbers was not large enough to reveal differences. In a study using climbers with abilities ranging from 3 to 8b, a significant negative correlation between self-reported redpoint climbing ability and climbing VO_2 was observed during climbs with 90° and 105° overhang; indicating the O_2 demand of climbing is lower in advanced climbers (Balas et al., 2014). It seems that results from studies investigating the influence of climber ability on climbing VO_2 are inconclusive and future research, using a wide range of abilities, is needed to clear up this these inconsistencies.

Ascent style: top rope versus lead and on-sight versus redpoint

A climbing route is ascended either by lead climb or on top rope. When performing a lead climb, a climber is attached to the rope that trails behind during the ascent and they routinely stop to clip quick draws to bolts (sport climbing) or place protection (traditional climbing), to both of which the climbing rope is passed through. These steps involve a pause in upward climbing and a sustained isometric gripping action of the non-clipping arm. While on lead climb, the climber must also support the weight of the suspended rope as well as the gear attached to the climbing harness. With top rope climbing, the climber is attached to the climbing rope that passes through an anchor at the top of the climb (hence the rope is above them) and is then secured by a belayer. Consequently, the risk of falling large distances is diminished and there is no need to clip bolts or place protection. As a result, the rate of top rope climbing is usually faster than lead climbing. Given the differences between lead climbing and top rope climbing it is plausible they may elicit different demands.

When comparing lead climbing to top rope climbing no differences in mean VO_2 (Dickson et al., 2012; Draper, Jones, Fryer, Hodgson, & Blackwell, 2010; Fryer et al., 2013) or peak VO_2 (Draper et al., 2010) were found despite lead climbing requiring more time to complete the route (Table 2.2). These findings were similar across climbing abilities (lead climb ability range: 6a–>7b) and during a variety of climbing grades (6a–7b) (Dickson et al., 2012; Draper et al., 2010; Fryer et al., 2013) (Table 2.2). When data were analysed at specific clipping points along the route there are conflicting results. For example, VO_2 was higher at certain points (bolts 1, 3 and 5 but not bolts 2, 4, 6 and 7) while climbing on top rope compared to lead climbing (Dickson et al., 2012), whereas Fryer et al. (2013) did not find any differences at any point during a climb. The elevated climbing VO_2 at particular bolts in top rope was attributed to a faster rate of climbing as stopping to clip bolts was not necessary (Dickson et al., 2012) (Table 2.2). However, if this was the case, differences in climbing VO_2 should have been observed at the other clipping positions.

Successfully ascending a route on the first attempt and without prior information/rehearsal is known as an on-sight. Ascending a route after having practiced or received information about the climbing route is known as a redpoint. On-sight attempts typically take longer and may be more stressful than a redpoint attempt, resulting in different physiological demands. When studied, mean climbing VO_2 between an on-sight lead climb and second lead climb were similar, despite the on-sight climb requiring significantly more time to complete (Draper, Jones, Fryer, Hodgson, & Blackwell, 2008) (Table 2.2).

In summary, it appears the style of ascent (lead climb vs. top rope) and familiarity with the route (on-sight vs. redpoint) has minimal influence on the oxygen demands of climbing.

Energy systems

The small to moderate increases in oxygen consumption during climbing in combination with increases in blood lactate concentration have traditionally been interpreted to mean the energy needs of sport climbing are predominantly met through anaerobic adenosine triphosphate (ATP) production (Booth et al., 1999). However, more recently, it has been suggested the main energy systems during indoor climbing were the aerobic and anaerobic alactic systems (Bertuzzi et al., 2007). The aerobic energy system likely makes two contributions: one to directly satisfy the energy demands of climbing and the second to aid in the resynthesis of high-energy phosphates. The latter is likely of significance when climbers are recovering on a route (Fryer et al., 2012). Although the anaerobic lactic system made the smallest energy contribution, it was significantly less in elite climbers (vs. recreational), and the relative energy contribution from the anaerobic lactic system tended (not significant) to increase as the difficulty of the route became harder (Bertuzzi et al., 2007).

Blood lactate response to climbing

A number of studies have assessed lactate responses to climbing with post-climbing blood lactate values ranging from 1.6 to 11.1 mmol•L^{-1} (Table 2.3). For comparison, incremental climbing tests to exhaustion have yielded peak blood lactate values of 10.2 mmol•L^{-1} (Booth et al., 1999; Espana-Romero et al., 2009). Higher post-climbing blood lactate values were found following climbs performed at a faster speeds (4.9–5.4 mmol•L^{-1} increase vs. 1.9 mmol•L^{-1} increase for faster vs. self-selected pace, respectively) (Rosponi, Schena, Leonardi, & Tosi, 2012). When climbers performed a submaximal route until (or near to) exhaustion blood lactate was higher (11.1 mmol•L^{-1}; mean climbing time: 24.9 min) (Sherk et al., 2011) than when the route was close to maximum climbing ability, and therefore shorter in duration than an easier climb (6.1 mmol•L^{-1}; 11.3 min) (Magalhaes et al., 2007; Watts, Newbury, & Sulentic, 1996). Collectively, findings from these latter two studies imply that the duration of climbing exerts an important influence on blood lactate responses to climbing. Other climbing variables, such as route difficulty, climber ability, and ascent style may also influence the lactate responses to climbing.

Route difficulty

When climbing route difficulty is increased by modifying steepness, blood lactate significantly increases (1.6, 2.4 and 3.2 mmol•L^{-1} for 90°/3+, 106°/5 and 151°/6. b+, respectively) (Mermier et al., 1997). As the time needed to climb each route was not reported this may have varied between routes and thus influenced blood lactate responses. However, when studies controlled for climbing time, blood lactate progressively increased in response to progressively steeper climbing angles (Fryer et al., 2011; Watts & Drobish, 1998) (Table 2.3). In these studies climbers performed the climbs in order of least steep to most steep, and as a result, the higher lactate values experienced at the steeper angles may have been partially due to elevated pre-climb lactate levels as well as residual fatigue from previous climbs.

As suggested, if climbing holds and their positions are maintained thus changes in steepness are responsible for increasing the grade of the climb, blood lactate increases. But if the steepness is modified by itself, while maintaining the climbing grade, blood lactate does not significantly change (de Geus et al., 2006). These findings point to climbing grade, rather than steepness, as having the larger influence on blood lactate responses. To confirm this notion, research needs to examine the blood lactate response to climbs of increasing grade while maintaining the climbing angle.

Table 2.3 Lactate reponses to climbing

Author	Participants	Experimental design/protocol	Lactate (mmol•L⁻¹)
Steepness of ascent and climbing route difficulty			
de Geus, Villanueva O'Driscoll, & Meeusen, 2006	15 M On-sight ability 7b–8a	Overhanging route: 120–135° Vertical route: 90° Overhanging traverse 135–180° Vertical traverse: 90°	6.2 (1.6) 6.0 (1.8) 5.6 (1.7) 4.8 (1.3)*
			* p<0.05, significantly different from overhanging route
		All routes were graded 7c, 13–17 m in length and had between 26 and 33 moves.	Lactate measured immediately post-climb
		Vertical route had significantly greater climbing time vs. overhanging route and vertical traverse (244 vs. 189 and 195 s)	
Fryer et al., 2011	10 (9 M, 1 F) Redpoint 6b+	91°, 5 100°, 5+ 110°, 6b+	Finger sample, toe sample 2.8 (0.7), 2.8 (0.7) 3.7 (1.1), 3.6 (1.1) 4.3 (1.0), 4.2 (1.2)
		Bouldering set on 4.03 m high wall, participants ascended and descended the route three times without rest. Angles performed in the order depicted above with 5 minutes of passive rest	Pre-values for finger and toe were: 1.8 (0.7) and 2.1 (0.7). Data above represents post-climb sample
Mermier, Robergs, McMinn, & Heyward, 1997	14 (9 M, 5 F) Ability unclear	Easy: 90°, 5.6 Moderate: 106°, 5.9 Difficult: 151°, 5.11+	1.6 (0.6)* 2.4 (0.7)* 3.2 (1.0)*
		3 × 5 minutes of climbing and lowering with 20 minutes rest. Each climb was performed on the same day from easiest to hardest (not randomised)	* p< 0.05, values were significantly different from one another

continued…

Table 2.3 continued...

Author	Participants	Experimental design/protocol	Lactate (mmol•L⁻¹)
Watts & Drobish, 1998	16 (9 M, 7 F) Completed a 1 credit climbing course and 10 days of climbing over the last year. Climbing grade ability unclear.	80° 86° 91° 96° 102° Treadmill run matching HR at 86° 5.7 for the least steep angle. 4 minutes at each angle, 6 minutes rest between, order not randomised, performed on a rock climbing treadmill	3.6 (1.2) 4.0 (1.3) 4.9 (1.6)* 5.1 (1.3)* 5.9 (1.2)* * $p<0.05$, significantly > preceding angle

Climber ability

Author	Participants	Experimental design/protocol	Lactate (mmol•L⁻¹)
Bertuzzi, Franchini, Kokubun, & Kiss, 2007	13 Elite (n=6): 7c–8b Recreational (n=7): 6a+–6c+	Recreational climbers (able to climb 6c+) Elite climbers (able to climb 7c) Easy route: 90°, 5+	4.4 (1.6) 2.4 (0.9)* * $p<0.05$, significantly < recreational climbers

Climbing speed

Author	Participants	Experimental design/protocol	Lactate (mmol•L⁻¹)
Rosponi, Schena, Leonardi, & Tosi, 2012	6 M On-sight: 7b+–8a	Self-selected pace (SS) Low speed (50% slower than SS) High speed (50% faster than SS) 13 m, 6a+, 10° overhang, TC, 5 minutes per speed including rapid lowering, minimum of 10 minutes in between speeds/ascents. Each speed completed twice, not randomised	Trial 1, Trial 2 1.9 (1.1)*, 1.9 (1.5)* 1.5 (1.7)*, 1.9 (1.6)* 4.9 (1.9), 5.4 (2.3) * $p<0.05$, significantly less than high speed

Ascent style: TR vs. LC; on-sight vs. redpoint

Author	Participants	Experimental design/protocol	Lactate (mmol•L⁻¹)
Dickson, Fryer, Blackwell, Draper, & Stoner, 2012	15 (14 M, 1 F) On-sight > 7b	LC TC 12.13 m, 7b, LC had a significantly greater climbing time (135.7 vs. 167.2) Not a within-subjects design	Pre, post, 5 min post, 10 min post, 15 min post 1.6 (0.5), 5.4 (1.4), 4.8 (1.4), 3.7 (1.2), 3.0 (1.0) 1.7 (0.3), 5.5 (1.0), 5.0 (1.3), 4.0 (1.0), 3.2 (0.7)

Study	Participants	Protocol	Results
Draper, Jones, Fryer, Hodgson, & Blackwell, 2008	10 M Lead 4+–5 traditional climbs	On-sight LC Redpoint LC 9.38 m, 5b. On-sight significantly greater climbing time than redpoint (213 vs. 199 s)	Data depicted in a graph. Immediately post-climb lactate was significantly less during the redpoint compared to on-sight
Draper, Jones, Fryer, Hodgson, & Blackwell, 2010	9 M Best sport lead 6a–6c	LC TR 9.38 m, 6a, 6 clips, 5° overhang during the first 2 m then vertical to the top. LC had significantly greater climbing time than redpoint (188 vs. 136 s)	Pre, post, 15 min post 1.5 (0.5), 3.1 (0.6), 1.2 (0.4) 1.5 (1.2), 2.5 (0.9)*, 0.8 (0.4)* * $p<0.05$, significantly difference from the same time point on lead
Fryer, Dickson, Draper, Blackwell, & Hillier, 2013	21 (18 M, 3 F) On-sight: 6b+–6c Redpoint: 6c+–7b	LC TR 6c, not a within-subjects design. Climbing time for lead and TC climbs were 109.9 and 163.7 s, respectively.	Pre, post, 5 min post, 10 min post, 15 min post 2.1 (0.4), 5.2 (1.1), 4.5 (1.3), 3.7 (1.2), 2.9 (1.0) 2.3 (0.7), 4.8 (0.8), 4.2 (1.1), 3/5 (1.2), 3.1 (1.0)

Maximal/graded climbing test

Study	Participants	Protocol	Results
Bertuzzi et al., 2012	11 Elite (n=6): 7c–8b Recreational (n=7): 6a+–6c+	'Fit climbing test' 10 m wall, 5+, 90° for the 1st 3 m, 110° for the last 7 m. Participants climbed up and down the route as fast as possible for 3 minutes.	7.8 (1.1) 7.4 (2.1) Values represent peak values post-climb

continued...

Table 2.3 continued...

Author	Participants	Experimental design/protocol	Lactate ($mmol \cdot L^{-1}$)
Booth, Marino, Hill, & Gwinn, 1999	7 (6 M, 1 F) On-sight 6b–7a	Graded climbing test 5c climbing route, TR, 24.	10.2 (0.6) 4.5 (0.5)
		Graded climbing test consisted of 3 trials of increasing velocity with 20 minutes recovery in between each. 5 minutes @ 8 m/min, 10 m/min and 12 m/min. Following 12 m/min 1 minute at 14 and 16 m/min	Climbing route represents 44% of graded test Lactate measured immediately post-climb
Espana-Romero et al., 2009	16 (8 M, 8 F) Also split into expert and elite	Men: on-sight 8a Women: on-sight 7a Expert (n=12): on-sight 7b Elite (n=4): on-sight 8b	8.8 (2.9) 13.6 (2.0)* 11.4 (3.0) 10.5 (5.1)
		Of the 16 participants data is displayed as a male and female split, as well as an elite and expert split. Climbing test is the same as Booth et al. 1999	* $p < 0.05$, significantly greater than men
Climbing route style			
Billat, Palleja, Charlaix, Rizzardo, & Janel, 1995	4 Regular climbers, 6 hours a week for 3 years.	Route 1: smaller holds Route 2: steeper, larger holds Both graded 7b	5.8 (1.0) 4.3 (0.8)
Recovery mode			
Watts, Daggett, Gallagher, & Wilkins, 2000	15 M Redpoint: 7b+–8c+	Active recovery: recumbent hand crank cycling, 25 weeks Passive recovery Not repeated measures	Pre, post, 10, 20 and 30 min post 2.5 (1.6), 5.7 (1.7)*, 3.8 (1.7)*, 2.5 (1.6), 2.3 (1.6) 3.5 (1.9), 6.8 (1.9)*, 5.5 (1.7)*, 4.3 (2.1)*, 3.5 (2.1) * $p < 0.05$, compared to pre-climb

Lactate sampling site

Draper, Brent, Hale, & Coleman, 2006	45 (31 M, 14 F) Participants had taken part in a climbing course at university or were regular climbers	Lactate Pro analysers at the ear Lactate Pro analysers at the finger Yellow Springs Instruments at the finger 9.38 m wall, 90°, 4	Pre, post, 5 minutes post 1.6 (0.6), 3.7 (1.4), 3.1 (1.4) 1.7 (0.6), 3.9 (1.4), 3.2 (1.3) 1.3 (0.4), 3.4 (1.3), 2.9 (1.3)
Fryer et al., 2011	10 (9 M, 1 F) Redpoint 6b+	91°, 5 100°, 5+ 110°, 6b+ Bouldering set on 4.03 m high wall, participants ascended and descended the route three times without rest. Angles performed in the order depicted above with 5 minutes of passive rest	Finger sample, toe sample 2.8 (0.7), 2.8 (0.7) 3.7 (1.1), 3.6 (1.1) 4.3 (1.0), 4.2 (1.2) Pre values for finger and toe were: 1.8 (0.7), and 2.1 (0.7). Data above represents post-climb sample

Descriptive response

Gajewski, Hübner-Woźniak, Tomaszewski, & Sienkiewicz-Dianzenza, 2009	21 M 5–8c	7a	Pre, 3 min post, 30 min post 1.8 (0.8), 6.4 (1.5), 2.3 (0.7)
Magalhaes et al., 2007	14 M Indoor climbers	Routes ranged from 6b–7b and were selected to be at the near maximum for each climber	6.1 (0.9) Value represents maximal blood lactate, lactate was measured at 3, 5, and 7 minutes post

continued…

Table 2.3 continued...

Author	Participants	Experimental design/protocol	Lactate (mmol•L⁻¹)
Sherk, Sherk, Kim, Young, & Bemben, 2011	10 M TC: 5+–7c	Climbers were assigned a route based on their reported climbing ability that ranged from 4+–5+	Pre, post 2.9 (0.6), 11.1 (1.0)* * p<0.05 significantly greater than pre
Watts, Newbury, & Sulentic, 1996	11 M On-sight: 7a+–8b	7a+, lead climbed and down climbed until falling 7.4 m vertical followed by 18.5 m overhanging semicircular arch followed by another 7.4 m vertical down climb	Pre, post 1.4 (0.8), 6.1 (1.4)* * p<0.05 significantly greater than pre. Values peaked immediately post but remained significantly higher than pre-values at 20 minutes post

Abbreviations: HR: heart rate, LC: lead climb, TC: top rope.

Climber ability

There is only one study examining the influence of climbing ability on blood lactate responses to climbing, and it found that recreational climbers experienced significantly higher post-climb blood lactate levels than elite climbers following an ascent of the same route (grade: 5+; climber ability: 6a–6c+ vs. 7c–8b+; 4.4 vs. 2.4 mmol•L^{-1}) (Bertuzzi et al., 2007). In the recreational climbers a significantly greater energy contribution was made by the glycolytic energy system, which was estimated from increases in blood lactate. The greater energy contribution by the glycolytic system was likely the result of the recreational climbers working relatively harder and may have contributed to the higher post-climb blood lactate levels. Another explanation for the different blood lactate responses between the recreational and elite climbers is climbing technique. Advanced climbers seem to spend more time resting on a route and this may reduce lactate production or improve lactate clearance, thus accounting for the lower post-climb lactate levels in elite climbers (Fryer et al., 2012). It is also plausible that elite climbers may have physiological adaptations that reduce lactate production or improve lactate clearance.

Ascent styles

Completing a lead climb or top rope had no significant effect on the post-climb blood lactate response (Dickson et al., 2012; Draper et al., 2008; Fryer et al., 2013); however, the lack of a within-subjects design and the small sample sizes of these studies make the interpretation of these findings challenging. Using a within-subjects crossover design, higher blood lactate levels were observed immediately following a lead climb (3.1 mmol•L^{-1}) compared to a top rope (2.5 mmol•L^{-1}) of the same route (6a) in experienced climbers (6a–6c) (Draper et al., 2010). Extra time, to clip the bolts, was required to complete the lead climb and would have resulted in more sustained isometric actions of the climbing musculature, which may have increased lactate production and/or reduced lactate removal. Additionally, post-climb lactate levels were significantly higher following an on-sight lead climb compared to a redpoint lead climb of the same route (approx. 3.9 vs. 3.1 mmol•L^{-1}) (Draper et al., 2008). The higher lactate values in response to the on-sight climb were attributed to significantly longer climb duration.

Physiological responses

Heart rate

Relative to the rise in climbing VO_2, heart rate (HR) demonstrates an exaggerated and disproportionate increase and when expressed relative to the maximum values obtained on a treadmill, climbing HR typically exceeds climbing VO_2 by 20–40 per cent (Table 2.2). Specifically, competition climbers experienced a climbing VO_2 equal to 61 per cent of treadmill VO_2max whereas HR reached 91 per cent of treadmill HR_{max} (Magalhaes et al., 2007) and climbing VO_2 in recreational climbers equalled approximately 70 per cent of treadmill VO_{2max} while climbing

HR fell between 83 and 90 per cent treadmill HR_{max} (Rodio, Fattorini, Rosponi, Quattrini, & Marchetti, 2008).

Although the exact mechanisms for the disproportionate rise in HR have yet to be determined, the repetitive and sustained isometric contractions of the forearm and arm musculature are widely accepted as key contributing factors. Isometric contractions reduce blood flow to the arm and forearm musculature. The resulting ischemia leads to metabolite accumulation and a muscle metaboreflex that in turn elevates sympathetic drive causing HR to increase disproportionately to the demands (Fryer et al., 2013; Sheel, 2004). The dependence on the upper body during climbing is also proposed to contribute to the inflated HR response as it results in greater sympathetic nervous system activation compared to lower body exercise (Fryer et al., 2013). Additionally, when the limbs of the upper body are used during climbing, they are often positioned above the heart. To overcome the forces of gravity and deliver blood to these muscles HR increases beyond the expected demand (de Geus et al., 2006). Anxiety, often related to falling, is associated with greater sympathetic nervous system activation and has been speculated to contribute to the HR response of climbing (Draper et al., 2008). However, anxiety was not a contributing factor to the exaggerated HR response of during indoor sport climbing (Fryer et al., 2013), but whether this holds true for outdoor climbing is unknown. The degree of difficulty of a climb and climbing ability are variables that appear to further modify climbing HR.

Route difficulty

Climbing grade (and thus route difficulty) is influenced by the steepness of a route and by the size, type and distance between holds. It has consistently been shown that as a climbing route becomes steeper HR increases (Balas et al., 2014; Mermier et al., 1997; Watts & Drobish, 1998); and this occurs without a concomitant rise in VO_2. On steeper routes self-selected climbing pace slows, consequently the climbing muscles perform isometric actions that are more sustained and this could produce a substantial rise in HR (Watts & Drobish, 1998). However, when climbing pace was maintained over climbs varying in steepness HR still tended to be higher during a steeper route (130 vs. 146 beats per minute (bpm) for 95° and 105°, respectively) (Balas et al., 2014). Thus, it is possible as a climb becomes steeper greater stress is placed on the muscles of the upper body, consequently increasing sympathetic drive and causing a subsequent increase in HR (Mermier et al., 1997).

As the routes in the above studies differed in steepness and in climbing grade it is unclear if one variable elicits a greater influence on HR. Other studies examining the influence of difficulty on the HR response to climbing have either increased the climbing grade (by making the holds smaller and farther apart) while maintaining steepness (Sheel et al., 2003) or maintained the climbing grade while increasing steepness (thus making the holds larger, more numerous, and closer together as the route becomes steeper) (de Geus et al., 2006). As HR did not increase when climbing grade was maintained (de Geus et al., 2006), but did when it was increased (Sheel et al., 2003), it appears that increasing the climbing grade, rather than steepness, exerts a greater influence on climbing HR.

Climbing ability

In comparison to elite climbers, recreational climbers experienced a significantly higher peak HR while climbing the same route (5+) in a similar time (Bertuzzi et al., 2007), which could be related to the recreational climbers climbing a route that was relatively more difficult. Additionally, for a given VO_2, HR during climbing (at a grade near or equal to maximum on-sight ability) exceeded that during treadmill running; with the difference being significantly higher in intermediate (6a) than advanced climbers (6c+) (Fryer et al., 2012) despite the climbing route being of similar relative difficulty. One explanation for the lower climbing HR in experienced climbers may be the greater amount of time resting on a climb (Fryer et al., 2012). More rest may lessen forearm blood flow occlusion thus reducing metabolite build-up and the involvement of the metaboreflex. It is also plausible training adaptations to the vasculature of the forearm muscles that improve metabolite clearance may have contributed to the lower climbing HR seen in more experienced climbers.

Vascular adaptations

Rock climbing involves repetitive isometric contractions of the forearm musculature, during which muscle blood flow is restricted and O_2 availability is reduced. These periods of ischemia and hypoxia are thought to stimulate adaptations to the local vascular bed (Thompson, Farrow, Hunt, Lewis, & Ferguson, 2014); consequently, rock climbers may have adapted vasculature, particularly in the upper body.

Climbers (>6a) exhibited a greater resting brachial artery diameter compared to non-climbers, perhaps allowing for enhanced forearm blood flow and oxygen delivery (Thompson et al., 2014). However, when brachial artery blood flow, blood flow velocity and diameter were assessed at the end of a continuous isometric protocol (Fryer, Stoner, Scarrott, et al., 2015) and following brachial artery ischemia with and without hand grip exercise (Thompson et al., 2014), the relative changes in these parameters were not different between non-climbers and climbers of different abilities. In these two studies, the absence of any differences between the climbers and non-climbers may be due to the non-climbing-specific protocols. During a climbing-specific, intermittent isometric endurance test until fatigue (10 s contraction phase: 3 s rest phase at 40 per cent maximum voluntary contraction), forearm blood flow during the three second rest periods was greater in elite climbers (≥7b) than non-climbers (Fryer, Stoner, Lucero, et al., 2015). Intermediate (6a) and advanced climbers (6c) also experienced higher forearm blood flow than the non-climbers, but the differences were not significant. Accompanying the higher forearm blood flow during the three second periods in the elite climbers was enhanced forearm muscle performance (as measured by force multiplied by the time to fatigue; force–time integral).

During an intermittent isometric endurance test until fatigue (10 s contraction phase: 3 s rest phase at 40 per cent MVC), intermediate (6c–7c) and advanced

(>7a) climbers demonstrated faster re-oxygenation (as measured by near infra-red spectroscopy) of the finger flexor musculature during the rest phase than non-climbers (MacLeod et al., 2007; Philippe, Wegst, Muller, Raschner, & Burtscher, 2012). Likewise, elite climbers ($\geq$7b) demonstrated greater re-oxygenation of the flexor carpi radialis muscle, but not the flexor digitorum profundus muscle, than non-climbers and intermediate climbers (6a) (Fryer, Stoner, Lucero, et al., 2015). In all three studies, faster re-oxygenation during the three second rest periods was associated with better performance in the intermittent isometric test. Adaptations to the forearm vasculature that improve muscle perfusion, such as an increase in capillary density, were proposed to account for the faster re-oxygenation and superior forearm muscle performance of the experienced climbers. To support this hypothesis, studies have shown enhanced capillary filtration capacity (which is indicative of a greater capillary density) in climbers (>6a) compared to non-climbers (Thompson et al., 2014). Elite climbers (7a–8a+), in comparison to controls, also demonstrated a higher forearm vascular conductance (Ferguson & Brown, 1997). The higher vascular conductance, which was attributed to enhanced vasodilator capacity of the forearm arterioles, could explain the greater forearm blood flow experienced by elite climbers during the short rest periods of climbing-specific tasks (Fryer, Stoner, Lucero, et al., 2015). In theory, faster re-oxygenation and increased forearm blood flow during short rest phases would result in a quicker restoration of phosphocreatine levels; a mechanism that would explain the improved performance on an intermittent isometric test and should be beneficial during competition climbing (Philippe et al., 2012). In addition to aiding re-oxygenation, a greater forearm blood flow could account for the previously mentioned lower post-climb lactate levels of experienced climbers in comparison to recreational climbers (Bertuzzi et al., 2007). Although the forearm adaptations of climbers appear to be associated with better performance during an isometric endurance test with a 10:3 s contraction:relaxation ratio, whether they contribute to differences in rock climbing ability is uncertain. For example, a 12.1:2.1 s contraction:relaxation ratio was observed for the dominant hand of experienced climbers (redpoint: 6a–7a+) when climbing a route graded 5+(Donath, Roesner, Schoffl, & Gabriel, 2013). Furthermore, during competition the contraction:relaxation ratio for competitive boulders was 7.9:0.6 s (White & Olsen, 2010). Thus, to better understand the differences between climbers and non-climbers future research needs to utilise contraction:relaxation ratios more representative of climbing.

Neuromuscular recruitment

Forearm muscle function, particularly that of the finger flexors, is critical to successful climbing (Watts et al., 1996). During a climb, the finger flexors are required to exert force under a variety of grip styles, each of which may place different demands on these muscles. When using electromyography (EMG) to examine the influence of different grip styles (four-finger crimp, pinch, open hand, and different two-finger pocket grips) during a two-move climbing sequence on the activation of the forearm muscles, all grip styles produced a higher forearm

EMG than a maximal handgrip exercise. The four-finger crimp (208 per cent of maximal handgrip EMG) and two-finger pocket with the fourth and fifth digits (222 per cent) grips yielded a higher EMG signal than a two-finger pocket with second and third digit (126 per cent). The two-finger pocket grip with fourth and fifth digits also yielded a higher EMG signal than an open-handed grip (143 per cent) (Watts et al., 2008). These results indicate that grip style influences activation of forearm musculature and suggests that climbers should utilise a variety of grip styles during training. The findings also question the utility of a standard handgrip task in assessing the functioning of the forearm muscles in climbers. As the climbing sequence was performed on a wall with an overhang of 45°, it is questionable if these findings apply to other routes.

To determine the importance of different muscle groups to indoor climbing performance of experienced climbers (7b), participants pre-fatigued one of four muscle groups (finger flexors, elbow flexors, lumbar flexors or shoulder adductors). To pre-fatigue the respective muscle groups, participants performed finger flexion, elbow flexion, lumbar flexion or shoulder abduction isometric exercises at 25 per cent of maximum voluntary contraction until force could no longer be maintained. In comparison to baseline climbing performance, the number of climbing moves was reduced when the finger flexors and elbow flexors were pre-fatigued, suggesting the functioning of these two muscles is critical to climbing performance (Deyhle et al., 2015). However, the route climbed was 40° overhanging, thus it is unlikely that these findings are applicable to climbing routes of different angles.

Recovery interventions

Blood lactate levels have been shown to remain significantly elevated for up to 30 minutes after indoor route climbing (Gajewski, Hübner-Woźniak, Tomaszewski, & Sienkiewicz-Dianzenza, 2009). As climbing competitions often involve climbing multiple routes with limited time available for recovery, identifying strategies that accelerate metabolic recovery could benefit performance.

Following a lead climb (7b), blood lactate levels returned to pre-climb levels sooner when climbers performed recumbent cycling compared to sitting (20 min vs. 30 min) (Watts et al., 2000). Similarly, when moderate to fast paced walking (for 90 s) was performed between five climbs, increases in blood lactate were lower than when climbers passively recovered between climbs (Draper, Bird, Coleman, & Hodgson, 2006). These finding suggest that active recovery strategies, such as walking and cycling, accelerate the clearance of lactate. However, as these studies did not incorporate a follow-up measure of performance, it is unclear if quicker lactate recovery aids subsequent climbing performance.

To address this shortcoming, climbers (6b–7b+) performed two climbs (6b) separated by 20 minutes, during which time participants used a different recovery method (seated rest, cycling, electromyostimulation of the forearm muscles or intermittent cold-water immersion of the arms). Reductions in blood lactate during the recovery period were greatest in response to cycling and were lowest following passive recovery (Heyman, B, Mertens, & Meeusen, 2009). Accompanying the greater reduction in blood lactate following cycling, was preservation in climbing performance during the second climb (as measured as time to exhaustion), implying that improved lactate clearance may assist subsequent climbing performance. Climbing performance was also maintained following cold-water immersion, which may be related to slower nerve impulse transmission, reduced muscle spasticity and an analgesic effect, all of which could delay fatigue during subsequent climbs. However, as blood lactate was not significantly reduced following the cold-water immersion, future research needs to confirm its effectiveness as a recovery strategy and any physiological mechanisms responsible for aiding climbing performance.

Summary

- Treadmill and climbing-specific VO_{2peak} are not related to climbing performance, but initial research suggests that VO_{2peak} achieved during upper body rowing or cycling may be related to climbing performance.
- Increases in climbing grade, by manipulating hold size and the distance between holds, elevates the physiological demands (i.e. VO_2, heart rate and blood lactate) of climbing more so than by increasing the steepness of a route.
- The styles of ascent (lead climb vs. top rope) and familiarity with the route (on-sight vs. redpoint) have minimal influence on the oxygen demands of climbing but do influence blood lactate responses.
- Forearm vascular adaptations in response to climbing allow for faster re-oxygenation of the finger flexor musculature and better endurance performance.
- The functioning of the finger and elbow flexors are important to climbing performance and a four-finger crimp and two-finger pocket (fourth and fifth digits) grip yield higher muscle activation than other grip styles (open hand and two-finger pocket with second and third digits).
- Active recovery strategies (e.g. walking and cycling) as well as cold-water immersion are effective at preserving subsequent climbing performance, irrespective of blood lactate removal.

Practical applications

- When assessing the aerobic fitness of climbers, protocols using upper body exercise such arm ergometry and rowing may be more beneficial.
- In instances in which recovery is important, but time for recovery is limited (e.g. competition climbing), climbers would benefit from using active recovery or cold water immersion strategies.
- To increase physiological stress (i.e. muscle activation, blood lactate) when training, climbers should incorporate a variety of grip styles and increase climb duration. The latter can be accomplished by ascending a longer route or by performing laps of a single route.

References

American College of Sports Medicine (2014). *ACSM's guidelines for exercise testing and prescription*. Philadelphia, PA: Wolters Kluwer/Lippincott Williams & Wilkins Health.

Aras, D., & Akalan, C. (2014). The effect of anxiety about falling on selected physiological parameters with different rope protocols in sport rock climbing. *Journal of Sports Medicine and Physical Fitness*, 54(1), 1–8.

Balas, J., Panackova, M., Strejcova, B., Martin, A. J., Cochrane, D. J., Kalab, M., … Draper, N. (2014). The relationship between climbing ability and physiological responses to rock climbing. *Scientific World Journal*, 678387.

Bertuzzi, R. C., Franchini, E., Kokubun, E., & Kiss, M. A. (2007). Energy system contributions in indoor rock climbing. *European Journal of Applied Physiology*, 101(3), 293–300.

Bertuzzi, R. C., Franchini, E., Tricoli, V., Lima-Silva, A. E., Pires, F. O., Okuno, N. M., & Kiss, M. A. (2012). Fit-climbing test: a field test for indoor rock climbing. *Journal of Strength and Conditioning Research*, 26(6), 1558–1563.

Billat, V., Palleja, P., Charlaix, T., Rizzardo, P., & Janel, N. (1995). Energy specificity of rock climbing and aerobic capacity in competitive sport rock climbers. *Journal of Sports Medicine and Physical Fitness*, 35(1), 20–24.

Booth, J., Marino, F., Hill, C., & Gwinn, T. (1999). Energy cost of sport rock climbing in elite performers. *British Journal of Sports Medicine*, 33(1), 14–18.

de Geus, B., Villanueva O'Driscoll, S., & Meeusen, R. (2006). Influence of climbing style on physiological responses during indoor rock climbing on routes with the same difficulty. *European Journal of Applied Physiology*, 98(5), 489–496.

Deyhle, M. R., Hsu, H. S., Fairfield, T. J., Cadez-Schmidt, T. L., Gurney, B. A., & Mermier, C. M. (2015). The relative importance of four muscle groups for indoor rock climbing performance. *Journal of Strength and Conditioning Research*, 29(7), 2006–2014.

Dickson, T., Fryer, S., Blackwell, G., Draper, N., & Stoner, L. (2012). Effect of style of ascent on the psychophysiological demands of rock climbing in elite level climbers. *Sports Technology*, 5(3–4), 111–119.

Donath, L., Roesner, K., Schoffl, V., & Gabriel, H. H. (2013). Work-relief ratios and imbalances of load application in sport climbing: another link to overuse-induced injuries? *Scandinavian Journal of Medicine & Science in Sports*, 23(4), 406–414.

Draper, N., Bird, E. L., Coleman, I., & Hodgson, C. (2006). Effects of active recovery on lactate concentration, heart rate and RPE in climbing. *Journal of Sports Science and Medicine*, 5(1), 97–105.

Draper, N., Brent, S., Hale, B., & Coleman, I. (2006). The influence of sampling site and assay method on lactate concentration in response to rock climbing. *European Journal of Applied Physiology*, 98(4), 363–372.

Draper, N., Dickson, T., Fryer, S., Blackwell, G., Winter, D., Scarrott, C., & Ellis, G. (2012). Plasma cortisol concentrations and perceived anxiety in response to on-sight rock climbing. *International Journal of Sports Medicine*, 33(1), 13–17.

Draper, N., Jones, G., Fryer, S., Hodgson, C., & Blackwell, G. (2010). Physiological and psychological responses to lead and top rope climbing for intermediate rock climbers. *European Journal of Sport Science*, 10(1), 13–20.

Draper, N., Jones, G. A., Fryer, S., Hodgson, C., & Blackwell, G. (2008). Effect of an on-sight lead on the physiological and psychological responses to rock climbing. *Journal of Sports Science and Medicine*, 7(4), 492–498.

Espana-Romero, V., Ortega Porcel, F. B., Artero, E. G., Jimenez-Pavon, D., Gutierrez Sainz, A., Castillo Garzon, M. J., & Ruiz, J. R. (2009). Climbing time to exhaustion is a determinant of climbing performance in high-level sport climbers. *European Journal of Applied Physiology*, 107(5), 517–525.

Ferguson, R. A., & Brown, M. D. (1997). Arterial blood pressure and forearm vascular conductance responses to sustained and rhythmic isometric exercise and arterial occlusion in trained rock climbers and untrained sedentary subjects. *European Journal of Applied Physiology and Occupational Physiology*, 76(2), 174–180.

Fryer, S., Dickson, T., Draper, N., Blackwell, G., and Hillier, S. (2013). A psychophysiological comparison of on-sight lead and top rope ascents in advanced rock climbers. *Scandinavian Journal of Medicine & Science in Sports*, 23(5), 645–650.

Fryer, S., Dickson, T., Draper, N., Eltom, M., Stoner, L., & Blackwell, G. (2012). The effect of technique and ability on the VO2–heart rate relationship in rock climbing. *Sports Technology*, 5(3–4), 143–150.

Fryer, S., Draper, N., Dickson, T., Blackwell, G., Winter, D., & Ellis, G. (2011). Comparison of lactate sampling sites for rock climbing. *International Journal of Sports Medicine*, 32(6), 428–432.

Fryer, S., Stoner, L., Lucero, A., Witter, T., Scarrott, C., Dickson, T., … Draper, N. (2015). Haemodynamic kinetics and intermittent finger flexor performance in rock climbers. *International Journal of Sports Medicine*, 36(2), 137–142.

Fryer, S., Stoner, L., Scarrott, C., Lucero, A., Witter, T., Love, R., … Draper, N. (2015). Forearm oxygenation and blood flow kinetics during a sustained contraction in multiple ability groups of rock climbers. *Journal of Sports Sciences*, 33(5), 518–526.

Gajewski, J., Hübner-Woźniak, E., Tomaszewski, P., & Sienkiewicz-Dianzenza, E. (2009). Changes in handgrip force and blood lactate as response to simulated climbing competition. *Biology of Sport*, 26(1), 13–21.

Heyman, E., De Geus, B., Mertens, I., & Meeusen, R. (2009). Effects of four recovery methods on repeated maximal rock climbing performance. *Medicine & Science in Sports & Exercise*, 41(6), 1303–1310.

Kenney, W. L., Wilmore, J. H., Costill, D. L., & Wilmore, J. H. (2012). *Physiology of sport and exercise*. Champaign, IL: Human Kinetics.

MacLeod, D., Sutherland, D. L., Buntin, L., Whitaker, A., Aitchison, T., Watt, I., … Grant, S. (2007). Physiological determinants of climbing-specific finger endurance and sport rock climbing performance. *Journal of Sports Sciences*, 25(12), 1433–1443.

Magalhaes, J., Ferreira, R., Marques, F., Olivera, E., Soares, J., & Ascensao, A. (2007). Indoor climbing elicits plasma oxidative stress. *Medicine & Science in Sports & Exercise*, 39(6), 955–963.

Mermier, C. M., Roberts, R. A., McMinn, S. M., & Heyward, V. H. (1997). Energy expenditure and physiological responses during indoor rock climbing. *British Journal of Sports Medicine*, 31(3), 224–228.

Michailov, M. L., Morrison, A., Ketenliev, M. M., & Pentcheva, B. P. (2014). A sport-specific upper-body ergometer test for evaluating submaximal and maximal parameters in elite rock climbers. *International Journal of Sports Physiology and Performance*, 10(3), 374–380.

Philippe, M., Wegst, D., Muller, T., Raschner, C., & Burtscher, M. (2012). Climbing-specific finger flexor performance and forearm muscle oxygenation in elite male and female sport climbers. *European Journal of Applied Physiology*, 112(8), 2839–2847.

Pires, F. O., Lima-Silva, A. E., Hammond, J., Franchini, E., Dal' Molin Kiss, M. A., & Bertuzzi, R. (2011). Aerobic profile of climbers during maximal arm test. *International Journal of Sports Medicine*, 32(2), 122–125.

Rodio, A., Fattorini, L., Rosponi, A., Quattrini, F. M., & Marchetti, M. (2008). Physiological adaptation in noncompetitive rock climbers: good for aerobic fitness? *Journal of Strength and Conditioning Research*, 22(2), 359–364.

Rosponi, A., Schena, F., Leonardi, A., & Tosi, P. (2012). Influence of ascent speed on rock climbing economy. *Sport Sciences for Health*, 7(2–3), 71–80.

Sheel, A. W. (2004). Physiology of sport rock climbing. *British Journal of Sports Medicine*, 38(3), 355–359.

Sheel, A. W., Seddon, N., Knight, A., McKenzie, D. C., & Warburton, D. E. (2003). Physiological responses to indoor rock-climbing and their relationship to maximal cycle ergometry. *Medicine & Science in Sports & Exercise*, 35(7), 1225–1231.

Sherk, V. D., Sherk, K. A., Kim, S., Young, K. C., & Bemben, D. A. (2011). Hormone responses to a continuous bout of rock climbing in men. *European Journal of Applied Physiology*, 111(4), 687–693.

Thompson, E. B., Farrow, L., Hunt, J. E., Lewis, M. P., & Ferguson, R. A. (2014). Brachial artery characteristics and micro-vascular filtration capacity in rock climbers. *European Journal of Sport Science*, 15(4), 296–304.

Watts, P., Jensen, R., Agena, S., Majchrzak, J. A., Schellinger, R., & Wubbels, C. (2008). Changes in EMG and finger force with repeated hangs from the hands in rock climbers. *International Journal of Exercise Science*, 1(2), 62–70.

Watts, P., Newbury, V., & Sulentic, J. (1996). Acute changes in handgrip strength, endurance, and blood lactate with sustained sport rock climbing. *Journal of Sports Medicine and Physical Fitness*, 36(4), 255–260.

Watts, P. B., Daggett, M., Gallagher, P., & Wilkins, B. (2000). Metabolic response during sport rock climbing and the effects of active versus passive recovery. *International Journal of Sports Medicine*, 21(3), 185–190.

Watts, P. B., & Drobish, K. M. (1998). Physiological responses to simulated rock climbing at different angles. *Medicine & Science in Sports & Exercise*, 30(7), 1118–1122.

White, D. J., & Olsen, P. D. (2010). A time motion analysis of bouldering style competitive rock climbing. *Journal of Strength and Conditioning Research*, 24(5), 1356–1360.

3 Economy in difficult rock climbing

Phillip (Phil) B. Watts

Efficiency is often stated as a component of the performance model for a variety of competitive or high-level physical activities. Measurement of true efficiency during human exercise requires assessment of the external work performed and direct measurement of the energy expenditure associated with the task. For human exertion, direct measurement of energy expenditure is impractical, thus energy expenditure is typically estimated from expired air analysis data and the term economy is substituted for efficiency. This chapter will review concepts and related research relative to assessment of economy during high-level rock climbing.

Efficiency versus economy

Efficiency is assumed to be an important component of the performance model for many competitive activities. By definition, efficiency is the ratio of external work performed relative to the energy expended during performance of a task. For human locomotion activities, the work performed is equal to $f \times d$ where $f =$ body mass and $d =$ distance of movement. When calculated in this manner, efficiency is expressed as a percentage value:

(Energy equivalent of Work Performed / Energy Expenditure) × 100

Direct assessment of energy expenditure during human movement is difficult due to technological constraints. For activities of sustained intensity, energy expenditure may be estimated through expired air measures and related to the total body oxygen uptake. This procedure of estimating energy expenditure is called indirect calorimetry. Contemporary portable expired air analysers have enabled indirect calorimetry for many human physical activities, including rock climbing.

When an indirect measure of energy expenditure is used in the equation for efficiency the resultant is commonly referred to as economy:

Economy = (Energy equivalent of Work Performed / Estimated Energy Expended) × 100

While not precisely synonymous, the terms economy and efficiency are often used interchangeably in general discussions. For the purposes of this chapter, the term economy will be used.

Indirect calorimetry and economy in rock climbing

A number of studies have reported measures of oxygen uptake during rock climbing though few have related oxygen uptake (VO_2) to work performed during an ascent since direct measurement of work performed is not possible during actual climbing. Reported values for average VO_2 during climbing range from 25 to 36 $ml \cdot kg^{-1} \cdot min^{-1}$ for sustained climbing of up to four minutes duration (Watts & Drobish, 1998; Watts, 2004; de Geus, O'Driscoll, & Meeusen, 2006; Draper, Jones, Fryer, Hodgson, & Blackwell, 2010). Generally, for sustained climbing of two minutes or longer, a plateau in VO_2 has been observed. Since these VO_2 values are likely below maximum VO_2 for fit climbers, it is suggested climbers can perform under steady-state metabolic conditions even on difficult routes. For such steady-state conditions, VO_2 may be used to estimate energy expenditure.

On the other hand, studies have reported significantly elevated post-exercise VO_2 and significant, though low, blood lactate accumulation, which suggest some mechanical energy is derived via non-oxidative metabolism during climbing (Watts et al., 2000; Bertuzzi, Franchini, Kokubun, & Kiss, 2007; España-Romero et al., 2012). None of these studies attempted to quantify the external work of the specific climbing task, thus calculation of economy is not possible from their data.

Rodio, Quattrini, Fattorini, Egidi, and Marchetti (2006) combined estimates of climbing and post-climbing energy expenditure to report a range of economy values (the authors used the term 'efficiency') of 8–20 per cent among 'expert' climbers. In this study a faster ascent was associated with better economy. Presumably this was due to less energy expended during static position support. Unfortunately, the authors did not clearly state how external work was measured, thus interpretation of their results is problematic.

In a theoretical work, Tosi, Ricci, Rosponi, and Schena (2011) described climbing efficiency as the ratio between mechanical gravitational work and total work performed. When their theoretical formula was applied to previously reported data of Booth, Marino, Hill, and Gwinn (1999), efficiency was estimated to be close to 20 per cent and similar to values for walking and running (Tosi et al., 2011).

Based upon their theoretical analysis, Tosi et al. (2011) concluded climbing efficiency would be related to speed of climbing up to a point since faster climbing would involve less time spent in static support. Their model also predicted a linear increase in power per unit of mass relative to speed of climbing. From a metabolic standpoint, this is confirmed by the research of Booth et al. (1999) and Watts et al. (1995) who found oxygen uptake in $ml \cdot kg^{-1} \cdot min^{-1}$ to increase linearly with climbing speeds between 8 and 12 $m \cdot min^{-1}$ on rock climbing treadmills. Thus, although the model of Tosi et al. (2011) predicts economy to be greater with faster climbing, the metabolic stress is higher.

According to Tosi et al. (2011), for terrain that requires a large isometric power, climbing fast should be more economical since the static support time would be minimized. For steep terrain where the work requirement for moving vertically is higher, the optimal climbing speed would be slower. This is supported by the findings of Watts and Drobish (1998) who measured energy expenditure through indirect calorimetry during climbing on a non-motorized climbing treadmill set at different angles. As the steepness of the terrain increased beyond vertical, climbing speed decreased while energy expenditure rate in kcals·min⁻¹ remained relatively constant.

There is a potential for error in the interpretation of real or theoretical static support data relative to economy and effective climbing. A recent study by Fryer et al. (2012) found advanced climbers (6a French rating) spent 39.7 per cent of climbing time in static support versus only 26.3 percent for intermediate climbers (6a). Although it would be tempting to say the advanced climbers in this study were less economical, the advanced climbers spent 25.09 per cent of climbing time resting the arms while rest time was only 2.38 per cent for the intermediate climbers. Clearly the metabolic consequence of static support time is variable in nature.

Training of economy

There is indirect evidence that economy of climbing is trainable through repetition of movement. España-Romero et al. (2012) reported climbing energy expenditures for nine climbers who completed ascents of the same route weekly for nine weeks. As with Rodio et al. (2006), the researchers did not assess the external work performed. However, since the specific terrain and body mass of the climbers did not change over the nine-week period, it may be assumed total external work remained consistent. Indirect calorimetry provided measures of energy expenditure during climbing and during a ten-minute period of post-climbing rest. Energy expenditure for climbing decreased with repetition of the route by ascent six and total energy expenditure (climbing + recovery) was significantly lower for ascent nine versus ascent 1. Recalling the formula for economy, energy equivalent of work performed divided by estimated energy expended, it may be seen that a decrease in energy expended for the same work performed results in greater economy. These results suggest economy is trainable and improves with repetition of specific climbing tasks.

Direct assessment of changes in external work performed has not been made in any of the reported energy expenditure studies. Due to the complex nature of outdoor climbing terrain and climber movement relative to the horizontal and vertical, along with the lack of a laboratory-based climbing ergometer, true measurement of external work remains elusive. Without measures of the external work, true determination of economy during climbing is not possible.

Anthropometry and economy

There are also complications with application of the concept of economy in climbing. As a first concern, climbing performance may be dependent upon the total work requirement – body mass times distance of movement. Thus, the external work of the task will vary with the mass of the climber and the distance travelled over the specific ascent route. Assuming identical lines of motion along a specific climbing route, a climber of low body mass would be expected to have lower energy expenditure than a climber with higher mass. This lower energy expenditure, however, should not be interpreted as greater economy since the total work performed would be less for the lighter climber. In such a case, perhaps the term energy conservation is more appropriate than economy.

Body mass may not directly affect climbing economy; however, there is an association between low mass and high-level climbing performance. Presumably this is due to the lower external work performed per specific route ascent for a lighter climber relative to a heavier climber. It may be assumed that muscle mass has potential to contribute to performance during climbing whereas, other than as a potential energy substrate, body fat does not contribute to force production and power generation. Thus, body weight attributed to fat has been considered a detriment in climbing.

Early research by Watts, Martin, and Durtschi (1993) found international-level competitive climbers to be small in stature with low body mass and percentage body fat. Twenty-one male climbers, with mean red-point ability of 5.13c/8b (YDS/French), had mean height, mass and percentage body fat of 1.78±0.06 m, 66.6±5.5 kg and 4.7±1.3 per cent. In the same study, 18 female climbers with mean red-point ability of 5.12c/7c had mean values of 1.65±0.04 m, 51.5±5.1 kg and 10.7±1.7 per cent for height, mass and percentage fat, respectively. These authors described the percentage fat levels in these athletes as 'extremely low' with possible negative health consequences.

More recent data seem to indicate a trend away from extreme mass reductions in high-level climbers. Magiera et al. (2013) reported mean values of 1.78±5.60 m, 68.8±5.0 kg and 10.4±3.3 per cent for height, mass and percentage fat in a group of 30 male climbers with a mean red-point ability level of 5.13b/8a. This percentage fat mean was more than 100 per cent higher than the earlier value for male competitive climbers reported by Watts et al. (1993).

España-Romero et al. (2009) also found higher percentage fat values of 25.2±3.6 per cent in nine female climbers (ability range = 5.11a/6c-5.12d/7c) and 13.3±3.3 per cent in ten male climbers (ability range = 5.11c/7a-5.13d/8b). The methodology for estimation of body fat may account for some of this difference. The percentage fat values reported by España-Romero et al. (2009) were derived via dual energy X-ray absorptiometry whereas other studies report values calculated from skinfold measures. Similar data have been reported by Kemmler et al. (2006) for a sample of twenty male climbers with abilities of 5.13b/8a or higher. In this sample, the climbers had a mean percentage fat of 11.0±1.8 per cent as determined via dual energy X-ray absorptiometry.

Watts, Joubert, Lish, Mast, and Wilkins (2003) compared anthropometry data for a large group of young competitive climbers (mean age of 13.5±3.0 years) with an age-matched group of 45 non-climbing children and youth. The climbers were significantly shorter and lighter than the non-climbers both in absolute values and relative to North American growth-development percentile norms. Percentage fat, measured via skinfolds, was 11.3 ± 6.6 per cent for the non-climbers and 7.8 ± 4.4 per cent for the climbers. No current research has reported long-term changes in anthropometry for rock climbers.

Currently available data support that highly successful climbers tend to be small with low body mass and percentage fat, though extremes do not seem to be the contemporary norm.

Geometric entropy and economy

Climbers may elect different strategies, body positions and movement patterns to complete the same route and thus affect the distance component of the external work formula. Cordier, France, Bolon, and Pailhous (1994) suggested there are two primary constraining factors which control a climber's movement path during an ascent. One constraint is external and influenced by the specific design of the climbing route. A second constraint is internal and dependent upon the climber's expertise and ability to produce effective sequences of movement. Within this concept, the first constraint is constant for a given route while factors related to the second constraint could vary and could influence economy.

The complexity of a climber's movement path during climbing has been described as geometric entropy. Cordier et al. (1994) and Sibella, Frosio, Schena, and Borghese (2007) described a method of quantifying geometric entropy through analysis of movement of a climber's centre of mass. A climber is video-recorded during an ascent and a mark at the centre of the climber's back, at waist level, is tracked via an automatic or manual digitization process to generate a two-dimensional line of motion (LM). The digital coordinates of the LM are used to determine a convex hull about the full movement range via special computer software. The geometric entropy (GE) quantity is calculated according to the formula:

$$GE = \ln((2*LM)/CH)),$$

where CH is the value of the convex hull about the line of motion (Sibella et al., 2007). Cordier et al. (1994) had seven climbers (three of 'average skill' and four of 'high skill') climb a set route ten times with a one minute rest between climbs. The researchers found geometric entropy to decrease with repetition of the climbing route and reach a plateau with the third repetition in the highly skilled climbers. Entropy also decreased in the average skill climbers with repetitions of the route; however, the decrease was more gradual.

Sibella et al. (2007) proposed that a lower geometric entropy during an ascent represented a higher level of 'fluency' of movement and greater economy. The term 'fluency' is not always well-defined in the scientific sense. Sibella et al. (2007) appear to use the term as classically defined where fluency reflects gracefulness and ease of movement or style. Others seem to define fluency as continuous movement unbroken by pauses. The fluency proposed by Sibella et al. does not consider non-movement pauses during an ascent which may or may not involve significant static muscular effort. Billat, Palleja, Charlaix, Rizzardo, and Janel (1995) found climbers to be dynamically moving 63 per cent of ascent time and in non-movement static support 37 per cent of ascent time on two routes. According to the previously discussed theoretical model of Tosi et al. (2011), such non-movement pauses would disrupt fluency and lower economy. However, it may not be universally assumed that pauses, and any subsequent effect on economy, would be less effective for a successful ascent. Some static positions during climbing are representative of resting and would be beneficial during ascent as shown by Fryer et al. (2012).

In an attempt to better assess fluency of movement during climbing, recent work by Seifert et al. (2014) provides some interesting new insights. This group collected data from an inertial measurement unit incorporating a triaxial accelerometer, triaxial gyroscope and triaxial magnetometer to calculate 'jerk' coefficients for hip trajectory and orientation of the hips during climbing. The jerk coefficient essentially describes movement from a stationary position, thus a high jerk coefficient would be interpreted as less fluid movement. These researchers found jerk coefficients for both hip trajectory and hip orientation to decrease with route repetition with an apparent plateau between repetitions three and four. Energy expenditure was not measured in this study, thus whether a decrease in the jerk coefficient would be associated with lower energy expenditure is not known.

Recently, Watts and co-workers have demonstrated a decrease in geometric entropy with repeated ascents of the same route and this decrease was associated with lower energy expenditure (Watts, España-Romero, Ostrowski, & Jensen, 2013). In this study, geometric entropy was significantly lower in ascents six through nine than during an on-sight ascent. The energy expenditure for climbing followed the same pattern and was significantly correlated with the change in entropy.

During on-sight ascents, Cordier et al. (1994) observed clusters of apparently non-fluid movement in the lines of motion of climbers. These clusters were termed 'complex nodes' and were interpreted as periods of 'searching' or route finding which could add to the total time spent in relatively static support or small exploratory body position changes without progression along the route. Such complex nodes are illustrated in Figure 3.1.

An abundance of these nodes could result in higher energy expenditure and lower economy for the same task. On the other hand, some complex nodes may reflect subtle movement during resting periods and it is not readily possible to differentiate whether the underlying movement is beneficial for the ascent or not.

Figure 3.1 from Watts et al. (2013) illustrates the line of motion for a climber during an on-sight (A1) and the ninth ascent (A9) of a route with an initial 6.5 m low level leftward traverse followed by a 6.8 m vertical ascent. Several complex nodes are indicated on the line of motion for the on-sight ascent. These nodes appear to be diminished in the ninth ascent of the route. Geometric entropy was reduced with route repetition for this climber and energy expenditure was 10.7 per cent lower in A9 versus the on-sight ascent.

While it is attractive to relate changes in geometric entropy to changes in efficiency or economy, much of any change in energy expenditure is likely due to

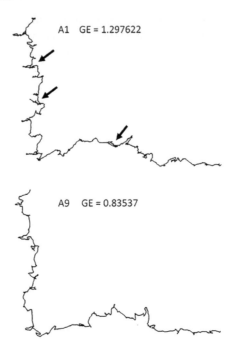

Figure 3.1 Line of Motion and Geometric Entropy (GE) for the same climber during an on-sight ascent (A1) and the ninth ascent (A9) of the same route

Arrows for A1 indicate apparent complex nodes of possible searching movement.

Source: Watts et al., 2013.

a reduced line of motion and subsequent reduction in the amount of external work performed. Still, a lower energy expenditure for the same route, regardless of the source, would likely have potential for resisting fatigue during climbing.

Cordier et al. (1994) point out that care must be taken when interpreting geometric entropy during climbing. While a higher entropy due to searching movements may be associated with less economical and less effective climbing, some very skilled climbers may exhibit high geometric entropy. A highly skilled climber will tend to have a smooth movement trajectory but will shift the centre of mass though a wide area with changes in body position. In particular, twists of the body contribute to a higher entropy calculation but may enable long reaches between holds while minimizing pulling force.

Relevance of economy

The relatively brief event times of climbing, and for competitive climbing in particular, may generate some doubt regarding the importance of true economy or efficiency. The risk of substrate depletion during climbing would be low due to the low total energy expenditure. High economy may be compromised in favour of other factors of performance such as optimal body position and static positions held while solving movement sequences and resting. A similar compromise is often seen when comparing middle-distance runners, with event times under five minutes, to marathon runners whose events last over two hours. Middle-distance runners typically have higher aerobic power but lower running economy than marathon runners. Economy for these athletes is compromised for faster running speed.

Whether improved economy of climbing is associated with increased force capability or increased resistance of fatigue in the specific musculature critical to performance is not known. Further research is necessary to answer the more applied questions regarding economy in difficult rock climbing.

Summary and practical applications

For climbing, minimizing the external work performed is likely more important than economy due to the potential impact on required muscular forces and resistance to muscular fatigue. The primary factors for reduction of the external work requirement (Force × Distance) of climbing include a relatively low body mass of the climber (Force) without compromise of muscular strength, a minimized line of motion of the ascent (Distance) with relatively low geometric entropy and a more fluid movement trajectory with fewer stops. Repetition of climbing-specific activity can reduce energy expenditure for the activity and possibly enable greater resistance to fatigue.

Highlights

- The degree of efficiency of rock climbing movement is the relationship of the total external work necessary to ascend a specific route relative to the metabolic energy expenditure associated with the ascent. When calculation of external work is not possible indirect means of assessment are used and the more appropriate term is economy.
- Economy may respond to climbing-specific training and technical practice, changes in body composition and increased route familiarity.
- It appears climbing economy may be sacrificed in some instances to enable effective performance on a given route.

References

Billat, V., Palleja, P., Charlaix, T., Rizzardo, P., & Janel, N. (1995). Energy specificity of rock climbing and aerobic capacity in competitive sport rock climbers. *Journal of Sports Medicine and Physical Fitness*, 35(1), 20–24.

Booth, J., Marino, F., Hill, C., & Gwinn, T. (1999). Energy cost of sport rock climbing in elite performers. *British Journal of Sports Medicine*, 33(1), 14–18.

Cordier, P., France, M. M., Bolon, P., & Pailhous, J. (1994). Thermodynamic study of motor behaviour optimization. *Acta Biotheoretica*, 42(2–3), 187–201.

de Geus, B., O'Driscoll, S. V., & Meeusen, R. (2006). Influence of climbing style on physiological responses during indoor rock climbing on routes with the same difficulty. *European Journal of Applied Physiology*, 98(5), 489–496.

de Moraes Bertuzzi, R. C., Franchini, E., Kokubun, E., & Kiss, M. A. P. D. M. (2007). Energy system contributions in indoor rock climbing. *European Journal of Applied Physiology*, 101(3), 293–300.

Draper, N., Jones, G. A., Fryer, S., Hodgson, C. I., & Blackwell, G. (2010). Physiological and psychological responses to lead and top rope climbing for intermediate rock climbers. *European Journal of Sport Science*, 10(1), 13–20.

España-Romero, V., Jensen, R. L., Sanchez, X., Ostrowski, M. L., Szekely, J. E., & Watts, P. B. (2012). Physiological responses in rock climbing with repeated ascents over a 10-week period. *European Journal of Applied Physiology*, 112(3), 821–828.

España Romero, V., Ruiz, J. R., Ortega, F. B., Artero, E. G., Vicente-Rodríguez, G., Moreno, L. A., ... & Gutierrez, A. (2009). Body fat measurement in elite sport climbers: comparison of skinfold thickness equations with dual energy X-ray absorptiometry. *Journal of Sports Sciences*, 27(5), 469–477.

Fryer, S., Dickson, T., Draper, N., Eltom, M., Stoner, L., & Blackwell, G. (2012). The effect of technique and ability on the VO_2–heart rate relationship in rock climbing. *Sports Technology*, 5(3–4), 143–150.

Kemmler, W., Roloff, I., Baumann, H., Schöffl, V., Weineck, J., Kalender, W., & Engelke, K. (2006). Effect of exercise, body composition, and nutritional intake on bone parameters in male elite rock climbers. *International Journal of Sports Medicine*, 27(8), 653–659.

Magiera, A., Roczniok, R., Maszczyk, A., Czuba, M., Kantyka, J., & Kurek, P. (2013). The structure of performance of a sport rock climber. *Journal of Human Kinetics*, 36(1), 107–117.

Rodio, A., Quattrini, F. M., Fattorini, L., Egidi, F., & Marchetti, M. (2006). Physiological significance of efficiency in rock climbing. *Medicina dello Sport*, 59(3), 313–317.

Seifert, L., Orth, D., Boulanger, J., Dovgalecs, V., Hérault, R., & Davids, K. (2014). Climbing skill and complexity of climbing wall design: assessment of jerk as a novel indicator of performance fluency. *Journal of Applied Biomechanics*, 30(5), 619–625.

Sibella, F., Frosio, I., Schena, F., & Borghese, N. A. (2007). 3D analysis of the body center of mass in rock climbing. *Human Movement Science*, 26(6), 841–852.

Tosi, P., Ricci, L., Rosponi, A., & Schena, F. (2011). A theory of energy cost and speed of climbing. *AIP Advances*, 1(3), 032169.

Watts, P. B. (2004). Physiology of difficult rock climbing. *European Journal of Applied Physiology*, 91(4), 361–372.

Watts, P. B., Clure, C. A., Hill, M. R., Humphreys, S. E., & Lish, A. K. (1995). Energy costs of rock climbing at different paces. *Medicine & Science in Sports & Exercise*, 27(5), S17.

Watts, P. B., Daggett, M., Gallagher, P., & Wilkins, B. (2000). Metabolic response during sport rock climbing and the effects of active versus passive recovery. *International Journal of Sports Medicine*, 21(3), 185–190.

Watts, P. B., & Drobish, K. M. (1998). Physiological responses to simulated rock climbing at different angles. *Medicine & Science in Sports & Exercise*, 30(7), 1118–1122.

Watts, P. B., España-Romero, V., Ostrowski, M., & Jensen, R. (2013). Change in geometric entropy and energy expenditure with repeated ascents in rock climbing (abstract). *Medicine & Science in Sports & Exercise,* 45, S5.

Watts, P. B., Joubert, L., Lish, A. K., Mast, J. D., & Wilkins, B. (2003). Anthropometry of young competitive sport rock climbers. *British Journal of Sports Medicine*, 37(5), 420–424.

Watts, P. B., Martin, D. T., & Durtschi, S. (1993). Anthropometric profiles of elite male and female competitive sport rock climbers. *Journal of Sports Sciences*, 11(2), 113–117.

Part II
Medicine

4 Sport climbing related injuries and overuse syndromes

Volker Rainer Schöffl and Andreas Schweizer

Rock climbing and its sub-disciplines, for example bouldering, competition climbing, sport climbing, are very popular in all age groups. An increasing number of indoor climbing gyms offer the possibility to perform the sport regularly independent from weather and daylight. As the sport applies high forces onto the fingers, new pathologies like closed finger flexor tendon pulley injuries and epiphyseal fractures of the fingers in young climbers occur. Also sport-specific overstrain syndromes have become known and should be known to physicians and therapists working in the field of sports medicine. An overview of the most common and most specific climbing related injuries as well as their diagnosis and treatment options are presented.

Introduction

Climbing is a popular sport nowadays, and interest in the medical aspects of it has arisen and several overview articles in general medical journals are available (Schöffl, 2008; Schweizer, 2012). Since the introduction of bolted routes (safe protection points with bolts every two to three metres) and the development of dedicated ropes allowing for dynamic and soft deceleration of falls, heavy injuries due to ground-drops have become very rarely (Schöffl, Morrison, Schöffl, & Küpper, 2012). The injury rates are at 0.079 per 1 000 hours for indoor climbing (Schöffl & Winkelmann, 1999b), at 0.2 per 1 000 hours of sport climbing (Neuhof, Hennig, Schöffl, & Schöffl, 2011), at 0.6 per 1 000 hours of mountaineering (Schussmann, Lutz, Shaw, & Bohn, 1990) and at 4.2 per 1 000 hours of rock climbing of all sub-disciplines (Backe, Ericson, Janson, & Timpka, 2009). Competition climbing also shows a small injury incidence (Schöffl & Küpper, 2006). The International Federation of Sports Competition Climbing (IFSC) reported about 0.29/1 000 h injuries in the complete 2012 World Cup series (Schöffl, Burtscher, & Coscia, 2013). These injury rates are lower compared to soccer playing with 31 per 1 000 hours (Junge & Dvorak, 2004), handball playing with 50 injuries per 1 000 hours (Wedderkopp, Kaltoft, Lundgaard, Rosendahl, & Froberg, 1997) or rugby playing with 286 injuries per 1 000 hours of sport (Gabbett, 2002).

In classical mountaineering, injuries are mostly due to ground-fall fractures and sprains of the lower extremities or the head and trunk (Schussmann et al.,

1990). In contrast, a fall in sport climbing is very common and inevitable when an athlete tries to complete a route at their performance limit. Because difficult routes often take place on steep or overhanging rock formations with rather small holds, they lead to a completely different injury pattern. Schöffl and colleagues mentioned that 67 per cent of 604 injuries concerned the upper extremities and shoulders whereas poly-traumas or fatal events accounted for less than 1 per cent (Schöffl, Hochholzer, Karrer, Winter, & Imhoff, 2003). In a more recent study of 911 climbing injuries, the same authors found 833 injuries (91.4 per cent) in the upper extremities. Finger injuries accounted for 52 per cent of all injuries (Schöffl, Popp, Küpper, & Schöffl, 2015). Injuries during bouldering also shifted more to the upper extremities (Josephsen et al., 2007) where more than 80 per cent of the injuries concerned the upper extremities. Of those, finger and shoulder joints were the most affected. Comparing outdoor to indoor climbing, it can be shown that the risk of injury in the former is a little bit higher, particularly for injuries to the knee, ankle and foot caused by down-jumps during bouldering (Schöffl et al., 2012).

Flexor tendon pulley injuries of the fingers due to 'crimping'

Among all finger injuries those concerning the flexor tendon sheath are the most common. The crimp grip position, which is commonly used by climbers up to 90 per cent of the time (Bollen, 1990b; Marco, Sharkey, Smith, & Zissimos, 1998), is a very specific position of the finger (Figure 4.1) resulting in very high loads onto the pulleys of the flexor tendon sheath, which are three to four times higher than the force acting at the fingertip (Schweizer, 2001). If a sudden load to the finger occurs as a consequence of a slipped-off foot or when the climber grasps to hold on very quickly during a dynamic move, one or more pulleys may disrupt (Figure 4.2) and a loud snapping sound can be noticed. Usually only one of the finger flexor tendon pulleys disrupts; the A2 pulley used to be 1.5 times more likely to be involved than the A4 pulley of either the ring or the middle finger. Other recent studies report a shift to more A4 versus A2 pulley injuries (Schöffl et al., 2015). This injury was first described by Bollen and Tropet in 1990 (Bollen, 1990a; Tropet, Menez, Balmat, Pem, & Vichard, 1990) in rock climbers and had not been described in the medical literature before. The climbers initially treated the injury by taping their fingers around the proximal phalanx without impairment of function (Bollen, 1990a).

The proximal interphalangela (PIP) joints are flexed more than 90° and the distal interphalangela (DIP) joints are hyper-extended; this way the thumb can also act as holding force. One-finger pocket (b) with typically complete flexed adjacent fingers increases the flexion force of a single finger to up to 50 per cent. The half/open crimp position (c) with PIP joints flexed to about 80° thereby generating most flexion torque. Squeezing and distorting the fingertips in crack (d) sometimes is the only way to hold on.

The diagnosis of a pulley disruption is based on the history (pop or snapping sound) and the clinical examination, where a painful flexor tendon bowstringing can be palpated during resisted finger flexion. The lift-off or bowstringing of the tendon can be visualised by ultrasonography (Klauser et al., 2002) or magnetic

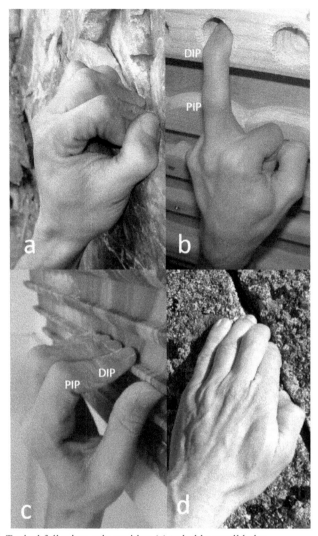

Figure 4.1 Typical full crimp grip position (a) to hold a small ledge

resonance imaging (MRI). The treatment recommendations are controversial as some hand surgeons still treat singular pulley disruptions with reconstruction (Moutet, Forli, & Voulliaume, 2004). However, most treat a single pulley disruption conservatively since Schöffl and Schöffl (2006) showed that with non-operative management no objective or subjective functional loss occurred. The non-operative treatment is generally functional. The healing time is between two and three months and full load bearing can be expected after four to six months.

To allow an adequate reposition of the tendon without compromising circulation within the finger we recommend to use a special pulley protection ring (Figure 4.2d) for the first two months after injury. It is formed in a way that the neuro-vascular

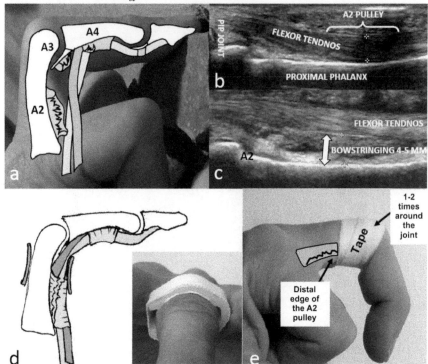

Figure 4.2 Finger flexor tendon sheath (a) with complete disruption of the A2 and the A3 pulley, partial disruption of the A4 pulley leading to bowstringing of the deep (FDP) and the superficial (FDS) flexor tendons

Ultrasonography of normal anatomy (b) and of a disrupted A2 pulley (c) with an apparent bowstringing of the flexor tendons. A pulley protection ring (d) brings the flexor tendon back to normal position. Properly applied pulley tape (e) prevents flexion of the PIP joint more than 80°.

bundles of the finger are not compressed. Thereafter a pulley protection tape (Figure 4.2e) is applied for 2–3 further months . To take strain off the healing pulley, it is applied around the PIP joint and inhibits flexion of that joint of more than 80° where pulley load becomes particularly high (Schöffl et al., 2009; Schweizer, 2001). With this treatment regimen we were able to reduce the initial bowstringing at the A2 pulley to about 50 per cent and at the A -pulley to about 40 per cent (Schneeberger & Schweizer, 2014). If, however, two or even more pulleys are disrupted, the amount of bowstringing increases substantially leading to a loss of active flexion range of motion of the finger where a reconstruction of the ligament has to be considered. The results of such interventions are generally good and do not differ considerably between different techniques (Arora et al., 2007; Schöffl, Küpper, Hartmann, & Schöffl, 2012). However, whether all these patients need a reconstruction at all is still being debated. We have seen a series of patients with multiple pulley ruptures who returned to their previous climbing level without restriction except for a small loss of flexion range of motion. It also needs to be considered that pulley reconstruction requires a rehabilitation time of several months.

Protective pulley tape around an intact pulley is very unlikely to be effective (Schweizer, 2000; Warme & Brooks, 2000). The main positive effect is that the PIP joint is not flexed more than 80–90° if the tape is applied close or even over the PIP joint itself. More important is the correct warming-up procedure and the avoidance of a pronounced crimp grip position. It has been shown that over the first 120 climbing moves, the amount of physiological bowstringing of the flexor tendons shows an increase of up to 30 per cent. Therefore, we recommend climbing about three to four routes with forty moves or eight to twelve boulder problems with increasing intensity (Schweizer, 2001). After a pulley injury, tape should be applied at either the distal end of the respective injured pulley (Schweizer, 2001) or as an H-tape at the level of the PIP joint (Schöffl, Einwag, Strecker, Hennig, & Schöffl, 2007). In some cases the left over trunk of the ruptured pulley can cause a tenosynovitis (flap irritation phenomenon) (Schöffl, Baier, & Schöffl, 2011).

Chronic tenosynovitis of the flexor tendons is the second most common finger problem in rock climbers. Clinically, the A2 or A4 pulleys are perceived painful upon palpating; sonographically, a synovitis or a scar formation and an alteration of the pulley similar to that of a trigger finger can be observed (Klauser, Frauscher, Gabl, & Smekal, 2005). Besides reduction of the training intensity and the strict prevention of the crimp grip position, local or systemic non-steroidal anti-inflammatory medications are possible. The condition can sometimes be very frustrating for the climbers because recurrent painful periods can last more than a year. Nevertheless, the prognosis is mostly good and operative treatment is rarely necessary. Newer therapeutic strategies also involve instillation of hyaluronic acid into the tendon sheath (Schöffl, Heid, & Kupper, 2012).

Injuries due to one and two finger pockets

In difficult sport climbing routes, very small holes (one or two-finger pockets), sometimes not deeper than just the distal phalanges, have to be held on to. In order to increase the strength of one finger, all other (not loaded) fingers are completely flexed into the palm while the load-bearing finger is nearly extended (Figure 4.3) which increases the maximum strength by up to 50 per cent (Schweizer, 2001). The common origins of the lumbrical muscle III and IV from two adjacent FDP tendons are moved apart and may suffer a strain or muscle tear (Figure 4.3). It usually happens when pulling a one-finger-pocket, resulting in a sharp sudden pain in the palm. Clinically, pain in the palm can be provoked when grasping a one or two-finger pocket but not when loading all fingers with a similar degree of flexion (Schweizer, Frank, Ochsner, & Jacob, 2003). It is very important to start with stretching exercises immediately, which are done in the same way as the injury was provoked but with much less load.

Crack climbing

Small cracks are climbed by jamming and distortion of only the fingers into the crack (Figure 4.1). If the climbers slip off the rock with their feet, suddenly high

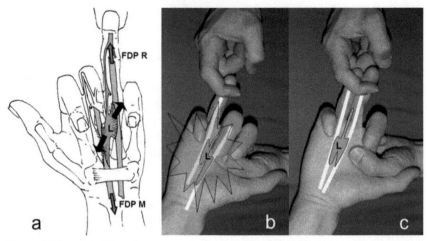

Figure 4.3 Lumbrical tears happen most often between the middle/ring and the ring/small fingers where the two heads of the common lumbrical muscle belly (L) are torn apart (a, b) during a one- or a two finger pocket. If the pain disappears while pulling both adjacent flexor tendons at the same excursion (c) the diagnosis of a lumbrical tear is likely

torsional forces are applied to the fingers which may lead to fractures, ligament tears or even dislocation of the finger joints. These mostly non-climbing-specific injuries can usually be treated by conservative means (taping, small splints) if only ligaments are concerned (be aware of impression fractures). Instability has to be assessed by a physician in order to decide what kind of tape or splint is needed (e.g. ulnar collateral ligament disruption of the thumb metacarpal phalangeal joint/skier's thumb).

The wrist

Falls onto the wrist or falls during rope climbing with a swing against the wall may lead to wrist injuries. Injuries to ligaments (scapholunate, triangular fibrocartilage) and particularly fractures of the scaphoid are very often only slightly painful. Frequently these injuries are seen only several months after the initial trauma. A ligamentous injury is quite difficult to treat at that late stage and the prognosis is much worse. Scaphoid fractures almost always turn into a non-union if left untreated and end up mostly in degenerative changes of the wrist. We recommend investigating a wrist thoroughly which has been painful for more than three weeks to exclude such an injury.

We observed indirect fractures of the hamulus ossis hamati. In one case this was the result of the pull of the FDP tendon during a repeated attempt of an under-cling grip on a difficult move. In this case the fatigue fracture was treated successfully with a splint in ulnar deviation of the wrist (Bayer & Schweizer, 2009). In another case we had to surgically reset the tip of the hamate due to ongoing pain with good result. Also, recently, stress-induced bone marrow oedema of the carpal bones was reported (Hochholzer & Schöffl, 2013).

The finger joints

Climbing leads to very high impact forces on the finger bones and joints with an impressive increase of the thickness of the cortices (Figure 4.4) (Hahn, Erschbaumer, Allenspach, Rufibach, & Schweizer, 2012). Whether rock climbing is leading to degenerative arthritis of the finger joint has been debated and investigated already by different authors (Bollen & Wright, 1994; Rohrbough, Mudge, Schilling, & Jansen, 1998; Sylvester, Christensen, & Kramer, 2006). They described radiographical changes of the finger joints of long-term climbers like osteophytes, subchondral sclerosis and joint space narrowing. Nevertheless, none of those authors could show clear evidence of an increased rate of degenerative arthritis. In these studies the radiographs were mostly performed in an anterior–posterior view. We conducted a study with anterior–posterior and the lateral views of the fingers in high level sport climbers (mean UIAA 10) (Allenspach, Saupe, Rufibach, & Schweizer, 2011). Almost all of the climbers had only little or no symptoms in the finger joints but 84 per cent showed osteophytes at the PIP joints and 68 per cent in the DIP joints, particularly in the lateral view (Figure 4.4). Six climbers (19 per cent) had signs of osteoarthritis (significant) whereas the age-matched non-climbing group had no signs of radiological changes in the finger joints. The oldest climbers performing

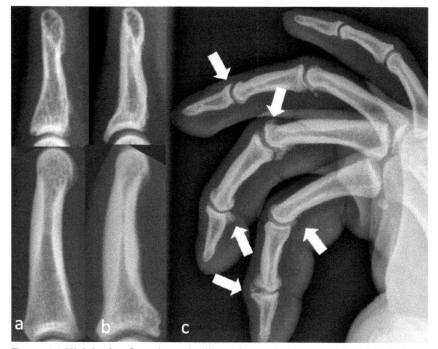

Figure 4.4 High load to finger bones leading to impressive increase of cortical thickness of the middle and distal phalanx (b) compared to non-climber's bones of the same age (a). Lateral view of the fingers of a 38-year-old world class boulderer (c). Almost every joint shows osteophytes and calcifications of the capsule. Joint space narrowing, a main sign of osteoarthritis, however, is not apparent

the sport at a high level are still not older than their early fifties. However, it seems that the changes observed happened through adaptations and do not show the same pattern of the common inherited degenerative arthritis (poly-arthrosis). We recommend to not use a pronounced crimp grip position with a flexion of the PIP joints to more than 80–90° and to try to keep the DIP joint always flexed to about 5–15°. This is also the position (85° flexion) where the PIP joint generates maximal flexion torque. By doing this, the joints are loaded in a midway position whereas the joint contact area remains as large as possible.

Fatigue fractures of the epiphysis of the base of the middle phalanx

The growth plates of the finger bones are not closed until the age of 17–19 years. They are the weakest structures of the finger and are most susceptible to injuries (Hochholzer & Schöffl, 2005). During full crimp grip position, a shift of the middle phalanx results proximally in a very high load to the dorsal part of the base of the middle phalanx. This may lead to a growth plate overload, consolidation and partial necrosis and finally to a growth plate fracture (fatigue fracture, Salter-Harris II fracture, Figure 4.5). A too early partial or complete closure of the growth

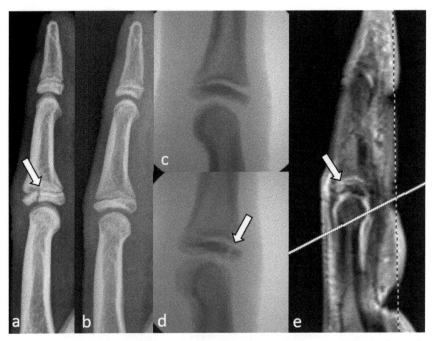

Figure 4.5 Epiphyseal fractures at the base of the middle phalanx due to crimp grip position in a 14-year-old climber (a). Strict avoidance of crimp grip lets the fracture heal out with slight joint surface incongruity but no axial deviation after 12 months. In lateral view of conventional radiographs the fracture line is often not visible (c). The same patient with an oblique view done under image intensifier makes the fracture visible (d). MRIs with in-plane slices of the epiphysis have high detectability of the fracture (e)

plate with an uneven or ceasing of further growth of the finger bone ending up in a considerable axial deviation or foreshortened finger may follow. As soon as pain without an obvious trauma in the PIP joints is apparent in an adolescent, the crimp grip position should not be tolerated at all until the pain disappears or the growth plates have closed at the age of 17–19 years. Regular radiological controls are mandatory. Be aware that the mostly oblique-oriented fracture lines are obscured and are not visible in conventional radiographs. These injuries are initially only detectable through MRI investigations (Bayer, Schöffl, Lenhart, & Herold, 2013). We recommend MRI analysis in all adolescent climbers with persistent finger pain and absent acute trauma for more than two weeks (Figure 4.5). The number of these epiphyseal injuries is rising. Out of 20 injured climbers of less than 14 years of age, 14 had epiphyseal fractures (Schöffl et al., 2015). Close medical observation of high intensity climbing adolescents is important, as well as information and education to the climbers, trainers and parents.

Neurological and other soft tissue problems of the upper extremities

Carpal tunnel syndrome, the most common nerve compression syndrome (Peters, 2001), is also the most common reason for surgical nerve decompression in climbers. But also the radial nerve at the elbow and proximal forearm may be an origin of pain (supinator-tunnel syndrome). Stretching exercises and deep friction massage of the supinator muscle are usually helpful; surgery is rarely necessary. Digital nerves can also be compressed but rather acutely (neuropraxia) when squeezed in cracks or holes, activating a sharp electrifying pain directly over the nerve with a hyposensibility and numbness distal to the injury. Symptoms usually disappear after a few weeks.

Ganglion cysts are found in climbers around the A1, A2 and A4 pulleys, are usually only a few millimetres large but rock hard and may provoke pain under direct pressure during climbing. Again, digital nerves may come under pressure from such a cyst which occasionally requires excision.

The most commonly disturbing pain in climbers around the elbow is radial and an ulnar epicondylitis, the latter being much more frequent. Infiltrations of any medication (Wolf, Ozer, Scott, Gordon, & Williams, 2011) did not have any effect in a recent study and, in particular, steroids should be avoided. An effective treatment option is active strengthening (Peterson, Butler, Eriksson, & Svärdsudd, 2011) of the elbow flexors. Apart from that, strengthening exercises for the antagonists of all flexor and internal rotators of the upper extremities are recommended to prevent muscular imbalance and overuse syndromes.

The shoulder joint

Although acute injuries of the shoulder in the sense of contusion, acromio-clavicular ligament sprains or dislocation caused by a fall or during a hard climbing move in an abducted and externally rotated shoulder may happen (Schweizer & Bircher, 2009), the majority of shoulder pathologies are due to repetitive overload injuries and micro-traumas and are probably the most common reason for surgical intervention in climbers (Schöffl, Popp, Dickschass, & Kupper, 2011).

The younger climbers often report a deep antero-superior shoulder pain which is mostly due to proximal biceps tendonitis in bicipital sulcus with a possible coexisting biceps tendon pulley lesion, a superior labrum lesion or subacromial bursitis. In a recent study, we found labrum tears being the most common condition in climbers and the fourth most common diagnosis in our injured climbers overall (Schöffl et al., 2015). MRI with intra-articular application of a contrast agent is the diagnostic tool of choice. If no higher grade of labrum tear exists and if the biceps tendon is not involved in the injury, initial treatment is conservative with improvement of active stability and centring of the gleno-humeral joint with physiotherapy and infiltration with corticosteroids. If the biceps tendon is ruptured within a SLAP lesion and/or intractable pain remains for several months, a biceps tenodesis and SLAP repair procedures are to be discussed, which are the most frequently performed procedures in younger and middle-aged climbers (Bircher, Thuer, Schweizer, & Bereiter, 2007; Popp & Schöffl, 2013; Schöffl et al., 2011). Most climbers return to their former climbing level.

Middle-aged climbers suffer from outlet impingement with rotator cuff tears, acromio-clavicular and less frequently from glenohumeral degenerative changes. In a retrospective survey Bircher et al. (2007) reviewed 20 climbers with operations being performed on 21 shoulder rotator cuff pathologies. In addition, an acromioplasty was performed in 17 shoulders and a biceps tenodesis of the long head of biceps in 15 cases. Rehabilitation was time intensive but the same climbing level was regained in almost all cases, after 12 months on average.

Preventive measures mean regular exercises of the antagonists of the shoulder internal rotators and flexors should be performed. Younger climbers should be advised not to regularly dangle their whole body weight (during recovery positions) with completely relaxed shoulder muscles.

Knee and hip

Almost 50 per cent of acute injuries involve the legs and feet. We have recently seen more climbers, especially boulderers, with femoro-acetabular impingement syndrome. Mostly conservative management is possible with physiotherapy and osteopathy. Sometimes intra-articular injections under fluoroscopic control are necessary and rarely an arthroscopic removal of the 'bulb' or a labrum repair is indicated. Due to the increasing number of boulderers, more and more injuries caused by heel hooking are presented. This technique puts extreme stress on the dorsal lateral structures of the leg, the biceps femoris, the popliteus, the posterior cruciate ligament and the knee collateral ligaments. Sometimes while heel hooking, climbers report a sudden snap with a loud 'cracking' sound. This is mostly caused by a change of the 'pivot' and the tractus iliotibialis suddenly moving over the lateral condyle (similar to the pivot shift sign in anterior cruciate injuries). We mostly perform MRI analysis to detect the exact injury; therapy is conservative if possible (Figure 4.6). Only rarely is a surgical repair necessary if a muscle is

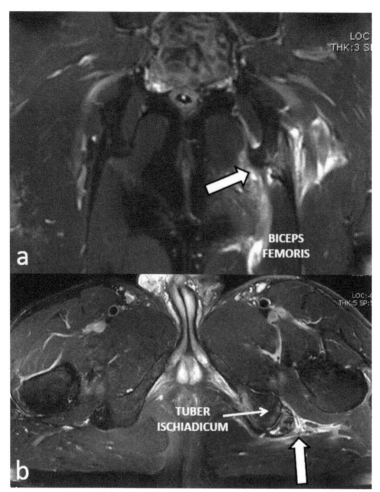

Figure 4.6 Proximal biceps femoris tendon/muscle avulsion injury during a foot-hook pull (knee flexion) with extensive contraction of the hamstring muscles which required operative refixation. The tear is visible in an MRI frontal (a) and axial (b) view indicated by arrows

completely torn off (e.g. biceps femoris on either side, the knee or the hip). Other knee injuries in climbers are anterior cruciate ligament disruption, meniscal tears or ruptures of the medial collateral ligaments, as the meniscus insertion and the knee ligaments are under extreme stress in the 'drop-knee' position.

The feet

Concerning acute injuries, the most frequent inciting factor for acute injury to the lower extremities in rock climbing is a fall (Mosimann, 2006). To further explain the different ways injuries occur while climbing, a differentiation between two different types of falls is necessary: a wall-collision fall and a ground fall (Hochholzer &

Schöffl, 2006). A wall-collision fall is one where the climber impacts the wall on a more or less vertical plane, while a ground fall is one where the climber impacts on a more or less horizontal plane. A ground fall from as little as 2–3 m high can lead to serious fractures of the calcaneus, talus and ankle joints (Schöffl & Küpper, 2013). Other ground fall injuries are sprains and ligament injuries (Backe et al., 2009; Nelson & McKenzie, 2009). One typical injury mechanism in indoor climbing is a fall onto the mattresses and the foot getting stuck in the intermediate section between two mattresses. Thus these gaps should be closed (Schöffl & Küpper, 2013).

Concerning chronic injuries, the majority of climbing foot injuries result from wearing climbing shoes unnaturally shaped or too small in size (Peters, 2001; van der Putten & Snijder, 2001). The shoe size reduction forces the foot to conform to the shoe and changes the biomechanical position of the foot within the shoe (Figure 4.7). The foot shortens through supination and contraction of the digits (Killian, Nishimoto, & Page, 1998; Peters, 2001). In front pointing the proximal and mostly all of the distal interphalangeal joints are flexed and the metatarsophalangeal joints are hyper-extended (crimping toes) (Schöffl & Winkelmann, 1999a). High ability climbers experience more foot deformities and injuries compared to climbers of lower ability due to the common practice of wearing climbing shoes sized smaller than normal street wear shoes (van der Putten & Snijder, 2001). Schöffl and Winkelmann (1999a) report an average (standard deviation) shoe size difference between normal shoes and climbing shoes of about 2.3 (0.73) continental sizes in high ability rock climbers. The suffering of pain while using their climbing shoes has been reported by 80–90 per cent of climbers, but they accept this discomfort for improved performance (Schöffl & Winkelmann, 1999a). Frequent problems are callosity (Figure 4.7), nail bed infections, pressure marks, neurologic complaints and subungual hematomas. In the long term, using tight fitting climbing shoes can lead to the development of a hallux valgus deformity (Schöffl & Winkelmann, 1999a; van der Putten & Snijder, 2001).

Through radiographic analysis of a standing climber within a climbing shoe and barefoot demonstrates how the climbing shoes forces the foot into a hallux valgus position. The hallux valgus angle increases from 14° barefoot to 21° within the shoe. In 53 % of the 354 long time high level climbers a hallux valgus, in 20% bilateral one was found. The general incidence in a group of male adults (age: 17–44) is only 4.5 per cent (Marcinko, 1994). Killian et al. (1998) found an average incidence of a hallux valgus of 34 per cent in climbers of all difficulty levels, but of 53 per cent of the group of climbers in the 5.12 range (UIAA 8+). Over recent years we have seen an increasing number of climbers with a hallux rigidus condition, to the extent of even requiring surgical therapy (cheilectomy or fusion) (Schöffl & Küpper, 2013).

Conclusion

Rock climbing and its sub-disciplines induce high forces onto the fingers with osseous and ligamentous adaptations not seen before in other activities. The upper extremities and particularly the fingers are prone to injury and overuse

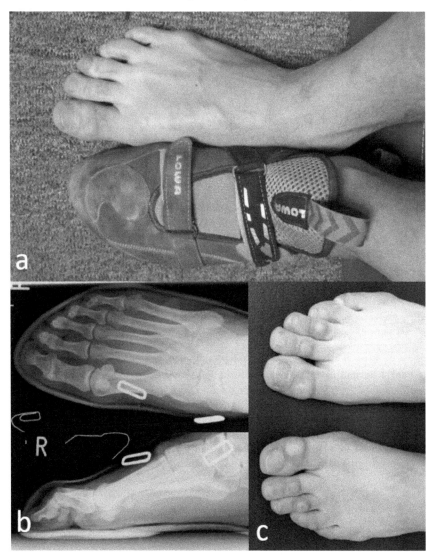

Figure 4.7 The shoe size reduction forces the foot to conform to the shoe and changes the biomechanical position of the foot within the shoe (a). Radiographs depicting the claw toe and forced hallux valgus position (b). 80–90 per cent of climbers are suffering pain while using their tight fitting climbing shoes; as a consequence a frequent problem is callosity around the toe joints (c)

syndromes. New pathologies like closed finger flexor tendon pulley injuries or lumbrical tears appear which can be treated mostly in a conservative manner with a good prognosis. More alarming are epiphyseal fractures of the fingers in young climbers which can result in early degenerative changes when not detected early and treated correctly, usually with no climbing for two to four months. After

10–20 years of intensive climbing a higher risk of degenerative changes of the finger joints is observed due to climbing-specific finger load (crimp grip position). Climbing wall and route setters may implement these findings for choosing more ergonomic climbing holds.

Summary

* Flexor tendon pulley injuries: can be treated mostly conservatively (pulley protection ring) if no relevant deficit of range of motion is apparent.
* Finger pain in adolescents: is mostly due to epiphyseal fractures; confirm the diagnosis with special MRI or with accurate image intensifier investigation. Stop climbing until consolidation.
* Crimp grip: is not completely avoidable in high level climbing; try to eliminate high load of the joint in its end position.
* Overuse syndromes: equilibrate joint forces by regularly exercising all antagonists, particularly at the shoulder, elbow and the trunk.

References

Allenspach, P., Saupe, N., Rufibach, K., & Schweizer, A. (2011). Radiological changes and signs of osteoarthritis in the fingers of male performance sport climbers. *Journal of Sports Medicine and Physical Fitness*, 51(3), 497–505.

Arora, R., Fritz, D., Zimmermann, R., Lutz, M., Kamelger, F., Klauser, A. S., & Gabl, M. (2007). Reconstruction of the digital flexor pulley system: a retrospective comparison of two methods of treatment. *Journal of Hand Surgery (European Volume)*, 32(1), 60–66.

Backe, S., Ericson, L., Janson, S., & Timpka, T. (2009). Rock climbing injury rates and associated risk factors in a general climbing population. *Scandinavian Journal of Medicine & Science in Sports*, 19(6), 850–856.

Bayer, T., Schöffl, V. R., Lenhart, M., & Herold, T. (2013). Epiphyseal stress fractures of finger phalanges in adolescent climbing athletes: a 3.0-Tesla magnetic resonance imaging evaluation. *Skeletal Radiology*, 42(11), 1521–1525.

Bayer, T., & Schweizer, A. (2009). Stress fracture of the hook of the hamate as a result of intensive climbing. *Journal of Hand Surgery (European Volume)*, 34(2), 276–277.

Bircher, H.-P., Thuer, C., Schweizer, A., & Bereiter, H. (2007). Shoulder injuries in sportclimbers. Presentation at the Congress of Swiss Orthopaedic and Trauma Society.

Bollen, S. R. (1990a). Injury to the A2 pulley in rock climbers. *Journal of Hand Surgery (European Volume)*, 15(2), 268–270.

Bollen, S. R. (1990b). Upper limb injuries in elite rock climbers. *Journal of the Royal College of Surgeons of Edinburgh*, 35(6 Suppl), S18–20.

Bollen, S. R., & Wright, V. (1994). Radiographic changes in the hands of rock climbers. *British Journal of Sports Medicine*, 28(3), 185–186.

Gabbett, T. J. (2002). Incidence of injury in amateur rugby league sevens. *British Journal of Sports Medicine*, 36(1), 23–26.

Hahn, F., Erschbaumer, M., Allenspach, P., Rufibach, K., & Schweizer, A. (2012). Physiological bone responses in the fingers after more than 10 years of high-level sport climbing: analysis of cortical parameters. *Wilderness & Environmental Medicine*, 23(1), 31–36.

Hochholzer, T., & Schöffl, V. (2006). *One move too many* (2nd ed.). Ebenhausen, Germany: Lochner Verlag.

Hochholzer, T., & Schöffl, V. (2013). Overuse bone marrow edema of the hands in sport climbers. *Sports Orthopaedics and Traumatology*, 29(3), 219–224.

Hochholzer, T., & Schöffl, V. R. (2005). Epiphyseal fractures of the finger middle joints in young sport climbers. *Wilderness & Environmental Medicine*, 16(3), 139–142.

Josephsen, G., Shinneman, S., Tamayo-Sarver, J., Josephsen, K., Boulware, D., Hunt, M., & Pham, H. (2007). Injuries in bouldering: a prospective study. *Wilderness & Environmental Medicine*, 18(4), 271–280.

Junge, A., & Dvorak, J. (2004). Soccer injuries. *Sports Medicine*, 34(13), 929–938.

Killian, R. B., Nishimoto, G. S., & Page, J. C. (1998). Foot and ankle injuries related to rock climbing. The role of footwear. *Journal of the American Podiatric Medical Association*, 88(8), 365–374.

Klauser, A., Frauscher, F., Bodner, G., Halpern, E. J., Schocke, M. F., Springer, P., ... zur Nedden, D. (2002). Finger pulley injuries in extreme rock climbers: depiction with dynamic US. *Radiology*, 222(3), 755–761.

Klauser, A., Frauscher, F., Gabl, M., & Smekal, V. (2005). High frequency sonography in the detection of finger injuries in sports climbing. *Sports Orthopaedics and Traumatology*, 21, 24–30.

Marcinko, D. E. (1994). *Hallux valgus: Morphologie, Klinik, operative Therapie*. Berlin, Germany: Ullstein Mosby.

Marco, R. A., Sharkey, N. A., Smith, T. S., & Zissimos, A. G. (1998). Pathomechanics of closed rupture of the flexor tendon pulleys in rock climbers. *Journal of Bone & Joint Surgery (American Volume)*, 80(7), 1012–1019.

Mosimann, U. (2006). Notfälle beim Eisklettern. *Bergundsteigen*, 4, 70–73.

Moutet, F., Forli, A., & Voulliaume, D. (2004). Pulley rupture and reconstruction in rock climbers. *Techniques in Hand & Upper Extremity Surgery*, 8(3), 149–155.

Nelson, N. G., & McKenzie, L. B. (2009). Rock climbing injuries treated in emergency departments in the U.S., 1990-2007. *American Journal of Preventive Medicine*, 37(3), 195–200.

Neuhof, A., Hennig, F. F., Schöffl, I., & Schöffl, V. (2011). Injury risk evaluation in sport climbing. *International Journal of Sports Medicine*, 32(10), 794–800.

Peters, P. (2001). Nerve compression syndromes in sport climbers. *International Journal of Sports Medicine*, 22(8), 611–617.

Peterson, M., Butler, S., Eriksson, M., & Svärdsudd, K. (2011). A randomized controlled trial of exercise versus wait-list in chronic tennis elbow (lateral epicondylosis). *Upsala Journal of Medical Sciences*, 116(4), 269–279.

Popp, D., & Schöffl, V. (2013). Shoulder SLAP and biceps tendon repair. *Minerva Ortopedica e Traumatologica*, 64, 247–263.

Rohrbough, J. T., Mudge, M. K., Schilling, R. C., & Jansen, C. (1998). Radiographic osteoarthritis in the hands of rock climbers. *American Journal of Orthopedics*, 27(11), 734–738.

Schneeberger, M., & Schweizer, A. (2014). Results of conservative treatment of closed finger flexor tendon pulley rupture with a pulley protection ring. IRCRA congress Pontresina, Switzerland.

Schöffl, I., Baier, T., & Schöffl, V. (2011). Flap irritation phenomenon (FLIP): etiology of chronic tenosynovitis after finger pulley rupture. *Journal of Applied Biomechanics*, 27(4), 291–296.

Schöffl, I., Einwag, F., Strecker, W., Hennig, F., & Schöffl, V. (2007). Impact of taping after finger flexor tendon pulley ruptures in rock climbers. *Journal of Applied Biomechanics*, 23, 52–62.

Schöffl, I., Oppelt, K., Jungert, J., Schweizer, A., Neuhuber, W., & Schöffl, V. (2009). The influence of the crimp and slope grip position on the finger pulley system. *Journal of Biomechanics, 42*(13), 2183–2187.

Schöffl, V. (2008). [Hand Injuries in Rock Climbing] Handverletzungen beim Klettern. *Deutsche Zeitschrift für Sportmedizin, 59*(4), 85–90.

Schöffl, V., Burtscher, E., & Coscia, F. (2013). Injuries and medical incidences during the IFSC 2012 Climbing World Cup Series. *Medicina Sportiva, 17*(4), 168–170.

Schöffl, V., Heid, A., & Kupper, T. (2012). Tendon injuries of the hand. *World Journal of Orthopedics, 3*(6), 62–69.

Schöffl, V., Hochholzer, T., Karrer, A., Winter, S., & Imhoff, A. (2003). [Finger problems in adolescent top level climbers – a comparison of the German junior national team with recreational climbers] Fingerschäden jugendlicher Leistungskletterer – Vergleichende Analyse der deutschen Jugendnationalmannschaft sowie einer gleichaltrigen Vergleichsgruppe von Freizeitkletterern. *Deutsche Zeitschrift für Sportmedizin, 54*, 317–322.

Schöffl, V., & Küpper, T. (2006). Injuries at the 2005 World Championships in Rock Climbing. *Wilderness & Environmental Medicine, 17*, 187–190.

Schöffl, V., & Küpper, T. (2013). Feet injuries in rock climbers. *World Journal of Orthopedics, 4*(4), 218–228.

Schöffl, V., Küpper, T., Hartmann, J., & Schöffl, I. (2012). Surgical repair of multiple pulley injuries – evaluation of a new combined pulley repair. *The Journal of Hand Surgery (American Volume), 37*(2), 224–230.

Schöffl, V., Morrison, A., Schöffl, I., & Küpper, T. (2012). Epidemiology of injury in mountaineering, rock and ice climbing. In D. Caine & T. Heggie (Eds.), *Medicine and Sport Science – Epidemiology of Injury in Adventure and Extreme Sports* (Vol. 58, pp. 17–43): Basel, Switzerland: Karger.

Schöffl, V., Popp, D., Dickschass, J., & Kupper, T. (2011). Superior labral anterior-posterior lesions in rock climbers—primary double tenodesis? *Clinical Journal of Sport Medicine, 21*(3), 261–263.

Schöffl, V., Popp, D., Küpper, T., & Schöffl, I. (2015). Injury distribution in rock climbers – a prospective evaluation of 911 injuries between 2009-2012. *Wilderness & Environmental Medicine, 26*(1), 62–67.

Schöffl, V., & Winkelmann, H. P. (1999a). [Foot deformations in sport climbers] Fußdeformitäten bei Sportkletterern. *Deutsche Zeitschrift für Sportmedizin, 50*, 73–76.

Schöffl, V., & Winkelmann, H. P. (1999b). Injury-risk on indoor climbing walls. *Sportverletzung Sportschaden: Organ der Gesellschaft fur Orthopadisch-Traumatologische Sportmedizin, 13*(1), 14–16.

Schöffl, V. R., & Schöffl, I. (2006). Injuries to the finger flexor pulley system in rock climbers: current concepts. *Journal of Hand Surgery (American Volume), 31*(4), 647–654.

Schussmann, L. C., Lutz, L. J., Shaw, R. R., & Bohn, C. R. (1990). The epidemiology of mountaineering and rock climbing accidents. *Wilderness & Environmental Medicine, 1*, 235–248.

Schweizer, A. (2000). Biomechanical effectiveness of taping the A2 pulley in rock climbers. *Journal of Hand Surgery (European Volume), 25*(1), 102–107.

Schweizer, A. (2001). Biomechanical properties of the crimp grip position in rock climbers. *Journal of Biomechanics, 34*(2), 217–223.

Schweizer, A. (2012). Sport climbing from a medical point of view. *Swiss Medical Weekly, 142*, w13688.

Schweizer, A., Bircher, H. P. (2009). Reposition of a dislocated shoulder under use of cannabis. *Wilderness & Environmental Medicine*, 20(3), 301–302.

Schweizer, A., Frank, O., Ochsner, P. E., & Jacob, H. A. (2003). Friction between human finger flexor tendons and pulleys at high loads. *Journal of Biomechanics*, 36(1), 63–71.

Sylvester, A. D., Christensen, A. M., & Kramer, P. A. (2006). Factors influencing osteological changes in the hands and fingers of rock climbers. *Journal of Anatomy*, 209(5), 597–609.

Tropet, Y., Menez, D., Balmat, P., Pem, R., & Vichard, P. (1990). Closed traumatic rupture of the ring finger flexor tendon pulley. *Journal of Hand Surgery (American Volume)*, 15(5), 745–747.

van der Putten, E. P., & Snijder, C. J. (2001). Shoe design for prevention of injuries in sport climbing. *Applied Ergonomics*, 32(4), 379–387.

Warme, W. J., & Brooks, D. (2000). The effect of circumferential taping on flexor tendon pulley failure in rock climbers. *American Journal of Sports Medicine*, 28(5), 674–678.

Wedderkopp, N., Kaltoft, M., Lundgaard, B., Rosendahl, M., & Froberg, K. (1997). Injuries in young female players in European team handball. *Scandinavian Journal of Medicine & Science in Sports*, 7(6), 342–347.

Wolf, J. M., Ozer, K., Scott, F., Gordon, M. J., & Williams, A. E. (2011). Comparison of autologous blood, corticosteroid, and saline injection in the treatment of lateral epicondylitis: a prospective, randomized, controlled multicenter study. *The Journal of Hand Surgery*, 36(8), 1269–1272.

5 High altitude medicine and cold effects in mountaineering

Jean Paul Richalet and Emmanuel Cauchy

Mountaineering exposes the human body to environmental constraints that may limit physical and cognitive performance and even threaten life. Altitude hypoxia and cold are the most prominent stresses encountered. Hypoxia will trigger numerous physiological responses: heart and ventilation accelerate and after a few days, red cell mass in the blood increases. These mechanisms of acclimatization help the organism to cope with hypoxia but physical and cognitive performance decrease as a function of altitude. Incomplete acclimatization may lead to acute mountain sickness and high altitude pulmonary or cerebral oedema. Prevention of these manifestations is based on slow ascent and limited exercise on the first days of exposure. Individual susceptibility to severe high altitude diseases can be evaluated by a hypoxic exercise test, especially for those who have never been exposed to high altitude. As body core temperature must be maintained around 37 °C in all circumstances, physiological mechanisms (shivering, cutaneous vasoconstriction) will be triggered when exposed to cold, but the most efficient response is behavioural (clothing, protection, activity). Inadequate exposure of extremities to cold may lead to frostbite, with several degrees of severity. Overall exposure of the body to cold may lead to hypothermia (core temperature below 35 °C), that can be life-threatening. Rewarming should be performed cautiously, when the risk of refreezing has been eliminated.

Introduction

This chapter deals with the specificities of mountaineering, in particular physiological and behavioural effects of altitude hypoxia. The authors provide practical applications for acclimatization to altitude and safety, including high altitude medicine, detection, prevention and treatment of acute mountain sickness, high altitude pulmonary oedema and high altitude cerebral oedema. This chapter also presents the effect of cold on the human body and the symptoms, prevention and treatment of frostbite and hypothermia.

Altitude effect

Physical characteristics

The physiological effects of altitude hypoxia on the human body are primarily determined by the value of oxygen pressure in the inspired air, given by the following equation:

$$PIO_2 = FIO_2 \times (P_B - PH_2O)$$

FIO_2 is the fraction of O_2 in inspired air, which is constant and equal to 0.2093 at all natural altitudes (hypobaric hypoxia). P_B is the barometric pressure. It decreases quasi-exponentially with increasing altitude. It also varies with the weather, the season and the latitude. PH_2O is the pressure of vapour in the inspired air: it does not change with altitude but varies with the body temperature (if body temperature is 37 °C, PH_2O is 47 mmHg).

Physiological effects

Altitude hypoxia is the unique 'extreme environment' to which the human body is able to adapt, or rather to 'acclimatize' (Richalet & Herry, 2006). A wide range of biological integrated mechanisms is triggered when an individual is acutely exposed to hypoxia. The immediate stimulation of peripheral chemoreceptors (carotid bodies) induces an increase in minute ventilation and heart rate, which, by accelerating the O_2 flux through the lungs and the circulation, partially compensate for the decrease in O_2 content in the blood.

With days of exposure to hypoxia, ventilation progressively increases (ventilatory acclimatization), while heart rate, especially maximal heart rate, decreases. After a few hours of exposure to hypoxia, erythropoietin is secreted by the kidneys, which will result, after five to seven days, in a progressive increase in red cell mass through bone marrow stimulation. A reduction of plasma volume is also observed in the first days, which may contribute to haemoconcentration. In parallel with hypoxemia, the hyperventilation induced by hypoxia leads to hypocapnia and alkalosis, which will be partially compensated by an increased urinary excretion of bicarbonates. Aerobic (i.e. oxygen dependent) physical performance, as evaluated by maximal O_2 consumption (VO_{2max}) decreases with increasing altitude, from altitudes as low as 600 m. With acclimatization, VO_{2max} might slightly increase but never reaches pre-exposure sea level values. Several physiological factors limit aerobic performance at altitude. Among the various successive steps of O_2 transport from ambient air to the mitochondria, the most probable limiting steps are blood oxygen transport (cardiac output and O_2 content) and diffusion at the pulmonary and the muscle levels. Briefly, the arterial O_2 content is reduced, due to a rapid decrease in arterial O_2 saturation from rest to exercise at a given altitude. The extraction of O_2 in the muscle is limited since the gradient of O_2 from the capillary to the mitochondria is reduced. The venous blood returning to the lungs is profoundly desaturated and the diffusion process in the lungs is limited so that the arterial blood does not fully receive the O_2 available in the alveoli.

Cognitive and behavioural effects

Cognitive impairment has been observed in acute exposure to hypoxia in various experimental or field conditions (Abraini, Bouquet, Joulia, Nicolas, & Kriem, 1998; Virués-Ortega, Buela-Casal, Garrido, & Alcàzar, 2004; Yan, 2014). However, the severity of symptoms depends on the level of altitude reached and the speed of ascent (i.e. the acclimatization). Up to 3500 m, minimal impairment has been reported, mainly reduced efficiency in complex tasks such as complex reaction time. From 3500 to 6500 m, working memory and learning might be impaired (Yan, 2014) (Table 5.1.). Above 6500 m, severe cognitive alterations can be observed and brain damage can be evidenced at magnetic resonance imaging (Table 5.1.). Somaesthetic illusions and visual and acoustic hallucinations have been reported at extreme altitudes, as well as impairment in codification and short-term memory (Virués-Ortega et al., 2004). Cognitive impairment can also be indirectly due to sleep disturbances, very frequent at high altitude, and symptoms of acute mountain sickness (headache, fatigue). Decision-making is altered above 6500 m, especially when the individual is left alone: this could explain part of the numerous accidents and deaths observed when climbing alone over 8000 m without supplementary oxygen (Abraini et al., 1998) (Table 5.1.).

Altitude-related diseases and treatments

To be fully effective, the mechanisms of adaptation to altitude hypoxia need a certain time, an 'acclimatization period'. During this early phase, symptoms of incomplete acclimatization may occur, namely acute mountain sickness (AMS), high altitude pulmonary oedema (HAPE) and high altitude cerebral

Table 5.1   Definition of altitude ranges

Altitude range	Definition	Effects
0–500 m	Near sea level	No effect on well-being or performance
500–2000 m	Low altitude	No effect on well-being, possible effect on performance, especially in highly trained athletes
2000–3000 m	Moderate altitude	Acute mountain sickness may occur in non-acclimatized lowlanders, significant decrease in aerobic performance
3000–5500 m	High altitude	Acute mountain sickness is frequent, pulmonary or cerebral edema are possible in susceptible subjects, aerobic performance is seriously decreased, even after acclimatization
Above 5500 m	Extreme altitude	Serious risk for health, no permanent residency possible, severe alteration of physical and mental performance

oedema (HACE) (Bärtsch & Swenson, 2013; Richalet & Herry, 2006). Other manifestations may occur, such as retinal haemorrhages, cerebral thrombosis or transient ischemic attacks, but the last two are relatively rare.

Symptoms of HACE are essentially neurological, with ataxia, neurological deficits and loss of consciousness. The best prevention of these pathological manifestations is a progressive ascent (less than 400 m of altitude between two consecutive nights) and the limitation of exercise during the first three days at altitude.

Acute mountain sickness

The main symptoms of AMS are headache, gastro-intestinal complaints (nausea, vomiting), insomnia, dizziness and fatigue. Around 25 per cent of persons going above 3000 m suffer from severe AMS. Symptoms generally appear after four to eight hours of exposure to hypoxia, after a rapid ascent above 3000 m, and disappear after two or three days. Peripheral oedema (face, ankles, wrist) may accompany the usual symptoms of AMS but may also appear without headaches. In some cases (individual susceptibility, rapid ascent to altitude, etc.), more severe conditions may occur: HAPE or HACE. They are life-threatening and necessitate a rapid re-oxygenation, mainly through descent to lower altitude (Bärtsch & Swenson, 2013; Richalet & Herry, 2006).

High altitude pulmonary oedema

Symptoms of HAPE are linked to an acute respiratory distress with dyspnoea, cough and thoracic discomfort. Subjects have great difficulty breathing and cannot perform any physical activity. Blue lips (cyanosis) and sometimes fever are associated with dyspnoea. The incidence is between 1 per cent and 2 per cent of persons going above 3000 m. If no treatment or re-oxygenation is available, the risk of death is around 40 per cent.

High altitude cerebral oedema

Symptoms of HACE are essentially neurological, with ataxia, neurological deficits and loss of consciousness. Symptoms may develop as an aggravation of AMS, with severe headache, resistant to any treatment, vomiting and fatigue. It may also appear with mood alterations (depression, aggressiveness) or with neurological symptoms such as difficulty of walking straight (ataxia) or speaking (aphasia) or disorientation. The incidence is around 0.5 per cent to 1 per cent of persons going above 3000 m. When loss of consciousness appears, death is observed in 60 per cent of cases.

Mechanisms of high altitude-related diseases

The causes of AMS, HAPE and HACE are not yet fully understood and still debated among specialists. The common mechanism of all forms of altitude-related diseases is the presence of oedema (under the skin: peripheral oedema; in the lung: HAPE; in the brain: HACE). The cause of headache is not clear: it might be a preliminary form of HACE with increase in brain pressure or might be similar to migraine. HAPE is multifactorial: there is an increase in the blood pressure in the pulmonary circulation, an increase in the permeability of capillaries and a decrease in the clearing of water that accumulates in the alveoli. Mechanisms of HACE are unclear but an increase in capillary permeability, a reduction in the metabolism of brain cells and distinctive anatomical features can be responsible for the development of HACE (Bärtsch & Swenson, 2013; Richalet & Herry, 2006).

Practical recommendations to prevent and take care of altitude-related diseases

Detection of high-risk subjects

Contrarily to what is often mentioned, severe AMS, HAPE and HACE may not be 'unpredictable'. Several risk factors have been identified in subjects more susceptible to developing these diseases (Richalet, Larmignat, Poitrine, Letournel, & Canouï-Poitrine, 2012). A recent epidemiological study performed on 1017 trekkers and climbers at high altitude have evidenced the following factors (Canouï-Poitrine et al., 2014; Coustet, Lhuissier, Vincent, & Richalet, 2015; Richalet et al., 2012):

- History of previous episodes of severe problems at high altitude: subjects who have already been sick have 13 times more chance of being sick than others when they return to high altitude.
- Rapid ascent: when the difference of altitude between two consecutive nights at the beginning of the stay over 3000 m is more than 400 m, the risk of being sick is multiplied by six.
- Subjects with history of migraine have four times more chance of being sick.
- Destinations such as Ladakh, Aconcagua or Mont Blanc increase the risk by a factor 2.4.
- Age under 46 years and being female increase the risk between 40 per cent and 80 per cent, depending on previous exposure to high altitude.
- Regular endurance training increases the risk by around 50 per cent: this means that training is not a protecting factor against severe AMS, HAPE or HACE, although it is mandatory to trek or perform an ascent at high altitude in good conditions.
- Physiological factors have been clearly identified, using a 'normobaric hypoxic exercise test' performed at 30 per cent of VO_{2max} at a simulated altitude equivalent to 4800 m.

Subjects with a low ventilatory response to hypoxia have 20 times more chance being sick. The test allows good detection of subjects that might be at risk of developing severe AMS, HAPE or HACE when they reach high altitude. It is particularly effective for a subject who has never been to high altitude beforehand (Richalet & Canouï-Poitrine, 2014; Richalet, Canouï-Poitrine, & Larmignat, 2013).

Prevention of high-altitude related diseases

Prevention measures derive from the risk factors identified above:

- Persons with a previous 'bad' experience at high altitude should be particularly careful and have good progressive acclimatization.
- The ascent should follow the golden rule: 'Do not go too high too fast': no more than 400 m between two consecutive nights at the beginning of the stay above 3000 m.
- Special attention should be paid when travelling to regions where the arrival at high altitude is rapid, without progressive acclimatization.
- Young, well-trained, very active subjects should be aware that endurance training does not protect against altitude problems!
- Individuals, who have never been to high altitude and have any doubt about their ability to adapt to this demanding environment, especially if they have any cardiovascular or respiratory disease, should attend a specialized consultation. Although it has been a controversial point for many years, it is now established that hypoxia exercise test can help to give specific, personalized advice before a sojourn at high altitude.
- Limit physical exercise in the first days of acclimatization, because when doing exercise at high altitude, the O_2 pressure in the blood drops, leading to increased risk of altitude diseases.
- When the overall risk has been identified as high during the consultation (taking into account all the risk factors mentioned above), or if the arrival or the climb at high altitude is too rapid so that the golden rule cannot be fulfilled, then only one preventive treatment is available: acetazolamide (Diamox). It has been shown to reduce by half the risk of developing severe symptoms at high altitude. The dose is half pill in the morning and half pill at noon, starting the day before reaching 3000 m and continuing until reaching the maximal altitude (maximum five days, during the acclimatization period). This molecule works by accelerating acclimatization (by increasing pulmonary ventilation and O_2 pressure in the blood). It is also slightly diuretic. It is well tolerated, but it should be prescribed by a medical doctor to be sure that there is no contra-indication to its use.

How should altitude-related illnesses be treated?

In the case of AMS, the first treatment consists of taking pain-releasing drugs, such as aspirin, paracetamol or ibuprofen. If it appears insufficient, rest is mandatory. If the symptoms do not resolve, then descent or O_2 inhalation or the use of a hyperbaric portable bag is necessary.

For HAPE, descent or any kind of re-oxygenation (O_2 inhalation, hyperbaric bag) should be provided as soon as possible. Medications should be started immediately with a drug to decrease pulmonary arterial pressure (calcium blocker or PDE5 inhibitor) and an anti-oedematous drug (corticosteroids).

HACE is a severe emergency condition and descent or any kind of re-oxygenation (O_2 inhalation, hyperbaric bag) should also be started as soon as possible. The only drugs that can be useful are corticosteroids that can be given orally if the subject is still conscious, otherwise intravenously (Bärtsch & Swenson, 2013; Richalet & Herry, 2006).

Cold effect

Physiological response to cold

Man is a homeothermic organism that needs to maintain his core temperature around 37 °C for optimal cellular metabolism. His preferred environmental temperature is rather tropical (around 27 °C) but he may adapt to extreme temperatures from -50 °C in polar regions to +40 °C in tropical regions. However, physiological mechanisms for temperature regulation are limited and the main process of adaptation to changes in ambient temperature is behavioural: clothes, heating, housing adaptations and so on (Cappaert et al., 2008; Mills, 1993; Richalet & Herry, 2006).

The physiological system involved in core temperature regulation comprises sensors (thermoreceptors located mainly in the skin and in the brain), control centres located in the hypothalamus and effectors through the extrapyramidal and autonomous nervous system. In steady-state conditions, the amount of heat produced by the body (due to cellular metabolism) is equal to the loss of heat through skin and pulmonary ventilation, so that core temperature is maintained constant, at around 37 °C. The heat flux through the body can be positive if heat is transferred from the ambience to the body or negative if heat is lost to the ambience. The mechanisms of heat transfer can be by conduction (contact of the skin with an object), convection (movement of fluid – air or water – around the body), radiation (especially from the sun) and evaporation of water (sweat) from the surface of the skin. The transfer mainly depends on the temperature difference between the skin and the external medium. The exchange of heat between the core (internal organs), the skin and the ambience is mainly related to the intensity of skin blood flow and therefore depends on the degree of vasodilation or vasoconstriction of the skin circulation, which is controlled by the sympathetic nervous system. Production of sweat by the eccrine glands will allow evaporation of sweat and consumption of calories by the skin to transform liquid water into vapour. Thermal shivering is another mechanism triggered by exposure to cold and consists of involuntary muscle contraction that contributes to heat production.

In the mountain environment, cold exposure might be extreme and loss of heat will be exacerbated by direct contact of the body with snow (conduction) and presence of wind (convection). The response will be essentially behavioural, by using adapted clothes to enlarge the thickness of the shell to protect the core from the outside temperature, and by avoiding exposure to violent winds. Skin vasoconstriction and shivering are the physiological responses to cold exposure. However, they are not sufficient to provide an adequate protection against cold.

When the mechanisms of temperature control are overtaken, two pathological conditions may affect either local parts of the skin (frostbite) or the body as a whole (hypothermia).

Frostbite

Frostbite affects mainly hands and feet but also the face (nose, chin, earlobes, cheeks and lips), buttocks/perineum (from sitting on metal seats) and penis (joggers) (Cauchy, Chetaille, Marchand, & Marsigny, 2001; McIntosh et al., 2011; McIntosh et al., 2014; Zafren, 2013).

When skin temperature drops, cutaneous blood flow is drastically reduced and skin cells become hypoxic and cold. When skin temperature reaches -2 °C, ice crystals slowly form in the extracellular fluid. Then endothelial cells are damaged, water comes out from the cells that become dehydrated and finally cells are disrupted. Vascular sludging occurs, blood viscosity rises and small vessels are occluded. When the tissue is rewarming, endothelial cells release inflammatory products that will aggravate tissue injury. Oedema will develop and extravasated fluid may accumulate in blisters. Red cell extravasation from vessels might produce haemorrhagic blisters.

The risk of amputation is particularly high when injuries occur in the austere environment, where resources are limited. The main reason for poor outcome in this environment is usually a delay in definitive care, which is often unavoidable. The emerging use of thrombolytics and iloprost offers the first major advances in the treatment of frostbite for decades and has reduced the rate of amputation (Cauchy, Cheguillaume, & Chetaille, 2011; Cauchy, Davis, Pasquier, Meyer, & Hackett 2016; Cauchy, Marsigny, Allamel, Verhellen, & Chetaille, 2000). The association of thrombolytics with iloprost seems to have a beneficial effect on stage 4. The use of intra-arterial thrombolytics in situ is also proposed by a few centres.

In the field, treatment of frostbite remains challenging for several reasons (Pasquier, Ruffinen, Brugger, & Paal, 2012; Zafren, 2013). First is the difficulty of assessing the severity of injury, a crucial determination that dictates management and evacuation decisions. Second is determining the time of onset of injury, duration of freezing and time since thawing in those who have spontaneously thawed. Other difficulties include the logistics of evacuation to an appropriate facility, and the presence of co-morbid conditions such as hypothermia, trauma or medical illness. In addition, treatment greatly depends on medical capabilities and available supplies. Finally, the most promising therapies for severe frostbite have been confined to hospital use and are unavailable, impractical or inappropriate for field use. Tragically, too many patients reach the hospital too late for successful use of medical therapy.

In the field and in hospital, evaluation of frostbite injury is based on presence or absence of perfusion and sensibility after rewarming, combined with extent of non-perfused tissue. For assessing perfusion, careful examination includes skin colour and temperature, pulse and capillary refill. Expedition basecamps or field clinics as well as hospitals may have fast-response infrared thermometers, pulse oximeters and even Doppler devices. Level of non-perfusion or discoloration can be described with the usual hand/foot anatomy of joints. Severity may be evaluated by a number of classification systems. A practical classification of frostbite injuries is proposed in Figure 5.1 (Cauchy et al., 2001) and is exemplified in Figures 5.2 to 5.5. At high altitude, the risk of poor outcome may increase due to hypoxemia (SpO_2 < 90 per cent, usually > 4500 m.), less vasodilation in the cold, dehydration. In the hospital setting, grading of frostbite severity is easier than in the field, due to the comfort and safety of the environment, availability of easy rapid rewarming, and observation over time. Although some practitioners obtain nuclear bone scans (Tc99m) on day 0, the literature suggests that scanning only on day 2–3 or later improves prognostication (Cauchy, Chetaille et al., 2000; Cauchy, Marsigny et al., 2000). A recent publication of frostbite management guidelines includes several important treatments for use in the field (Cauchy et al., 2016). For example, the victim should rehydrate orally with warm fluids and

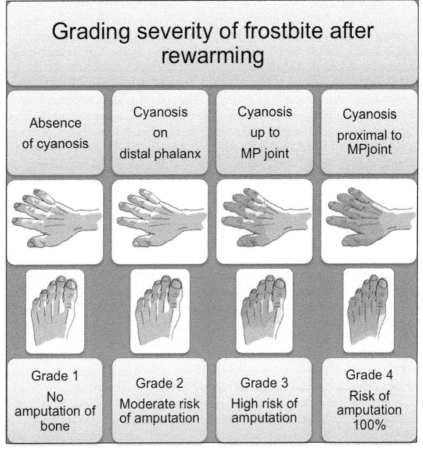

Figure 5.1 Grading severity of frostbite and bone amputation risk after rewarming

Source: Cauchy et al., 2001

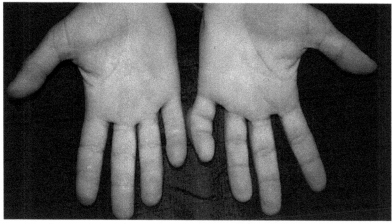

Figure 5.2 First-degree frostbite: no lesion after rapid rewarming

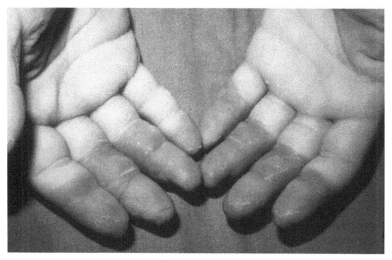

Figure 5.3 Third-degree frostbite: lesions with hemorrhagic blisters on intermediate and distal phalanges

the injured extremity should be rewarmed by immersion in a 37–39 °C water bath for one hour if there is low risk of refreezing. In order to treat hyperviscosity and inflammation, the guidelines recommend 12 mg/kg/day of ibuprofen, and others recommend aspirin (250 mg/day). If blisters appear, a dressing is suggested. Systemic antibiotics should be considered for severe frostbite (grade 3–4) in special circumstances. Others have suggested that for foot frostbite, anti-coagulants should be considered to avoid the complications of thrombosis and phlebitis, especially if the victim is non-ambulatory.

Recently, two new ideas for field treatment have been suggested but not yet studied: pre-hospital distal sympathetic nerve block, and increased oxygenation (O_2 inhalation or hyperbaric bag) for frostbitten patients who are at high altitude,

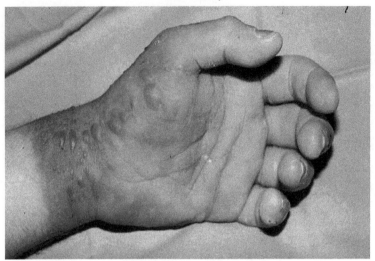

Figure 5.4 Fourth-degree with extended lesions up to carpus

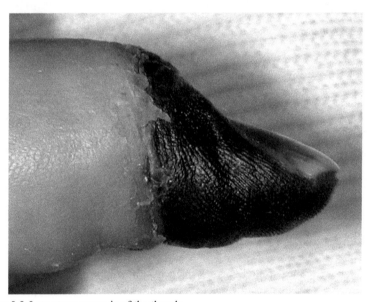

Figure 5.5 Late stage necrosis of the thumb

or hypoxic for any reason (SpO_2 <90 per cent, usually > 4500 m) (Cauchy, Leal, Magnan, & Nespoulet, 2014; Pasquier et al., 2012).

Hypothermia

Hypothermia is defined by a decrease in core temperature below 35 °C. Mild hypothermia is considered between 35 °C and 32 °C (stage I), moderate hypothermia between 32 °C and 28 °C (stage II), severe hypothermia between 28 °C and 24 °C (stage III), malign hypothermia with cardiac arrest between 24 °C and 13 °C (stage IV) and irreversible hypothermia below 13 °C (stage V). It is due to a deficit in the balance between heat production and heat loss in cold environments (Mills, 1993; Mohr, Jenabzadeh, & Ahrenholz, 2009).

Hypothermia is a life-threatening condition and should be recognized rapidly at the site of the accident in field conditions (avalanche or crevasse) and properly managed.

Mild hypothermia is characterized by shivering, tachycardia, tachypnoea and peripheral vasoconstriction. Diuresis is increased, which will lead to hypovolemia. In moderate hypothermia, shivering disappears, bradycardia and respiratory depression occur, consciousness is altered, pupils dilate. Severe hypothermia is associated with altered electrocardiographic activity, coma and apnoea. Pulmonary oedema often may occur. Below 20 °C, the electroencephalogram is flat and the reflexes disappear.

Measuring core temperature is important but frequently difficult to perform in field conditions. Oesophageal measurement is the gold standard, epitympanic thermometers are more accurate and more practical to use than rectal or oral thermometers, but imprecise in the case of cardiac arrest. Management of a hypothermic patient will depend on the degree of hypothermia, the duration of exposure to cold and the eventual presence of associated injuries (traumatic or medical) (Brugger et al., 2013; Zafren et al., 2014).

Insulation by all available means (blankets, clothing, chemical heat packs) is recommended but rewarming should not be initiated before the patient is transported to a medical unit with appropriate facilities for monitoring. Too rapid rewarming of extremities and rough movements can lead to 'core temperature after drop' due to a further decrease in core temperature and associated clinical deterioration. When peripheral tissues are warmed, vasodilation allows cooler blood in the extremities to circulate back to the heart and may provoke cardiac arrhythmias.

Mild hypothermia can be easily managed by passive external rewarming and rehydration with warm fluids. More severe hypothermia will necessitate more active management in hospital emergency units, with perfusion of warm fluids, extracorporeal membrane oxygenation or cardiopulmonary bypass. Potassium concentration in the plasma will be a good prognosis marker: when the value is above 12 mmol/L, resuscitation may be discontinued.

At high altitude, hypothermia can be aggravated by hypoxia and exhaustion; in any case, descent to lower and warmer altitudes is mandatory to prevent further degradation (Brugger et al., 2013; Zafren et al., 2014).

Practical recommendations

The influence of air temperature and wind speed should be taken into account by using the wind-chill index, as wind, by accelerating convection heat loss, aggravates the risk of cold injuries (Table 5.2).

Prevention of frostbite is essential and is based on adequate clothing and protection against cold and wind. Shoes must not be too tight in order to facilitate

Table 5.2 Wind-chill index chart. Felt temperatures for various ambient temperatures (T) and wind speed (S). For example, for an ambient temperature of −4°C and a wind speed of 30 km/h, a subject feels an outside temperature of −20°C. Zone I (clear): range of speeds and temperatures where adapted clothing is sufficient to allow a normal physical activity without high risk. Zone II (mild grey): range of speeds and temperatures where polar clothing, intense physical activity and limited time of exposure to cold can prevent hypothermia. Zone III (dark grey): exposure, even short, is not recommended, due to high risk of cold injuries.

T (°C) / S (km.h⁻¹)	4	2	−1	−4	−7	−9	−12	−15	−18	−21	−23	−26	−29	−32	−34
8	3	0	−3	−6	−9	−11	−14	−17	−21	−24	−26	−29	−32	−35	−37
15	−2	−6	−9	−13	−16	−19	−23	−26	−29	−33	−36	−39	−43	−47	−50
22	−6	−9	−12	−17	−21	−24	−28	−32	−35	−40	−43	−46	−50	−54	−57
30	−8	−11	−16	−20	−23	−27	−32	−36	−39	−43	−47	−51	−55	−60	−63
40	−9	−14	−18	−22	−26	−30	−34	−38	−42	−47	−51	−55	−59	−64	−67
50	−11	−15	−19	−24	−28	−32	−36	−41	−44	−49	−53	−57	−62	−66	−70
58	−12	−16	−20	−25	−29	−33	−37	−42	−45	−51	−55	−59	−64	−68	−72
65	−12	−17	−21	−26	−30	−34	−38	−43	−47	−52	−56	−60	−65	−70	−74

blood circulation into extremities. Gloves should be of good insulating quality and two pairs of gloves should always be available. Using sunglasses with lateral protection against wind will prevent cornea frostbite.

Clothing should be multi-layered since the air captured between the layers is the best insulating material: an internal layer will allow evaporation of sweat with minimal absorption, a middle layer will provide insulation, and a removable external layer that is wind and water resistant will allow evaporation of moisture. Toes, fingers, ears and skin should be protected. Remove wet clothing as soon as practical and replace with dry, clean items.

Hydration and diet should be adequate, with regular fluid intake during climbing activities, if possible with warm fluids. It should be taken into account that thirst is often blunted in cold and hypoxic conditions.

Rewarming of patients with frostbite or hypothermia should always be performed with caution, taking into account that the risk of refreezing can be extremely deleterious.

Summary

- Regulation of body (core) temperature is extremely important for homeostasis and cell metabolism.
- Physiological responses to cold exposure (vasoconstriction, shivering) have limited effects; the most efficient response to cold is behavioural (exercise, clothing, protection).
- Frostbite can be avoided by using adequate protection (shoes, gloves, glasses). Local rewarming should be initiated when the risk of refreezing is absent.
- The severity and prognosis of hypothermia depend on the core temperature. Rewarming should be performed in hospital facilities when hypothermia is severe.

References

Abraini, J. H., Bouquet, C., Joulia, F., Nicolas, M., & Kriem, B. (1998). Cognitive performance during a simulated climb of Mount Everest: implications for brain function and central adaptive processes under chronic hypoxic stress. *Pflugers Arch*, 436, 553–559.

Bärtsch, P., & Swenson, E. R. (2013). Clinical practice: acute high-altitude illnesses. *New England Journal of Medicine*, 368, 2294–2302.

Brugger, H., Durrer, B., Elsensohn, F., Paal, P., Strapazzon, G., Winterberger, E., ... Boyd, J. (2013). Resuscitation of avalanche victims: evidence-based guidelines of the international commission for mountain emergency medicine (ICAR MEDCOM): intended for physicians and other advanced life support personnel. *Resuscitation*, 84(5), 539–546.

Canouï-Poitrine, F., Veerabudun, K., Larmignat, P., Letournel, M., Bastuji-Garin, S., & Richalet, J. P. (2014). Risk prediction score for severe high altitude illness: a cohort study. *PLoS One*, 9(7), e100642.

Cappaert, T. A., Stone, J. A., Castellani, J. W., Krause, B. A., Smith, D., & Stephens, B. A. (2008). National Athletic Trainers' Association position statement: environmental cold injuries. *Journal of Athletic Training*, 43, 640–658.

Cauchy, E., Cheguillaume, B., & Chetaille, E. (2011). A controlled trial of a prostacyclin and rt-PA in the treatment of severe frostbite. *New England Journal of Medicine*, 364, 189–190.

Cauchy, E., Chetaille, E., Lefevre, M., Kerelou, E., & Marsigny, B. (2000). The role of bone scanning in severe frostbite of the extremities: a retrospective study of 88 cases. *European Journal of Nuclear Medicine*, 27, 497–502.

Cauchy, E., Chetaille, E., Marchand, V., & Marsigny, B. (2001). Retrospective study of 70 cases of severe frostbite lesions: a proposed new classification scheme. *Wilderness & Environmental Medicine*, 12, 248–255.

Cauchy, E., Davis, C., Pasquier, M., Meyer, E. F., & Hackett, P. (2016). Proposal for a novel treatment pathway for management of severe frostbite in the austere environment. *Wilderness & Environmental Medicine*, in press.

Cauchy, E., Leal, S., Magnan, M. A., & Nespoulet, H. (2014). Portable hyperbaric chamber and management of hypothermia and frostbite: an evident utilization. *High Altitude Medicine & Biology*, 15, 95–96.

Cauchy, E., Marsigny, B., Allamel, G., Verhellen, R., & Chetaille, E. (2000). The value of technetium 99 scintigraphy in the prognosis of amputation in severe frostbite injuries of the extremities: a retrospective study of 92 severe frostbite injuries. *Journal of Hand Surgery (American Volume)*, 25, 969–978.

Coustet, B., Lhuissier, F.J., Vincent, R., & Richalet, J. P. (2015). Electrocardiographic changes during exercise in acute hypoxia and susceptibility to severe high altitude illnesses. *Circulation*, 131, 786–794.

McIntosh, S. E., Hamonko, M., Freer, L., Grissom, C. K., Auerbach, P. S., Rodway, G. W., ... Johnson, E. (2011). Wilderness medical society practice guidelines for the prevention and treatment of frostbite. *Wilderness & Environmental Medicine*, 22(2), 156–166.

McIntosh, S. E., Opacic, M., Freer, L., Grissom. C.K., Auerbach, P. S., Rodway, G. W., Cochran, A., ... Hackett, P. H. (2014). Wilderness Medical Society practice guidelines for the prevention and treatment of frostbite: 2014 update. *Wilderness & Environmental Medicine*, 25(4 Suppl), S43–54.

Mills, W. J Jr. (1993). Summary of treatment of the cold injured patient. 1980. *Alaska Medicine*, 35, 50–53.

Mohr, W. J., Jenabzadeh, K., & Ahrenholz, D. H. (2009). Cold injury. *Hand Clinics*, 25, 481–496.

Pasquier, M., Ruffinen, G. Z., Brugger, H., & Paal, P. (2012). Pre-hospital wrist block for digital frostbite injuries. *High Altitude Medicine & Biology*, 13, 65–66.

Richalet, J. P., & Canouï-Poitrine, F. (2014). Pro: hypoxic cardiopulmonary exercise testing identifies subjects at risk for severe high altitude illnesses. *High Altitude Medicine & Biology*, 15, 315–317.

Richalet, J. P., Canouï-Poitrine, F., & Larmignat, P. (2013). Acute high altitude illnesses (letter). *New England Journal of Medicine*, 369, 1664–1665.

Richalet, J. P., & Herry, J. P. (2006). *Médecine d'altitude et des sports de montagnes*. Paris, France: Masson.

Richalet, J. P., Larmignat, P., Poitrine, E., Letournel, M., & Canouï-Poitrine, F. (2012). Physiological risk factors of severe high altitude illness: a prospective cohort study. *American Journal of Respiratory and Critical Care Medicine*, 185, 192–198.

Virués-Ortega, J., Buela-Casal, G., Garrido, E., & Alcàzar, B. (2004). Neuropsychological functioning associated with high-altitude exposure. *Neuropsychology Review*, 14, 197–224.

Yan, X. (2014). Cognitive impairments at high altitudes and adaptation. *High Altitude Medicine & Biology*, 15, 141–145.

Zafren, K. (2013). Frostbite: prevention and initial management. *High Altitude Medicine & Biology*, 14, 9–12.

Zafren, K., Giesbrecht, G. G., Danzl, D. F., Brugger, H., Sagalyn, E. B., Walpoth, B., ... McDevitt, M. (2014). Wilderness Medical Society practice guidelines for the out-of-hospital evaluation and treatment of accidental hypothermia: 2014 update. *Wilderness & Environmental Medicine*, 25(4), S66–S85.

6 Hypoxic training

Grégoire Millet and Olivier Girard

Historically, altitude training emerged in the 1960s and was limited to the 'Live High Train High' method for endurance athletes looking to increase their haemoglobin mass and oxygen transport capacity. This 'classical' method was complemented in 1990s by the 'Live High Train Low' method where athletes benefit from the long hypoxic exposure and from the higher intensity of training at low altitude. Innovative methods were recently proposed, 'resistance training in hypoxia' and 'repeated sprint training in hypoxia' presumably with peripheral adaptations postponing muscle fatigue. Another point of interest is the potential physiological differences between 'real altitude' (hypobaric hypoxia) and 'simulated altitude' (normobaric hypoxia) and the clinical significance of this difference. The panorama of the hypoxic methods is now wider than in the past. Mountaineers are recommended to use the 'traditional' methods while climbers would benefit using the 'innovative' methods.

Hypoxia

Introduction and definition

For 60 years, 'altitude training' has been associated with endurance sports. As an illustration, a MEDLINE database search found ~1 000 entries using the search words 'ALTITUDE or HYPOXIA and ENDURANCE'. However, only 50 entries came up when, for instance, 'ALTITUDE or HYPOXIA and TEAM SPORTS' was used instead.

While mountaineering is highly aerobic by nature it also requires producing some high-intensity short actions. Conversely, climbing is a short-duration sport activity requiring exceptional neuromuscular qualities (strength and flexibility).

Hypoxia is defined as any combination of reduced barometric pressure (BP), and/or a reduced inspired fraction of oxygen (F_IO_2), which ultimately results in an inspired partial pressure of oxygen (P_IO_2) less than 150 mmHg (Conkin & Wessel, 2008). Acute patho-physiological responses to hypoxia or adaptations to hypoxic training can be investigated using two different types of exposure: hypobaric hypoxia (HH; $F_IO_2 = 20.9\%$; BP < 760 mmHg) or normobaric hypoxia (NH; $F_IO_2 < 20\%$; BP = 760 mmHg) (Conkin & Wessel, 2008).

The aim of this chapter is not to detail the pathophysiological responses to high altitude (see Chapter 5) but rather to highlight the latest hypoxic/altitude training methods to improve fitness in both mountaineers and climbers. After a brief overview of the history of altitude training, we will detail the 'classical' methods' primarily implemented to improve O_2 transport capacity and introduce the 'recent' methods developed partly in our laboratory in Lausanne and now used beyond the spectrum of endurance sports. One major point of interest is the potential physiological differences between 'real altitude' (HH) and 'simulated altitude' (NH) and the clinical significance of such differences. For each altitude intervention, we will highlight the main adaptive mechanisms, the potential beneficial and deleterious effects, and the applicability of research findings to best prepare athletes. From a practical perspective, we will also discuss how mountaineers and climbers can optimize their preparation by means of pre-acclimatizing to high altitude, improving their aerobic fitness and/or increasing their muscular power. Finally, promising innovative perspectives regarding the integration of the various types of hypoxic interventions will be proposed.

Historical perspectives

Pioneer investigations on human responses to high altitude were conducted more than a century ago (Barcroft, 1911). The well-described hypoxia-induced decrease in working capacity was reported as early as in the 1950s, while the potential for using chronic altitude exposure ('Live High Train High' method; LHTH) for performance enhancement in trained endurance athletes was described later, after the Mexico City Olympic games in 1968. Historically, the LHTH method is the first one used by athletes. Thus it is paradoxical that LHTH is now probably the less known method with several key questions still unanswered (Lundby, Millet, Calbet, Bartsch, & Subudhi, 2012).

Intermittent hypoxic exposure (IHE) has been studied for medical purposes since the 18th century, mainly in the Ukraine and Russia (Serebrovskaya, 2002). The first published evidence regarding the usefulness of intermittent hypoxic training (IHT) for increasing exercise capacity dates back to the early 1930s in military aviation staff. In particular, IHT and IHE have been widely studied for their therapeutic benefits in the ex-USSR, while scientists in Western countries were more concerned with their potential deleterious effects on health (e.g. sleep apneas, oxidative stress ...). The benefits of IHT for athletic performance improvement (e.g. 'Live Low Train High' method; LLTH) have been studied more recently (Roskamm et al., 1969) and the wider use of IHT to a large scale by the athletes was related to the emergence of various normobaric hypoxic devices (e.g. hypoxic chambers, hypoxic tents).

The 'Live High Train Low' (LHTL) method was introduced in the early 1990s (Levine & Stray-Gundersen, 1997). While first efforts used the terrestrial/natural way (e.g. living in HH and driving to the valley for training at lower altitude), the development of hypoxic facilities has prompt the implementation of LHTL camps using NH exposure (i.e. nitrogen houses, O_2-filtration chambers/tents or

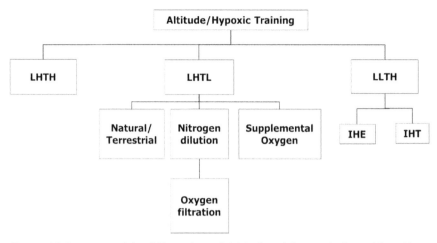

Figure 6.1 Panorama of the different hypoxic/altitude training methods used by athletes in the late 2000s

Source: Wilber, 2007.

breathing hypoxic mixtures with a mask) (Rusko, Tikkanen, & Peltonen, 2004). The main advantage of using NH is to reduce travel times and to make individual adjustments.

The panorama of the hypoxic methods existing towards the end of the 2000s is displayed in Figure 6.1 (Wilber, 2007).

In the 2000s, we suggested combining hypoxia and normoxia during interval-training sessions (IHIT, intermittent hypoxia interval training) (Roels et al., 2005). We (Millet, Faiss, & Pialoux, 2012) also challenged the 'equivalent air altitude model' (Conkin & Wessel, 2008) and the fact that the decrease in P_IO_2 is the only factor influencing the physiological responses to hypoxia. More recently, we introduced a new efficient method for improving the ability to repeated maximal intensity exercise bouts (repeated sprint training in hypoxia; RSH) (Faiss, Leger, et al., 2013). Resistance training in hypoxia (RTH) was also proposed with or without vascular occlusion (Friedmann et al., 2003) with the purpose of promoting hypertrophy and power production, yet with unclear benefits in the available literature. Finally, we proposed combining different methods for maximizing the benefits and reducing the main drawbacks of each one (Millet, Roels, Schmitt, Woorons, & Richalet, 2010). For example, by combining LHTL and RSH ('Live High Train Low and High'; LHTLH), where athletes live high and train low except for few intense workouts at altitude, additional benefits regarding both aerobic fitness and repeated-sprint ability have been reported in team sport players (Brocherie, Millet, et al., 2015). The usefulness of the combination of LHTH and high-intensity training near sea level ('Live High Train High and Low'; LHTHL) was also demonstrated in swimmers (Rodriguez et al., 2015).

All these recent improvements in hypoxic methods were validated with a new nomenclature differentiating LLTH interventions: IHE (intermittent hypoxic

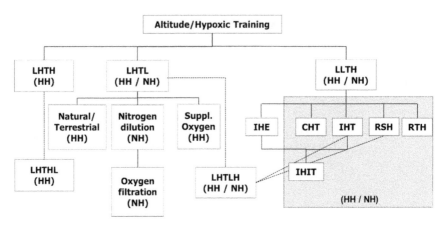

Figure 6.2 Panorama of the different hypoxic/altitude training methods used by athletes in 2015

exposure), CHT (continuous hypoxic training); interval training (IHT; interval training in hypoxia) and RSH (repeated sprint training in hypoxia) (Millet, Faiss, Brocherie, & Girard, 2013), while the addition of RTH is now seen in Figure 6.2.

Figure 6.2 summarizes the current (in 2015) panorama of all altitude/hypoxic training methods available and used by a wide range of endurance (cycling, distance running, triathlon …: LHTH, LHTL, LHTHL), intermittent sports' (football, rugby, tennis…: RSH, RTH, LHTLH) or power (middle-distance, judo) athletes. Beyond the specific use of hypoxia exposure to acclimatize to high altitude, both mountaineers and climbers will undoubtedly benefit from integrating some of these hypoxic methods within their training regimen.

Table 6.1 Historical perspectives on the implementation of altitude/hypoxic training methods

Interventions	Acronyms	Date	Targeted athletes	Publication years
Live High Train High	LHTH	1960s	Endurance trained	(Dill & Adams, 1971)
Intermittent hypoxic training	IHT	1960s	Endurance trained	(Roskamm et al., 1969)
Live High Train Low	LHTL	1997	Endurance trained	(Levine & Stray-Gundersen, 1997)
Resistance training in hypoxia	RTH	2000s	Power trained	(Friedmann et al., 2003)
Repeated sprint training in hypoxia	RSH	2013	Team/racquet sports	(Faiss, Leger, et al., 2013)
Live High Train Low and High	LHTLH	2015	Team/racquet sports	(Brocherie, Girard, Faiss, & Millet, 2015)
Live High Train High and Low	LHTHL	2015	Endurance trained	(Rodriguez et al., 2015)

Table 6.1 shows the date of introduction for each method. It makes clear that the 'classical' ones (LHTH, IHT and LHTL) have been very recently complemented by several other means. It widens the clinical uses of hypoxia in the sports area.

Differences between 'real altitude' (HH) and 'simulated altitude' (NH)

The 'equivalent air altitude model' (Conkin & Wessel, 2008) suggests that HH and NH can be used interchangeably. The alveolar pressure in O_2 (P_AO_2 in mmHg) is calculated as follows:

$$P_AO_2 = FiO_2 \times (BP - 47)$$

in mmHg, where FiO_2 is the inspired fraction of O_2 and BP is the barometric pressure. At sea level, in normoxia, the pressure in O_2 is ~150 mmHg with FiO_2 = 20.93 % in normoxia and BP = 760 mmHg.

One may decrease P_AO_2 either by reducing BP (by travelling to altitude or being in a hypobaric chamber; HH where F_IO_2 = 20.9 % and BP < 760 mmHg) or by reducing the fraction (e.g. concentration) of O_2 (NH where F_IO_2 < 20 % and BP = 760 mmHg) (Conkin & Wessel, 2008).

Practically, a first means of reaching an altitude of 3500 m requires travelling to mountains (for example, at Jungfraujoch, Switzerland) where F_IO_2 is 'normal' at 20.93 % but BP lowered ('real altitude') to 420–430 mmHg, inducing a PO_2 of 91–94 mmHg (instead of 150 mmHg at sea level). Otherwise, simulating the same altitude using hypoxic devices located at sea level would require a FiO_2 of ~13 %. If the chamber is located at altitude, where BP is decreased, then the reduction in FiO_2 is smaller. For example, for simulating an altitude of 3500 m, FiO_2 will be 15 % at the French Nordic Ski Center in Prémanon located at 1150 m and ~16 % at the Sports Center 'Le Signal' in the ski resort of Les Saisies at 1650 m.

Regarding the main effect of altitude training, that is the improvement in O_2 transport capacity, it seems that, for the same PiO_2, both the decrease in O_2 flux to the tissues and the erythropoietic responses leading to the increase in haemoglobin mass (Hbmass) are similar (Saugy et al., 2014).

However, various biological markers such as ventilation, fluid balance, acute mountain sickness (AMS), nitric oxide (NO) metabolism (Faiss, Pialoux, et al., 2013) and sport performance support the notion that *hypobaric hypoxia induces different physiological responses compared to normobaric hypoxia*, as reviewed in Millet et al. (2012). In particular with evidence of HH being a more severe environmental condition than one at sea level atmospheric pressure, different (larger) physiological adaptations are associated with natural compared to artificial altitude. It is beyond the scope if this chapter to detail each response. However, this is of importance for mountaineers for sleep quality and pre-acclimatization.

Sleep

Recently, Saugy et al. (2014) showed that breathing frequency was higher and arterial O_2 saturation lower at a real altitude of 2250 m compared to when this altitude was simulated in a normobaric hypoxic chamber (Figure 6.3).

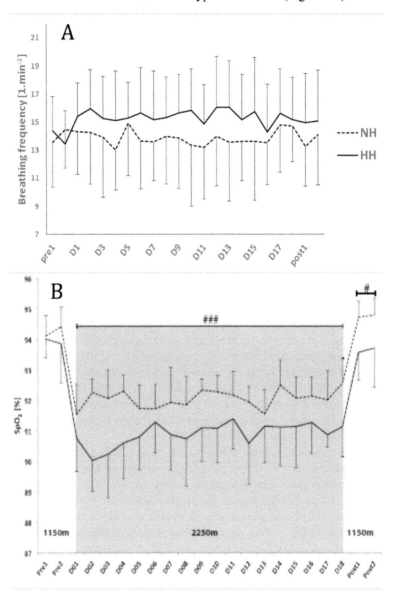

Figure 6.3 Nightly pattern of A) breathing frequency, and B) O2 saturation (SpO₂) in 'real altitude' (HH) versus 'simulated altitude' (NH) at 2250 m during 18 days of LHTL training. The grey area shows the nights in altitude

Source: Saugy et al., 2014.

In athletes, this difference in ventilatory pattern may influence their sleep quality and their recovery. In fact, despite the same ambient PO_2, a higher hypopnea index and increased heart rate (HR) values occurred in HH (Saugy et al., 2014).

Acute mountain sickness and pre-acclimatization

The second important difference between HH and NH is the prevalence and severity of AMS symptoms. 'Real altitude' induces a higher severity of symptoms than 'simulated hypoxia' (Roach, Loeppky, & Icenogle, 1996). Reasons are still unclear, and different hypotheses have been raised, for example indirect consequences of the gas density inducing the ventilatory pattern, back-diffusion in N_2, direct effects on central nervous system, haemodynamic NO-dependent regulation (Loeppky et al., 2005).

One of the key practical questions for mountaineers concerns the optimal strategy of pre-acclimatization prior to travel to high altitude. With acclimatization, AMS symptoms are ameliorated (or even eliminated), while physical performance is improved when compared to that at the time of arrival at altitude. Acclimatization – at least during the early stages – is mainly driven by ventilatory acclimatization. This is manifested in a progressive increase in the hypoxic ventilatory response, as evidenced by a decrease in end-tidal CO_2 ($PetCO_2$) and an increase in arterial O_2 saturation while at altitude (Fulco, Beidleman, & Muza, 2013).

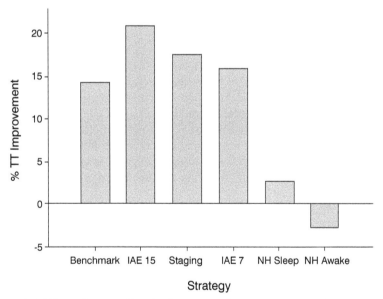

Strategy

Figure 6.4 Effect of pre-acclimatization on performance (expressed as percentage improvement compared to non-acclimatized subjects) at a real altitude of 4300 m (Fulco et al., 2013). Benchmark: time trial (TT) performance improved by 14 % while living continuously at 4300 m and the improvement was similar with different HH pre-acclimatization strategies. Conversely, NH pre-acclimatization did not induce any performance enhancement, when compared to non-acclimatized subjects

Although there is no direct comparison between HH and NH exposure relating to a pre-acclimatization period preceding a high-altitude ascent, the current literature supports that 'NH treatment provides little useful benefit during subsequent HH residence' (Figure 6.4).

These authors concluded that 'Overall, pre-acclimatization strategies using HH are much more effective than those using NH' and that 'NH and HH clearly cannot be used interchangeably and are not as effective as pre-acclimatization strategies to reduce AMS and improve exercise performance during subsequent HH residence' (Fulco et al., 2013; Fulco et al., 2011).

Current hypoxic methods

Live High Train High

The LHTH method aim is primarily to enhance O_2 transport capacity by increasing the number of red blood cells and the Hbmass. Two important questions are: 1) what is the appropriate altitude? and 2) what is the optimal duration of an altitude stay? The combination of altitude level and exposure duration allows the 'hypoxic dose' to be defined, which is useful when comparing the hypoxic stimulus between studies (Chapman et al., 2014; Wilber, Stray-Gundersen, & Levine, 2007).

Altitude level

The rate of erythropoietin (EPO) formation in response to acute hypoxic exposure seems proportional to the level of hypoxic stress (Eckardt et al., 1989). Owing to the flat shape of the oxyhaemoglobin dissociation curve above 60 mmHg (e.g. at lower altitude), changes in arterial pressure in O_2 (P_aO_2) may not have a large effect on arterial saturation in O_2 (S_aO_2). It is known that P_aO_2 values below 60 mmHg are reached from altitudes of about 2500 m (Anchisi, Moia, & Ferretti, 2001). Due to the combined effect of altitude- and exercise-induced desaturation, it is therefore proposed that the optimal altitude is slightly below this altitude (2200–2500 m). This was confirmed with athletes (Figure 6.5) (Chapman et al., 2014).

In 'endurance' sports, the choice of optimal altitude of residence for both LHTH and LHTL is now well-defined and ranges between 2200 and 2500 m (Chapman et al., 2014; Millet & Schmitt, 2011). Although a clear erythropoietic response has been observed below 2000 m in some studies (Garvican-Lewis, Halliday, Abbiss, Saunders, & Gore, 2015), it is generally believed that altitudes below 2000 m should not be used (Wilber, 2007). Higher altitudes (> 2800 m) are not recommended either as sleep perturbation and alteration in the autonomic nervous control are likely to blunt positive adaptations (Girard et al., 2013).

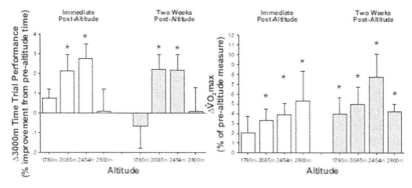

Figure 6.5 Change in 3 km running time trial performance (left panel) and in maximal oxygen consumption (ΔVO_{2max}) (right panel) immediately (post-) and two weeks after four-week LHTL altitude training camps held at 1780 m, 2085 m, 2454 m and 2800 m

Source: Chapman et al., 2014.

Exposure duration

The increase in Hbmass for altitudes between 2200 and 3000 m is strongly related to the total exposure duration. There is a general agreement that ~300 hours of exposure to hypoxia should be used in order to observe a mean Hbmass increase of 3–4 % (Saunders, Garvican-Lewis, Schmidt, & Gore, 2013). The increase in Hbmass has been estimated to range between 1.0 % and 1.1 % for every 100 h of exposure, independent of the type of altitude (i.e. LHTH (> 2100 m), or LHTL (~3000 m)) (Gore et al., 2013). However, in elite endurance athletes with already elevated initial Hbmass before embarking an altitude camp, the chances of observing a meaningful increase in Hbmass are smaller (Robach & Lundby, 2012). Hence, with larger Hbmass (16–18 g·kg⁻¹) and $\dot{V}O_{2max}$ (80–85 mL·min⁻¹·kg⁻¹) values (Heinicke et al., 2001) compared to athletes engaged in other sport disciplines such as the team-sport players (9–13 g·kg⁻¹ and 55–65 mL·min⁻¹·kg⁻¹) (Wachsmuth et al., 2013), room for Hbmass improvement is narrower in endurance athletes.

To conclude (Bergeron et al., 2012), LHTH may increase sea level performance in some, but not all, individuals (Girard et al. 2013). Athletes should live at an altitude between 2200 and 2500 m. The duration of exposure should not be less than two weeks, ideally four weeks.

Live High Train Low

The main idea behind the use of LHTL is to benefit from the altitude-induced augmentation of red blood cell mass (and thus O_2 carrying capacity), while avoiding the problems associated with reduced VO_{2max} and training intensity at altitude by training near sea level. This reduction in VO_{2max} in altitude is well described (Wehrlin & Hallen, 2006) and has been estimated between 7 and 9 % for every additional 1000 m of altitude ascent above sea level (Robergs,

Quintana, Parker, & Frankel, 1998; Wehrlin & Hallen, 2006). This decline in VO_{2max} has been observed at altitudes as low as 580 m (Gore et al., 1997) and is highly variable between athletes. Compared to their less aerobic-fit counterparts, endurance athletes with a higher aerobic profile will suffer a larger decline in VO_{2max} at altitude (Woorons, Mollard, Lamberto, Letournel, & Richalet, 2005). This is mainly because of the larger decrease in arterial O_2 saturation (Robergs et al., 1998) in high calibre endurance-trained athletes.

To date, over 70 scientific publications (for review, see Millet et al., 2010; Richalet & Gore, 2008) have confirmed the efficiency of LHTL for sea-level performance improvement. However, the nature of the main underlying mechanisms – the 'central theory' (e.g. increased Hbmass and improved O_2 transport capacity) (Levine & Stray-Gundersen, 2005) versus the 'peripheral theory' (e.g. improved muscular efficiency with angiogenesis or better buffering capacity) (Gore & Hopkins, 2005) – is still debated. Recent investigations strongly challenge the central theory as performance changes were not related to changes in VO_{2max} or Hbmass in elite swimmers (Rodriguez et al., 2015).

The main recommendations for LHTL are the use of an optimal altitude for residence between 2200 and 2500 m to provide an optimal erythropoietic effect and up to 3100 m for non-haematological (e.g. pH regulation and muscle buffer capacity; economy) parameters (Millet et al., 2010). While positive adaptations can already be visible after two weeks (200 h) of exposure, the optimal duration of an LHTL altitude intervention appears to be four weeks (400 h) for inducing accelerated erythropoiesis and ~18 days (300 h) for peripheral adaptations. A key parameter is the daily exposure duration with a minimum of 12 h/day, but ideally 14–18 h/day.

Intermittent hypoxic exposure

Intermittent hypoxic exposure (IHE) has been proposed with prolonged exposures (60–90 min) or by switching between breathing (9–12 % O_2) hypoxic and normoxic air during short (5–10 min) periods. It seems quite clear (Lundby et al., 2012; Tadibi, Dehnert, Menold, & Bartsch, 2007) that IHE induces minimal benefits on performance at sea level. It is also doubtful that IHE is an efficient pre-acclimatization strategy.

Intermittent hypoxic training

Interval training in hypoxia (performed below or near peak power output) has been investigated in-depth. For a long time, it was thought that adding the stress of hypoxia during 'aerobic' interval training would potentiate greater performance improvements compared to similar training at sea level (Millet et al., 2010). IHT presents the advantages of minimal travel, relatively low expense and causing limited disruption to the athletes' normal training environment and lifestyle. Another advantage is also to avoid the deleterious effect –decreased muscle excitability– of an extended stay in altitude. However, to date, there is a consensus that the effects of training cannot be distinguished from those of hypoxia. As such, it seems that after decades of research 'IHT does not increase exercise performance at sea level in endurance athletes any more than simply training at sea level' (Faiss, Girard, & Millet, 2013; Lundby et al., 2012).

Therefore we are not recommending IHT as an important component of the preparation of mountaineers. In order to increase VO_{2max} more efficiently, we would instead recommend performing high-intensity interval training (HIIT) at sea level in combination with RSH.

Repeated sprint training in hypoxia

RSH is a new hypoxic method (Faiss, Leger, et al., 2013; Faiss et al., 2014; Millet et al., 2013) developed in Lausanne. It was in fact initiated from the work conducted by Professor Hoppeler in the 2000s (Vogt et al., 2001) showing that up-regulation of several genes' mRNA was observed only when exercise was at high intensity and high altitude (and not with lower intensity hypoxic exercise) (Vogt et al., 2001).

Following RSH, fatigue development during repeated sprints with incomplete recoveries until exhaustion is postponed (Faiss, Leger, et al., 2013). RSH is currently considered an innovative training strategy in intermittent sports (team and racket sports). RSH efficiency likely relates to the compensatory vasodilatory effects on fast twitch (FT) fibres' behaviour leading to an improved O_2 extraction by these fibres. Greater amplitudes of muscle blood perfusion variations post-RSH suggesting enhanced muscle blood flow supported the above hypothesis of a greater O_2 utilization by FT after this particular intervention (Faiss et al. 2013). Physical activities involving extensive recruitment of FT would benefit more from using RSH routines. Because upper-arm muscles contain a high proportion of FT (Klein, Marsh, Petrella, & Rice, 2003), it is anticipated that RSH would be a promising strategy for climbers, but its efficiency still needs to be endorsed in this population.

Resistance training in hypoxia

Resistance exercise in hypoxia was originally investigated using blood flow restriction by vascular occlusion through the use of a cuff applied proximally to a limb in order to partially limit the arterial inflow (Takarada et al., 2000). More recently, resistance training in systemic hypoxia (e.g. breathing a hypoxic air mixture) has been investigated with contrasting outcomes (Scott, Slattery, Sculley, & Dascombe, 2014). In a pioneering study (Friedmann et al., 2003), it was shown that low-intensity resistance training (6 x 25 reps at 30 % of one repetition maximum, three times a week for four weeks) induced similar strength gains when training was conducted in hypoxia or in normoxia. Contrastingly, others (Manimmanakorn, Hamlin, Ross, Taylor, & Manimmanakorn, 2013) have reported a larger increase in maximal strength and hypertrophic responses in the hypoxic training group. To date, it seems that moderate to severe hypoxia (FiO_2 between 12 and 16 %) and a high metabolic stress (e.g. short recovery periods: 30 s and 60 s for 20–30% and 60–70% of 1 repetition maximal) are needed for inducing any superior physiological adaptations – and eventually physical performance – with RTH compared to similar resistance training in normoxia (Scott et al., 2014).

Combination of hypoxic methods

A promising way of optimizing hypoxic training is to combine methods (LHTH and LHTL), potentially inducing 'central' adaptations (e.g. increase in Hbmass and VO_{2max}) and those (RSH and RTH) producing mainly 'peripheral' adaptations (muscle efficiency). Brocherie, Millet, et al. (2015) demonstrated that combining LHTL and RSH in elite team-sport players induced both a significant enhancement in Hbmass but also larger improvement in sports-specific physical performance (aerobic fitness, repeated-sprint ability). Rodriguez et al. (2015) have shown that LHTH combined with high-intensity training at sea level is an efficient method in swimmers.

Practical applications

A broad range of hypoxic methods, targeting different mechanisms (Table 6.2), could be used by mountaineers and climbers to improve several aspects of their performance. Recommendations on how to optimize the benefits of these various altitudes' methods are offered in Table 6.3. Mountaineers are recommended to use mainly LHTH and LHTL methods in 'real altitude' and eventually to combine with RTH. Climbers will benefit from delayed muscle fatigue from RSH and RTH.

Summary

- Altitude/hypoxic training embraces a large range of different methods.
- 'Traditional' methods ('Live High Train High' and 'Live High Train Low') with prolonged hypoxic exposure aim principally to increase oxygen transport capacity.
- Recent innovative methods ('repeated sprint training in hypoxia' and 'resistance training in hypoxia) induce peripheral muscle adaptations, postponing fatigue.
- There are physiological differences between 'real altitude' (hypobaric hypoxia) and 'simulated altitude' (normobaric hypoxia), with higher effectiveness in HH for pre-acclimatization to altitude.
- Mountaineers are recommended to use the 'traditional' methods while climbers would likely benefit using the 'innovative' methods.

Table 6.2 Main hypoxic methods and associated mechanisms

Methods	Physiological mechanisms						Preparation for		
	O2 transport Hbmass	Hypertrophy/ increased strength	Capillarization	Oxidative capacity	Buffering capacity	Decrease fatigability	Competition at altitude	Competition at sea level	Training
LHTH	+++	−	+	++	+	+	+++	+	+
LHTL	+++	−	++	++	++	++	++	+++	+++
IHT	+	−	+	+	++	+	+	+	+
RSH	−	+	++	++	+++	+++	+	+++	+++
RTH	−	++	−	−	+	++	−	−	++
LHTLH	+++	+	++	++	+++	+++	+++	+++	++

+++: major effect; ++: important effect; +: moderate effect; −: negligible effect

Table 6.3 Practical recommendations for the different hypoxic methods

Methods	Recommendations					
	Minimal altitude	*Optimal altitude*	*Minimum duration*	*Ideal duration*	*Training intensity*	*Sports*
LHTH	1800 m	2200–2500 m	12 days	4 weeks	Aerobic + sprints	Endurance
LHTL	2200 m	2200–3000 m	12 days (10 h/d)	4 weeks (> 16h/d)	Aerobic first then more intense	All
IHT	2000 m	2500–3500 m	6 sessions	3–4 weeks	Second threshold	Lactic (?)
RSH	2500 m	3000–4000 m	4 sessions	Blocks of 8 sessions	Sprints	Intermittent (team/combat/racquet)
RTH	3000 m	4000–5000 m	6 sessions	Blocks of 8 sessions	?	Power and strength
LHTLH	2000 m	2800–3000 m	12 days	3 weeks	Aerobic + sprints	Intermittent (team/combat/racquet)

References

Anchisi, S., Moia, C., & Ferretti, G. (2001). Oxygen delivery and oxygen return in humans exercising in acute normobaric hypoxia. *Pflügers Archive*, 442(3), 443–450.

Barcroft, J. (1911). The effect of altitude on the dissociation curve of blood. *Journal of Physiology*, 42(1), 44–63.

Bergeron, M. F., Bahr, R., Bartsch, P., Bourdon, L., Calbet, J. A., Carlsen, K. H., ... Engebretsen, L. (2012). International Olympic Committee consensus statement on thermoregulatory and altitude challenges for high-level athletes. *British Journal of Sports Medicine*, 46(11), 770–779.

Brocherie, F., Millet, G. P., Hauser, A., Steiner, T., Rysman, J., Wehrin, J. P., & Girard, O. (2015). 'Live High-Train Low and High' hypoxic training improves team-sport performance. *Medicine & Science in Sports & Exercise*, 47(10), 2140–2149.

Chapman, R. F., Karlsen, T., Resaland, G. K., Ge, R. L., Harber, M. P., Witkowski, S., ... Levine, B. D. (2014). Defining the 'dose' of altitude training: how high to live for optimal sea level performance enhancement. *Journal of Applied Physiology*, 116(6), 595–603.

Conkin, J., & Wessel, J. H., 3rd. (2008). Critique of the equivalent air altitude model. *Aviation, Space, and Environmental Medicine*, 79(10), 975–982.

Eckardt, K. U., Boutellier, U., Kurtz, A., Schopen, M., Koller, E. A., & Bauer, C. (1989). Rate of erythropoietin formation in humans in response to acute hypobaric hypoxia. *Journal of Applied Physiology*, 66(4), 1785–1788.

Faiss, R., Girard, O., & Millet, G. P. (2013). Advancing hypoxic training in team sports: from intermittent hypoxic training to repeated sprint training in hypoxia. *British Journal of Sports Medicine*, 47 Suppl 1, i45–i50.

Faiss, R., Leger, B., Vesin, J. M., Fournier, P. E., Eggel, Y., Deriaz, O., & Millet, G. P. (2013). Significant molecular and systemic adaptations after repeated sprint training in hypoxia. *PLoS One*, 8(2), e56522.

Faiss, R., Pialoux, V., Sartori, C., Faes, C., Deriaz, O., & Millet, G. P. (2013). Ventilation, oxidative stress, and nitric oxide in hypobaric versus normobaric hypoxia. *Medicine & Science in Sports & Exercise*, 45(2), 253–260.

Faiss, R., Willis, S., Born, D. P., Sperlich, B., Vesin, J. M., Holmberg, H. C., & Millet, G. P. (2014). Repeated double-poling sprint training in hypoxia by competitive cross-country skiers. *Medicine & Science in Sports & Exercise*, 47(4), 809–817.

Friedmann, B., Kinscherf, R., Borisch, S., Richter, G., Bartsch, P., & Billeter, R. (2003). Effects of low-resistance/high-repetition strength training in hypoxia on muscle structure and gene expression. *Pflügers Archive*, 446(6), 742–751.

Fulco, C. S., Beidleman, B. A., & Muza, S. R. (2013). Effectiveness of preacclimatization strategies for high-altitude exposure. *Exercise and Sport Sciences Reviews*, 41(1), 55–63.

Fulco, C. S., Muza, S. R., Beidleman, B. A., Demes, R., Staab, J. E., Jones, J. E., & Cymerman, A. (2011). Effect of repeated normobaric hypoxia exposures during sleep on acute mountain sickness, exercise performance, and sleep during exposure to terrestrial altitude. *American Journal of Physiology – Regulatory, Integrative and Comparative Physiology*, 300(2), R428–436.

Garvican-Lewis, L. A., Halliday, I., Abbiss, C. R., Saunders, P. U., & Gore, C. J. (2015). Altitude exposure at 1800 m increases haemoglobin mass in distance runners. *Journal of Sports Science and Medicine*, 14(2), 413–417.

Girard, O., Amann, M., Aughey, R., Billaut, F., Bishop, D. J., Bourdon, P., ... Schumacher, Y. O. (2013). Position statement—altitude training for improving team-sport players' performance: current knowledge and unresolved issues. *British Journal of Sports Medicine*, 47 Suppl 1, i8–i16.

Gore, C. J., & Hopkins, W. G. (2005). Counterpoint: positive effects of intermittent hypoxia (live high:train low) on exercise performance are not mediated primarily by augmented red cell volume. *Journal of Applied Physiology*, 99(5), 2055–2057; discussion 2057–2058.

Gore, C. J., Little, S. C., Hahn, A. G., Scroop, G. C., Norton, K. I., Bourdon, P. C., ... Emonson, D. L. (1997). Reduced performance of male and female athletes at 580 m altitude. *European Journal of Applied Physiology and Occupational Physiology*, 75(2), 136–143.

Gore, C. J., Sharpe, K., Garvican-Lewis, L. A., Saunders, P. U., Humberstone, C. E., Robertson, E. Y., ... Neya, M. (2013) Altitude training and haemoglobin mass from the optimised carbon monoxide rebreathing method determined by a meta-analysis. *British Journal of Sports Medicine*, 47(Suppl. 1), i31–i39.

Heinicke, K., Wolfarth, B., Winchenbach, P., Biermann, B., Schmid, A., Huber, G., ... Schmidt, W. (2001). Blood volume and hemoglobin mass in elite athletes of different disciplines. *International Journal of Sports Medicine*, 22(7), 504–512.

Klein, C. S., Marsh, G. D., Petrella, R. J., & Rice, C. L. (2003). Muscle fiber number in the biceps brachii muscle of young and old men. *Muscle Nerve*, 28(1), 62–68.

Levine, B. D., & Stray-Gundersen, J. (1997). 'Living high-training low': effect of moderate-altitude acclimatization with low-altitude training on performance. *Journal of Applied Physiology*, 83(1), 102–112.

Levine, B. D., & Stray-Gundersen, J. (2005). Point: positive effects of intermittent hypoxia (live high:train low) on exercise performance are mediated primarily by augmented red cell volume. *Journal of Applied Physiology*, 99(5), 2053–2055.

Loeppky, J. A., Roach, R. C., Maes, D., Hinghofer-Szalkay, H., Roessler, A., Gates, L., ... Icenogle, M. V. (2005). Role of hypobaria in fluid balance response to hypoxia. *High Altitude Medicine & Biology*, 6(1), 60–71.

Lundby, C., Millet, G. P., Calbet, J. A., Bartsch, P., & Subudhi, A. W. (2012). Does 'altitude training' increase exercise performance in elite athletes? *British Journal of Sports Medicine*, 46(11), 792–795.

Manimmanakorn, A., Hamlin, M. J., Ross, J. J., Taylor, R., & Manimmanakorn, N. (2013). Effects of low-load resistance training combined with blood flow restriction or hypoxia on muscle function and performance in netball athletes. *Journal of Science and Medicine in Sport*, 16(4), 337–342.

Millet, G., & Schmitt, L. (2011). *S'entraîner en altitude: mécanismes, méthodes, exemples, conseils pratiques*. Paris: De Boeck Supérieur.

Millet, G. P., Faiss, R., Brocherie, F., & Girard, O. (2013). Hypoxic training and team sports: a challenge to traditional methods? *British Journal of Sports Medicine*, 47 Suppl 1, i6–i7.

Millet, G. P., Faiss, R., & Pialoux, V. (2012). Point: hypobaric hypoxia induces different physiological responses from normobaric hypoxia. *Journal of Applied Physiology*, 112(10), 1783–1784.

Millet, G. P., Roels, B., Schmitt, L., Woorons, X., & Richalet, J. P. (2010). Combining hypoxic methods for peak performance. *Sports Medicine*, 40(1), 1–25.

Richalet, J. P., & Gore, C. J. (2008). Live and/or sleep high:train low, using normobaric hypoxia. *Scandinavian Journal of Medicine & Science in Sports*, 18 Suppl 1, 29–37.

Roach, R. C., Loeppky, J. A., & Icenogle, M. V. (1996). Acute mountain sickness: increased severity during simulated altitude compared with normobaric hypoxia. *Journal of Applied Physiology*, 81(5), 1908–1910.

Robach, P., & Lundby, C. (2012). Is live high-train low altitude training relevant for elite athletes with already high total hemoglobin mass? *Scandinavian Journal of Medicine & Science in Sports*, 22(3), 303–305.

Robergs, R. A., Quintana, R., Parker, D. L., & Frankel, C. C. (1998). Multiple variables explain the variability in the decrement in VO_{2max} during acute hypobaric hypoxia. *Medicine & Science in Sports & Exercise*, 30(6), 869–879.

Rodriguez, F. A., Iglesias, X., Feriche, B., Calderon-Soto, C., Chaverri, D., Wachsmuth, N. B., ... Levine, B. D. (2015). Altitude training in elite swimmers for sea level performance (Altitude Project). *Medicine & Science in Sports & Exercise*, 47(9), 1965–1978.

Roels, B., Millet, G. P., Marcoux, C. J., Coste, O., Bentley, D. J., & Candau, R. B. (2005). Effects of hypoxic interval training on cycling performance. *Medicine and Science in Sports and Exercise*, 37(1), 138–146.

Roskamm, H., Landry, F., Samek, L., Schlager, M., Weidemann, H., & Reindell, H. (1969). Effects of a standardized ergometer training program at three different altitudes. *Journal of Applied Physiology*, 27(6), 840–847.

Rusko, H. K., Tikkanen, H. O., & Peltonen, J. E. (2004). Altitude and endurance training. *Journal of Sports Sciences*, 22(10), 928–944.

Saugy, J. J., Schmitt, L., Cejuela, R., Faiss, R., Hauser, A., Wehrlin, J. P., ... Millet, G. P. (2014). Comparison of 'live high-train low' in normobaric versus hypobaric hypoxia. *PLoS One*, 9(12), e114418.

Saunders, P. U., Garvican-Lewis, L. A., Schmidt, W. F., & Gore, C. J. (2013). Relationship between changes in haemoglobin mass and maximal oxygen uptake after hypoxic exposure. *British Journal of Sports Medicine*, 47 Suppl 1, i26–30.

Scott, B. R., Slattery, K. M., Sculley, D. V., & Dascombe, B. J. (2014). Hypoxia and resistance exercise: a comparison of localized and systemic methods. *Sports Medicine*, 44(8), 1037–1054.

Serebrovskaya, T. V. (2002). Intermittent hypoxia research in the former Soviet Union and the Commonwealth of Independent States: history and review of the concept and selected applications. *High Altitude Medicine & Biology*, 3(2), 205–221.

Tadibi, V., Dehnert, C., Menold, E., & Bartsch, P. (2007). Unchanged anaerobic and aerobic performance after short-term intermittent hypoxia. *Medicine & Science in Sports & Exercise*, 39(5), 858–864.

Takarada, Y., Takazawa, H., Sato, Y., Takebayashi, S., Tanaka, Y., & Ishii, N. (2000). Effects of resistance exercise combined with moderate vascular occlusion on muscular function in humans. *Journal of Applied Physiology*, 88(6), 2097–2106.

Vogt, M., Puntschart, A., Geiser, J., Zuleger, C., Billeter, R., & Hoppeler, H. (2001). Molecular adaptations in human skeletal muscle to endurance training under simulated hypoxic conditions. *Journal of Applied Physiology*, 91(1), 173–182.

Wachsmuth, N., Kley, M., Spielvogel, H., Aughey, R. J., Gore, C. J., Bourdon, P. C., … Garvican-Lewis, L. A. (2013). Changes in blood gas transport of altitude native soccer players near sea-level and sea-level native soccer players at altitude (ISA3600). *British Journal of Sports Medicine*, 47 Suppl 1, i93–99.

Wehrlin, J. P., & Hallen, J. (2006). Linear decrease in .VO_{2max} and performance with increasing altitude in endurance athletes. *European Journal of Applied Physiology and Occupational Physiology*, 96(4), 404–412.

Wilber, R. L. (2007). Application of altitude/hypoxic training by elite athletes. *Medicine & Science in Sports & Exercise*, 39(9), 1610–1624.

Wilber, R. L., Stray-Gundersen, J., & Levine, B. D. (2007). Effect of hypoxic 'dose' on physiological responses and sea-level performance. *Medicine & Science in Sports & Exercise*, 39(9), 1590–1599.

Woorons, X., Mollard, P., Lamberto, C., Letournel, M., & Richalet, J. P. (2005). Effect of acute hypoxia on maximal exercise in trained and sedentary women. *Medicine & Science in Sports & Exercise*, 37(1), 147–154.

Part III
Biomechanics

7 Postural regulation and motion simulation in rock climbing

Franck Quaine, Lionel Reveret,
Simon Courtemanche and Paul G. Kry

The objective of this chapter is to understand the biomechanics of rock climbing based on the forces applied at each support. The mechanical principles of rock climbing biomechanics are presented first and adapted with different climbing devices used to measure the contact forces. A computational method is presented to overcome the need for a climbing device equipped with three dimensional (3D) force sensors. A simulation method of 3D climbing movements is developed. The first part of this chapter describes the role of limbs in postural regulation during climbing. Notably, supporting forces depend on the posture of the climber, the number of supports and the climbing wall inclination. We discuss the transition between static postures and movement with dynamic motion of the limbs. The second part of the chapter focuses on the kinematics of rock climbing and introduces a modelling technique for estimating the support forces thanks to motion capture analysis.

Introduction

Rock climbing is a physical activity performed against gravity, in which the forces applied on the holds allow the climber to maintain balance and safely progress on the rock climbing support (e.g. cliff or artificial wall). The hands and feet provide points of contact with which the climber can interact with the environment, through application of accurate forces. The climber's objective is to move limbs to catch next holds with the hands or feet, while maintaining balance. In essence, a rock climbing motion is successful if the climber manages the supporting forces in order to grasp the target hold without falling. Postural stability is thus an important determinant of success. Postural stability is dependent on various parameters, including the climber's skills and mechanical constraints related to the support surface (e.g. support configuration, hold size and shape).

Gray (1944) was the first to propose a biomechanical model of a body balance during a quadrupedal posture on a vertical supporting frame. He demonstrated that maintenance of balance is achieved through normal (i.e. vertical) and tangential (i.e. horizontal) forces at the supports because the vertical projection of the centre of mass lies outside the contact area of the supports.

This situation is often encountered in rock climbing, specifically when the surface of the holds is reduced. Hence, the supporting forces are not solely the normal opposite reaction forces to the body weight, but include the tangential forces, which depend on the body position. Moreover, McIntyre and Bates (1982) analysed ladder ascent and demonstrated that the function of the arms was to control proximity of the body to the ladder, while the legs counteract the weight of the worker. According to this, it is possible to adapt the forces applied at the arms by adopting the position that gives the vertical projection of the centre of mass closer to the contact area of the supports.

A number of experimental studies aimed to characterize the mechanical determinants of the postural stability during rock climbing through analysis of supporting force variations. When one of the limbs was to be moved from a stable quadrupedal posture, the climber had to share the supporting forces on the three remaining supports to avoid loss of balance. Tests were performed in a laboratory environment for different climbing situations (e.g. tilt, hand or foot movement, initial posture, type of holds, etc.) mimicking real rock climbing. For this purpose, artificial climbing walls equipped with instrumented climbing holds were used.

In this chapter, we introduce the mechanical principles of equilibrium in rock climbing, the climbing devices used to measure forces at the holds, and display results concerning the analysis of posture-kinetic coordination and prediction of optimal timing through internal torque optimization in rock climbing.

Mechanical principles of equilibrium in rock climbing

During bipedal standing, postural balance requires the vertical projection of the centre of mass to lie in the base of support. On a vertical wall, the climber's centre of mass is often located outside the narrow base of support, which corresponds to the holds' contact surface (Quaine, Martin and Blanchi, 1997). This specific situation requires the climber to apply accurate supporting forces at the holds in order to counteract the body weight moment around the foot contacts.

The principles of Newtonian mechanics are useful to study the supporting forces. The external forces acting on the whole body are the weight of the climber and the reaction forces at the holds.

The climber's equilibrium is governed by two general equations for the translation and rotation, as follows:

$$\sum \overrightarrow{Fext} = m\overrightarrow{a_{CG}} \tag{1}$$

and

$$\sum \overrightarrow{\tau Fext_{/LF}} = I_{/LF}\overrightarrow{\alpha_{CG/LF}} \tag{2}$$

stating that in a laboratory reference system $(LF, \vec{i}, \vec{j}, \vec{k})$ with the origin at the left foot (LF) the sum of the external forces given by Eq.1 equals the product of the mass (m) of the climber by the linear acceleration of its centre of mass (a_{CG}), and the sum of the moment reactions in Eq.2 about the left foot hold equals the product of the inertial moment of the body ($I_{/LF}$) by the angular acceleration of the centre of mass ($\overrightarrow{\alpha_{CG/LF}}$) respective to the left foot hold (*LF*). In this expression, it was assumed that no torque was exerted by the hands and the feet around the holds.

Including the forces and moments at each support from 1 to 4, Eq.1 and Eq.2 give:

$$(1) \Leftrightarrow \begin{cases} \sum_1^4 \overrightarrow{Fi} = m\overrightarrow{a_{iCG}} \\[2mm] \sum_1^4 \overrightarrow{Fj} = m\overrightarrow{a_{jCG}} \\[2mm] \sum_1^4 \overrightarrow{Fk} + \overrightarrow{W} = m\overrightarrow{a_{kCG}} \end{cases}$$

and

$$(2) \Leftrightarrow \begin{cases} \sum_1^4 \overrightarrow{\tau Fk_{/LF}} + \sum_1^4 \overrightarrow{\tau Fj_{/LF}} + \overrightarrow{\tau W_{/LF}} = \overrightarrow{\tau i_{/LF}} \\[2mm] \sum_1^4 \overrightarrow{\tau Fk_{/LF}} + \sum_1^4 \overrightarrow{\tau Fi_{/LF}} + \overrightarrow{\tau_{LF} W} = \overrightarrow{\tau j_{/LF}} \\[2mm] \sum_1^4 \overrightarrow{\tau Fi_{/LF}} = \overrightarrow{\tau k_{/LF}} \end{cases}$$

.

The vector $\overrightarrow{W}$ represents the weight of the climber.

When the climber stops his ascent at a resting point in order to analyse the rock above him to think about his next moves, or to recover from fatigue, the projection of Eq.1 and Eq.2 along each axis in static condition gives:

$$(1) \Leftrightarrow \begin{cases} Fi1 - Fi2 - Fi3 + Fi4 = 0 \\ -Fj1 + Fj2 - Fj3 + Fj4 = 0 \\ Fk1 + Fk2 + Fk3 + Fk4 - W = 0 \end{cases}$$

and

$$(2) \Leftrightarrow \begin{cases} \tau Fk1_{/LF} + \tau Fk2_{/LF} + \tau Fj3_{/LF} - \tau Fj2_{/LF} - \tau W_{/LF} = 0 \\ \tau W_{/LF} - \tau Fi2_{/LF} - \tau Fi3_{/LF} = 0 \\ \tau Fi2_{/LF} - M\tau i1_{/LF} = 0 \end{cases} \quad (3)$$

In this model, Quaine et al. (1997) call the normal forces (i.e. $\overrightarrow{Fk}$) 'antigravitational forces' since they directly opposed the body weight, whereas the tangential ones (i.e. $\overrightarrow{Fi}, \overrightarrow{Fj}$) were termed 'stabilizing forces' since they controlled the body position and opposed the destabilizing body weight moment expressed around the left foot hold contact.

Hence, the biomechanical model shows that climbers deal with two types of mechanical constraints: they must be able to share their body weight on the holds, while controlling the rotational movement. In order to reduce rotational moments, climbers can adopt climbing positions that position the body closest to the wall (e.g. 'frog' or 'drop-knee' position).

The climbing devices used to measure forces at the holds

Rock climbing device at Joseph Fourier University (Grenoble, France)

The pioneers in measuring and analysing climbing forces were Rougier, Billat, Merlin and Blanchi (1991). They proposed a device enabling the study of posturo-kinetic coordination for climbers thanks to an artificial climbing frame called a 'climbing ergometer'. Their results were interesting since they demonstrated that when moving a limb, the novice climbers displayed more diagonal force distribution than a contralateral transfer of forces characterized by the expert climbers. Unfortunately, these results were not sufficient to deeply understand postural stability since they only accounted for the normal forces at the holds and thus nothing was known about the tangential forces at the supports.

This original device was improved by replacing the initial one dimensional (1D) normal force transducer by 3D sensors (Quaine and Martin, 1999; Noe, Quaine and Martin, 2001). The climbing holds were fastened to each transducer, allowing independent measurement of the forces applied to each support in the three dimensions of space in the laboratory reference system (Figure 7.2). For all the experiments, the same holds were used for right and left sides. Holds were symmetrical (8 cm width and a 1 cm deep), enabling a wedging type of support for the feet and a crimp grip position of the fingers. The signals from the transducers were amplified (PM Instrumentation, ref 1965, Orgeval, France) and recorded on a personal computer. The sampling frequency was 100 Hz. Data were filtered with a second-order Butterworth filter (10 Hz low pass cut-off frequency).

Postural regulation in rock climbing

In this section, we present the main results concerning the effect of body position and tilt of the climbing support on the supporting forces. The aim is to explain the climber's adjustments to voluntary hold release by comparing the applied forces of a stable four-point-support posture to a three-point-support posture in different quasi-static conditions, to lead to an understanding of the mechanical events associated with supporting-force management in rock climbing. Results reported in this section were obtained thanks to the device at Joseph Fourier University.

Effect of body position (Quaine et al., 1997)

Two positions were tested: an imposed position with the trunk far from the supporting wall that is difficult to maintain, and an optimized position with the trunk close to the wall. The imposed position was related to the posture spontaneously adopted by beginners, whereas the optimized posture corresponded to skilled behaviour. The optimized position is named 'frog position' and is used to rest on a vertical slab. It allows the body's centre of gravity to be placed closer to the wall and thus reduces the body weight moment around the foot contacts. For each position, the climbing frame was adjusted to the anthropometry of the climbers. The width between the holds corresponded to that of the shoulders, and the distance between the lower and the upper holds was adjusted while a subject stood on the experimental device with the upper arms and thighs horizontal. The task involved releasing a specified hold and maintaining the three-point-support posture without any change in the initial position. Hence, the subjects were asked to reduce the amplitude of the movement in order to minimize the centre of mass shifts. The subject went from a four-support to a three-support stable position. Only the data from trials involving right foot displacements are reported here.

Typical force variations are reported in Figure 7.1 for the imposed position. During quiet four-point-support standing, and for both postures, support forces displayed similar results. Antero-posterior forces at the hands opposed those at the feet. Lateral forces at the hands were opposed, as were those for the feet. The climber pulled backwards with upper limbs and pushed forward with lower limbs. The tangential force values were 1.4 times lower in the optimized position than in the imposed position. Hence, the forces applied at the arms are drastically reduced when the posture is close to the wall, permitting less fatigue. This is concordant with the results given in Balas (2014), which showed that skilled climbers placed higher loading on foot holds, which was associated with lower physiological demands.

The important implication for coaches, trainers and climbers is that significant supporting force magnitude reduction may be achieved with adapted posture. Coaches should create specific exercises with beginners in order to teach the technical aspects of vertical wall climbing that reduce the tangential forces by adopting positions closest to the wall.

In the tripedal posture, normal and tangential forces have to be redistributed on the three remaining supports after the right foot has been released. In the imposed position, the normal force lost at the right foot was transferred to the contralateral limbs and did not change on the ipsilateral support. The tangential forces collapsed on the ipsilateral support and were transferred to the contralateral side. Conversely, a different pattern was observed in the optimized position since the normal and tangential forces did not reduce on the ipsilateral hold. It appears that the force transfers differ according to the difficulty of the position: the contralateral distribution of the reaction forces was observed for an imposed position, while a more homogeneous distribution occurred during an optimised position.

These results indicate that efficiency in balancing in rock climbing implies a more homogeneous force sharing on the remaining supports, especially for the

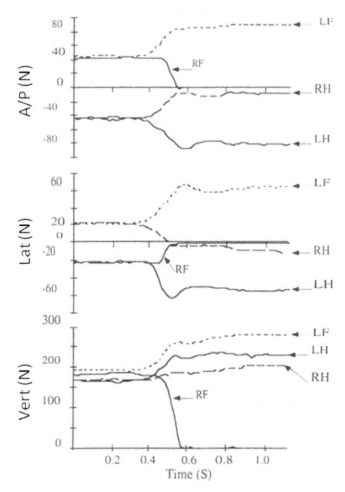

Figure 7.1 Typical force variations following a right-foot release in the imposed position. RH and LH correspond to right and left hand, RF and LF to the right and left foot

Source: Adapted from Quaine et al., 1997.

tangential forces. The results given by Testa, Martin and Debû (2003) reinforce this statement. They analysed children and adolescents posture-kinetic control during rock climbing. They observed that tangential forces were progressively involved in controlling equilibrium in children (8–10 years) and adolescents (10–15 years). They proposed that a progressive 3D control of force variations emerges in adolescents. Bourdin, Teasdale, Nougier, Bard and Fleury (1999) used the tangential forces to control the initial position. They studied the organization of reaching and grasping movements in rock climbing. They observed that climbers delayed adjustments in hand configuration until the target hold has been reached, whatever the initial position. They concluded that only the target hold acts as a mechanical stop for the climber without any requirement to reduce the hand velocity at the impact.

It can be proposed that on a vertical wall, the main action of the upper limbs is to stabilize and control the posture of the climber, while the lower limbs counterbalance the body weight. The tangential forces are necessary to counteract the backwards body weight moment. Releasing a hold induces a force transfer onto the remaining supports according to the difficulty of the posture. Postures close to the wall are characterized by a more homogeneous force sharing pattern on the three remaining supports.

Effect of the tilt of the climbing support (Noe et al., 2001 and Noe, 2006)

Using a similar methodology, the aim of these studies was to understand mechanisms of equilibrium in overhanging positions, which are frequently observed during rock climbing. For quadrupedal postures in cats (Macpherson, 1988) and humans (Gelat, Caron, Metzger and Rougier, 1992), it is well known that diagonal force transfer is characteristic of positions where the centre of mass projection is within the support surface area. By contrast, the contralateral transfer is related to positions with no supporting base (Quaine et al., 1997). In rock climbing, overhanging wall inclination is very interesting for biomechanical analysis since it engenders a significant base of support in which the centre of mass can be potentially projected.

The works of Noe et al. (2001) and Noe (2006) studied the effect of wall inclination on postural regulation in rock climbers. Two positions have been tested. The first one was the reference vertical position, with the climbing device set vertically. The second position was overhanging: the climbing device had been adjusted so that the wall was inclined 10° to the vertical. The climbers were asked to adopt the least constraining position with their forearms placed vertically. They all adopted the same position, with the trunk close to the plane of the holds. From a stable quadrupedal posture, the subjects were instructed to release a specified hold and to maintain the tripedal position for a few seconds.

Developing Eq.2 for the overhanging position gives supplementary moment components associated to the tilt of the support, as:

$$(2) \Leftrightarrow \begin{cases} \tau Fk1_{/LF} + \tau Fk2_{/LF} + \tau Fj3_{/LF} -)\tau Fj2_{/LF} - \tau W_{/LF} = 0 \\ \tau W_{/LF} - \tau Fi2_{/LF} - \tau Fi3_{/LF} - \tau Fk3_{/LF} - \tau Fk2_{/LF} = 0 \\ \tau Fi2_{/LF} - \tau Fi1_{/LF} + \tau Fj2_{/LF} - \tau Fj3_{/LF} = 0 \end{cases} \tag{4}$$

Comparing terms in Eq.3 and Eq.4 demonstrates that expression of the moment around the antero-posterior axis ($\overrightarrow{\tau i_{/LF}}$) did not change, whereas the moments around the lateral and vertical axes ($\overrightarrow{\tau j_{/LF}}$ and $\overrightarrow{\tau k_{/LF}}$) were created by two supplementary forces, the vertical and antero-posterior components at the hand holds, respectively. These terms are displayed on Figure 7.2.

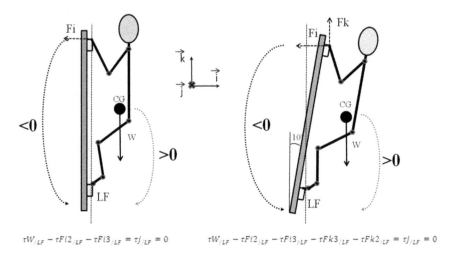

$$\tau W_{/LF} - \tau Fi2_{/LF} - \tau Fi3_{/LF} = \tau j_{/LF} = 0 \qquad \tau W_{/LF} - \tau Fi2_{/LF} - \tau Fi3_{/LF} - \tau Fk3_{/LF} - \tau Fk2_{/LF} = \tau j_{/LF} = 0$$

Vertical support   Overhanging support

Figure 7.2 Schematic representation of the moments at work in a vertical and an overhanging posture. Moment components about the left foot hold (LF) around the lateral axis in the reference system (. Clockwise moments were negative and counterclockwise moments were positive. On the vertical support, the positive moment of the body weight (W) applied to the centre of gravity (CG) is counterbalanced by the negative moment of the antero-posterior force applied at the hand. On the overhanging support (10° tilt), both the vertical and antero-posterior hand forces create a negative moment which counterbalances the positive moment induced by the body weight

In the overhanging position, the analysis of the tangential forces at the hands showed that the magnitude was less important than in the vertical position. This is related to the reduced backwards destabilizing body weight moment induced by the support base in the overhanging case. Normal forces analysis indicated that most of the body weight was supported by the foot holds in the vertical position, and by the hand holds in the overhanging position. Noe et al. (2001) concluded that the biomechanical action of the hands increased in overhanging positions. The hands were thus involved in counterbalancing the body weight with normal forces while stabilizing the body weight moment with tangential forces. This result explains the higher physiological activity reported by several authors for climbing in overhanging positions (Watts and Drobish, 1998; Balas 2014).

After the limb release, supporting forces have to be shared on the remaining holds. In the overhanging position, changes involved less extensive contralateral force transfers compared to those observed in the vertical position. This pattern enables the climbers to use extensively the hand holds in order to maintain balance. One explanation given by Noe et al. (2001) is that this pattern reinforces safety by using the arm supports more efficiently.

Eq.1 and Eq.2 demonstrate that the climber may be considered as a statically over-determined system with more unknown forces than equations. This makes the problem under-determined in the sense that more than one force combination on the holds will produce the whole body equilibrium. Eq.3 and Eq.4 show that a link between the hand forces and the body weight moment is noted, but the model does not show any obvious link between the tangential and normal forces applied on the holds. Currently, the parameters used by the climbers to share the supporting force between the feet and hand holds and between the tangential and normal components remain unknown. Further studies focusing on the 'drop-knee' or 'Egyptian' positions may be useful to better understand this sharing pattern. These positions are frequently used in climbing and according to the biomechanical principles presented here, we may assume that these positions reverse in part the mechanical action of the feet versus the hands. However, before conclusions can be drawn, tangential and normal force analysis must be conducted in these positions.

As a conclusion, monitoring supporting forces during rock climbing highlights the mechanical adaptations that rock climbers make in different situations. It increases knowledge concerning postural regulation in order to ensure performance and safety. This methodology is relevant and adapted to rock climbing analysis, and further studies could be conducted to understand the effect of the level of expertise, the type of rock climbing shoes or the type of holds.

However, despite the widespread use of this methodology, one of the major limitations is that it requires a climbing wall equipped with 3D force sensors at each hold. This reduces considerably the potential application of this approach to specific laboratory tasks, which may be considered as only approximately representative of actual rock climbing. One solution to go further is to use inverse dynamics coupled with optimization procedures to assess the forces at the holds without the use of a measuring device. This is presented in the second part of this chapter.

Estimation of contact forces from kinematics and its application in climbing

The estimation of multiple contact forces from kinematic data alone is a fundamentally ill-posed problem. For a person hanging on a bar with both hands, the observation of only the body pose alone does not reveal if the person is using strong forces and torques on the left arm only, or the right arm only, or, most likely, a balance between left and right arms. A common practice to solve for the ambiguity of contact forces is to minimize the internal torques and the external contact forces under the constraint of the classical dynamics equations. This approach has been used in robotics for the control of autonomous robots (Righetti, Buchli, Mistry, Kalakrishnan and Schaal, 2013), in computer graphics for the creation of 3D animation (Wei and Chai 2010), and in biomechanics for the evaluation of effort in sit-to-stand with one arm tasks (Robert, Causse and Monnier, 2013). We present here the application of this optimality criterion to climbing through two experiments. The first experiment quantitatively evaluates the estimation of contact forces from kinematics by comparison with data collected for nine climbers on a three metre high climbing wall instrumented with six gauges. The computational method for predicting contact forces allows one to drive a physical simulation of 3D climbing motion. A second experiment on a ten metre high indoor wall compares the result of such a simulation with real performance.

General principle

We first review the general principle of the method to highlight its critical parameters. For a detailed explanation of the equations, we refer the reader to Robert et al. (2013) for a general presentation and Courtemanche (2014) for the specific implementation used here. The posture of the body is parameterized with a set of n+6 degrees of freedom (DOF), with n=43 for the joints (we applied standard biomechanical constraints such as 1 DOF at knees and elbows) and 6 DOFs for the root body. Every DOF is actuated by muscle torques, except the 6 DOF of the root body, which are unactuated. The equations of motion are thus split between actuated DOFs and non-actuated DOFs. Conceptually, the root position and orientation are actuated through contact with the environment. Rotations are parameterized using exponential maps to avoid Euler angles issues (gimbal lock) or the normalization and double coverage issues of unitary quaternions. This leads to two sets of linear equations, one set relating the 6 DOFs of the body root with external contact forces, and another set relating the internal torques to the forces and torques applied on the root joint.

When more than one contact is established, these equations cannot be solved. There are more unknowns than equations, meaning there exists several valid combinations of internal torques and external contact forces. To obtain a unique solution, we therefore design two quadratic energy terms for torques and contact forces, which we minimize under the constraint of the equations of motion. This introduces two sets of weighting factors for torques and contact forces in the optimization. The choice of these weighing factors has a direct impact on the result of the optimization. Robert et al. (2013) proposed a list of values for weighting factors used to predict contact forces and internal torques for the similar problem of a sit-to-stand with one arm task. We discuss here the relevance of choices of parameters when applied to data for climbing through the evaluation on an instrumented wall.

Comparison of contact force predictions and measurements from an instrumented wall

The climbing wall structure on which the hold sensors are mounted (Figure 7.3) is a square of 2.5 metres wide, with a negative slope of four degrees. It consists of a torsion box forming a grid of six by six cells. Each cell can be filled with a hold and a 6D sensor (force and torque). A total of six sensors have been used for the capture sessions, along with 24 infra-red cameras. Calibration of the motion capture system and the sensors has been described in Aladdin and Kry (2012).

Nine climbers participated in the data capture process: two beginners, two intermediate climbers, and five expert climbers. The beginners were men climbing for the first or second time. The intermediate climbers were women climbing at a level between 5.10d and 5.11b. The expert climbers were men with best redpoint

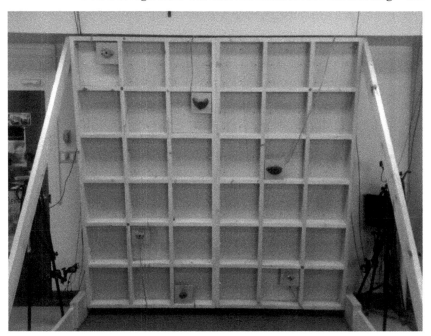

Figure 7.3 The instrumented bouldering wall used for the data capture. The holds are mounted on 6D force sensors. On each side of the wall one can see the tripods on which four of the 24 OtpiTrack cameras are mounted

ascent from 5.13a to 5.14a. A total of 172 recordings were captured. In order to perform the motion analysis presented below, a selection was done to refine these raw data. The selection process consisted of two main steps detailed in Courtemanche (2014). First, sequences in which joint velocities exceed 100 rad/s were removed, in order to discard obvious recording failures. Second, trajectories were cleaned with a Blackman filter to compute the linear acceleration of body segments. Sequences where the body acceleration changed sign twice in less than 150 ms are removed. This last step prevented the inclusion of shaking body segments, which occurs when markers are mislabelled. After data cleaning and avoiding trials with too much noise, a set of 15 trials was selected.

The motion capture data was used as input to compute the contact forces by optimization as presented in previous section. This estimation was compared to contact forces measured on the sensors. To simplify computation, we approximated contacts as point contacts only and thus considered that only forces, and no torques, were applied at the contact. The holds were considered as plain grips concentrated at a single point of contact. In the optimization process, to obtain the force contacts value from the kinematic data only, Robert et al. (2013) derived a set of weighing factors for the internal torques from the literature. We compared this set of parameters with two other sets: one set of uniform weights and one set derived from maximal values recorded by the force sensors. Figure 7.4 illustrates the results for the three sets of parameters.

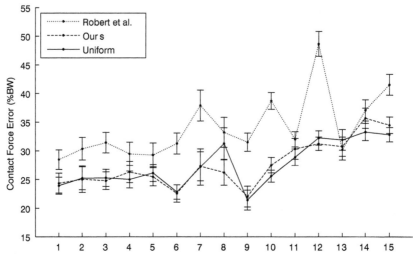

Figure 7.4 Results for average prediction of contact forces along each sequence of 15 performers as percentage of body mass with 95 per cent confidence interval. Each curve corresponds to a choice of weighing torque factors, from Roberts et al. (2013), from maximal torques measured during the recording, and from a uniform set of values. Results from Roberts et al. (2013) are the top curve. Our results using maximal torques as weights and uniform values are below. These two later results do not show significant difference

The average quality of the contact force prediction is between 20 and 30 per cent of the performer body weight (BW). Results suggest that the choice of weights is specific to the activity as a uniform set of parameters provides better results than the parameters used in Robert et al. (2013) for a different task. This suggested to us that we investigate more specific parameters for optimization. To this end, we used the value of real contact forces measured by the sensor to perform a standard inverse dynamics computation on the performers' data. This provided the values of internal joint torques out of which we retained the maximal magnitude as an indicator of weighing factor. Like in Robert et al. (2013), the rationale is that larger maximal torques must correspond to smaller weighing factors to let the minimization produce solutions with increased internal torque values. This choice of parameters allows us to significantly improve the prediction of contact forces for one performer only, and does not yet generalize to parameters specific to climbing.

We observed that the prediction of contact forces could be improved by setting the ankle weight to zero. This means that the value of the predicted joint torque at the ankle is not bounded in the optimization. In comparison to uniform weights, suppressing the ankle cost significantly reduced the error for 3 of the 15 sequences. Measured as a percentage of body weight, the error dropped from 25 per cent to 21 per cent, 25 per cent to 23 per cent, and 34 per cent to 28 per cent in these sequences as illustrated in Figure 7.5.

Inspecting the frame of maximal improvement for one of these sequences (sequence 15), the motion performed by the climber at this instant was to move his

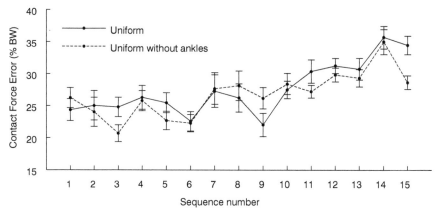

Figure 7.5 Contact force prediction with no constraint on ankle joint torques

centre of mass closer to the wall in order to load his right foot and to unload his left hand for reaching the final hold. At this instant, the dorsiflexion maximum angle is reached when the foot moves up, leading to the ability of the climber to generate as much passive plantarflexion torques as desired, and therefore bypassing totally the need to minimize it. Conversely, sequence 9 saw its prediction results made worse with ankle torque weights set to zero. At the beginning and at the middle of this sequence, which are the most torque intensive periods, the torques are almost equally distributed between the right ankle, the right knee, the right hip, the lumbar joint, and the right shoulder, showing that for energetic motions, the limiting weights play a more important role than for easy motions.

As a conclusion, this approach of computing contact forces from inverse dynamics cannot be considered a complete replacement of hardware force sensors because we observed an average accuracy of about 25 per cent of the body weight. In the next section, we present a way to make use of this technique to simulate 3D climbing motion on a bouldering wall. We compare this generated motion to the performance of a real subject.

Motion simulation in rock climbing

The input to the simulation consists of a set of holds located on a wall and a discrete sequence of postures of an anthropomorphic mannequin using these holds to perform a complete climbing route. Motion planning is thus constrained as the interpolation between these poses. Between poses, the spatial interpolation follows a straightforward linear scheme for hand and foot positions using a cubic spline interpolation for the root joint position and a spherical interpolation for the orientation of the joints. The parameter left free is the timing of these interpolations, that is, how fast transitions between poses occur.

We apply here the hypothesis of optimal torque described in the previous section to solve for this free timing parameter and generate simulated motion. Between poses, the transition duration is broken down into a set of three units whose individual time can vary. Along with the spatial interpolation between poses, duration values given to these segments create full body kinematic trajectories of the limbs, similar to virtual motion capture trials. Using the previously described method, contact forces and internal torques are automatically derived from the kinematic hypothesis. Among all the possible values of timing segments, an overall optimization thus selects the ones that correspond to the sum of least internal torques.

We perform two sets of experiments of this simulation technique. A first experiment on the instrumented wall allows quantitative comparison between the generated timing and the timing measured from motion capture. Figure 7.6 illustrates two results of this first experiment for one of the sequences.

The results in Figure 7.6 are given for different sets of initial values chosen for the optimization of timing segments. Different constant values have been tested. A constant value means an equal duration between identified poses was used. For completeness, initialization from the ground truth value has also been tested and reported. This sensitivity analysis illustrates the stability of the optimization.

A second experiment was performed on a full size indoor climbing wall. Ground truth timing was extracted from a temporal analysis of the video by an expert user identifying key moments in the performance, corresponding to stable static poses. The 3D locations of the holds were extracted from straightforward geometric calibration as the wall is strictly flat and vertical. The poses and the corresponding positions of the hands and feet have been manually identified from video. Given how the hands and feet are set on the holds, a standard inverse kinematics procedure generated a full body pose and thus the required sequence of input body poses of the virtual climber. To achieve as realistic as possible poses, the centre of mass is constrained to stay 10 cm away from the wall while joint orientations are minimized to match a given rest pose and the hands and feet locations on holds.

Figure 7.7 presents the timing optimization in this case. The previous experiment was limited to a very short sequence of poses. It can be noticed here that the optimization follows the overall pattern of the ground truth timing but at a much faster rate. One likely interpretation of this underestimation of timing is related to the fact that the optimization is only focused on minimal torques. As such, it does not account for the decision time made by the climber to choose grasps, whereas this decision time is zero for the virtual climber as it is only the sequence of poses which is provided as an input to the method. As a practical application of this technique, this method could be used as an initial evaluation of the complexity for a route with a given set of holds. After optimization, locations in the climbing sequence that have lower time intervals might indicate easy situations, while those with higher times might reflect more complex parts of the route.

Practical applications

This chapter described knowledge about rock climbing biomechanics. Both normal and tangential forces applied on the holds are relevant in order to characterize the postural control in rock climbing. On a vertical support, the upper limbs mainly act as whole body stabiliser, whereas the lower limbs counteract vertical collapsing. A link between the horizontal force values and the couple due to the body weight

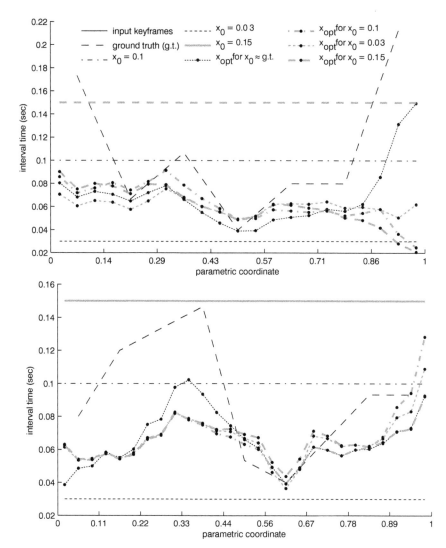

Figure 7.6 Sensibility analysis for timing prediction (two examples)

Horizontal axis is the spatial progression along the wall, normalized as a parametric coordinate.
Vertical axis indicates durations. Each curve is a timing hypothesis for an example progression.
Each point on a curve gives how much time is spent at this given position in the overall progression.
Plain vertical lines indicate key input poses along the progression. Between these poses, three steps
are considered, whose timing may differ, as well as time spent at key poses. Ground truth for timing
is given as a dashed line and is obtained from motion capture data. Flat horizontal dashed lines
correspond to sensitivity analysis of the overall optimization to the initial values chosen for timing
intervals. They are arbitrarily set initially equal at each progression step, hence the horizontality.
Solid curves indicate the result of the optimization for these chosen initial values.

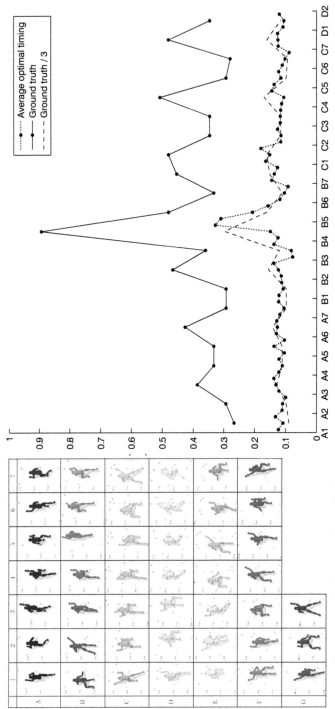

Figure 7.7 Timing optimization for a large climbing wall, and on the left, the given input poses

with respect to the feet was shown. Moving a limb involves the same pattern of normal and horizontal forces exerted by the limbs, the less extensive contralateral transfer being observed in easier positions.

To overcome for the need to use a climbing device equipped with 3D force sensors, a computational method is presented. The method is based on inverse dynamics coupled with the minimization of the internal torques and external forces. Predicted contact forces accuracy is about 25 per cent of the body weight. This method allows a physical simulation of 3D climbing motion on a bouldering wall and a complete climbing route.

Summary

- Force measurements reveal important information about posture during climbing.
- The role of the upper limbs is to stabilize and control the body position in rock climbing.
- Equilibrium is easier to maintain in overhanging positions than on a vertical wall.
- Inverse dynamics of captured climbing motion can provide approximations of contact forces with an accuracy up to 25 per cent of body weight.
- Hypothesis on timing of climbing movements can be simulated through optimization.

References

Aladdin, R., Paul Kry, P. (2012). *Static pose reconstruction with an instrumented bouldering wall*. In Proceedings of the 18th ACM symposium on Virtual Reality Software and Technology, pp. 177–184.

Balas, J. (2014). The effect of climbing ability and slope inclination on vertical foot loading using a novel force sensor instrumentation system. *Journal of Human Kinetic*, 44(1), 75–81.

Bourdin C., Teasdale N., Nougier V., Bard C., Fleury M. (1999). Postural constraints modify the organization of grasping movements. *Human Movement Sciences*, 18, 87–102.

Courtemanche, S. (2014). *Analysis and Simulation of Optimal Motion in Rock Climbing* (PhD Thesis, Grenoble University, Grenoble).

Gelat, T., Caron, O., Metzger, T., Rougier, P. (1992). Human posturokinetic strategies from a horizontal quadrupedal stance. Temporal and biomechanical aspects. *Gait and Posture*, 2(4), 221–226.

Gray, J. (1944). Studies in the mechanics of the tetrapod skeleton. *Journal of Experimental Biology*, 20, 88–116.

Macpherson, J. M. (1988). Strategies that simplify the control of quadrupedal stance. I. Forces at the ground. *Journal of Neurophysiology*, 60(1), 204–217.

McIntyre, D. R., Bates, B. T. (1982). Effects of rung spacing on the mechanics of ladder ascent. *Journal of Movement Study*, 8, 55–72.

Noe, F. (2006). Modifications of anticipatory postural adjustments in a rock climbing task: the effect of supporting wall inclination. *Journal of Electromyography and Kinesiology,* 16(4), 336–341.

Noe, F., Quaine, F., Martin, L. (2001). Influence of steep gradient supporting walls in rock climbing: biomechanical analysis. *Gait and Posture,* 13, 86–94.

Quaine, F., Martin, L. (1999). A biomechanical study of equilibrium in sport rock climbing. *Gait and Posture,* 10, 233–239.

Quaine, F., Martin, L., Blanchi, J. P. (1997). The effect of body position and number of supports on wall reaction forces in rock climbing. *Journal of Applied Biomechanics,* 13, 14–23.

Righetti, L., Buchli, J., Mistry, M., Kalakrishnan, M., Schaal, S. (2013). Optimal distribution of contact forces with inverse dynamics control. *International Journal of Robotics Research,* 32(3), 280–298.

Robert, T., Causse, J., Monnier, G. (2013). Estimation of external contact loads using an inverse dynamics and optimization approach: general method and application to sit-to-stand maneuvers. *Journal of Biomechanics,* 46(13), 2220–2227.

Rougier, P., Billat, R., Merlin, M., Blanchi, J. P. (1991). Conception d'un système pour étudier la relation posturo-cinétique dasn un plan vertical: application sur une population de grimpeurs. *I.T.B.M.,* 12, 568–580.

Testa, M., Martin, L., Debû, B. (2003). 3D analysis of posturo-kinetic coordination associated with a climbing task in children and teenagers. *Neuroscience Letters,* 336, 45–49.

Watts, P. B., Drobish, K. M. (1998). Physiological responses to simulated rock climbing at different angles. *Medicine and Science in Sports and Exercise,* 30(7), 1118–1122.

Wei, X., Chai, J. (2010). VideoMocap: modeling physically realistic human motion from monocular video sequences. *ACM Transactions on Graphics,* 29, 42.

8 Grip capabilities of climbers' hands and fingers

Laurent Vigouroux

This chapter summarizes the data and knowledge available from the literature on the grip capacity of climbers. Several studies have been conducted over the last decades to determine the maximum grip capacity and the forearm muscle fatigue of rock climbers compared to non-climbers and/or according to the grip technique used, for example crimp or slope. These studies have shown that compared to non-climbers, climbers can exert higher forces during fingertip tasks and are more resistant to forearm muscle fatigue. The differences in grip performance observed with the use of crimp and slope grips seem to depend on hold characteristics rather than on biomechanical configuration. In addition, biomechanical models have allowed the forces withstood by tendons and ligaments while gripping a hold as well as the specific muscle capacities of climbers to be estimated. These estimations have shown that the strong forces exerted on the musculoskeletal systems of the hand and finger lead to an important risk of pulley rupture. Expert climbers show a highly specific muscular adaptation, which demonstrates a major increase in finger flexor strength and, conversely, a reduction/conservation of finger extensor and wrist muscle strength. More generally, this chapter points to the need for developing new training tools and programmes which take into account individual climber's physiological characteristics.

Introduction

One of the many original aspects of sport climbing and rock climbing is the intense use of the upper limbs (fingers, hands, forearms and arms) to balance and displace the entire body on various wall inclinations ranging from vertical to full overhang profiles (Watts & Drobish, 1998). As a consequence of this vertical quadrupedal locomotion, the practice of climbing generates high forces on fingertips, on forearm muscles and on ligaments, which have to be maintained up to several minutes (Mermier, Robergs, McMinn, & Heyward. 1997; Noé Quaine, & Martin, 2001; Quaine, Martin, Leroux, Blanchi, & Allard, 1996). Expert climbers therefore develop unusual prehensile capabilities, which are highly specific and differ from other sporting populations who train their hands differently (Cutts & Bollen, 1993; Shea, Shea, & Meals, 1992). Although rock climbing has evolved over the century, little is known about the hand–finger performance of climbers and their specific hand muscle capabilities. This lack of knowledge is also due to the fact that measuring grip performance and estimating hand muscle capacity requires the use of complex testing procedures and complex biomechanical models. Because of these challenges, the design of training exercises and training programmes as well as the prevention of pathologies is currently quite empirical. For example, to expand the finger performance, the majority of climbers use 'hangboard' exercises which consist of supporting the entire body weight using only their hands to grasp various types of holds. While this kind of exercise has obvious advantages to improve the force exerting capacity and fatigue resistance of the finger flexors, it cannot be used to strengthen other specific hand muscles. Moreover, to use this specific tool, too little knowledge about climber forearm muscles and climber forearm physiology is available for trainers to modulate the intensity of the training adequately and in a controlled manner. This lack of knowledge has led to many empirical beliefs and unfounded, sometimes contradictory, ideas, which hampers the sophisticated development of a climber's capacities.

This chapter aims at providing an overview of the scientific knowledge currently available on the grip capabilities of climbers. The first part covers the specific capabilities of climbers with respect to fingertip force exertion in terms of maximum performance and fatigue. The second part deals with the specific muscle forces exerted while squeezing a climbing hold and the consequences on the risks of injury. Finally, an analysis of the adaptations of the hand and finger muscles resulting from several years of climbing is presented and discussed. More generally, this chapter aims to provide quantitative data that could be used to optimize training programmes for climbers and to improve the prevention of pathologies resulting from climbing as well as rehabilitation.

Grip forces developed by climbers: maximum performance and effect of fatigue

Sport climbing consists of displacing the body along a wall and requires griping holds with one's fingers using each hand alternately. This effort involves intense, intermittent and static exercise using the forearm muscles (Quaine, Vigouroux, & Martin, 2003a). For the hardest routes, the available holds mainly require the use of the fingertips only, with the grip contact force applied on the entire surface or only part of the fingertip pulp. The greater the overhang of the climbing wall, the greater the forces required for the hands to support the body (Noé et al., 2001). At the very high skill level, the body weight has to be supported by selected fingers only. The ability to generate force at the fingertip and reduce inherent muscle fatigue as much as possible is crucial in order to maintain contact with the holds and ensure the success of an ascent (Watts et al., 1996).

To generate fingertip force on a hold, a countless number of joint positions and finger combinations can be used. However, among the numerous possible grip techniques, climbers mainly use two types of finger positions: the slope grip and the crimp grip (Figure 8.1). The crimp grip, which involves a hyper-extension of distal interphalangeal (DIP) joints combined with major flexion of the proximal interphalangeal (PIP) joints, is used to grasp sharp holds with a depth that is shorter than the length of the distal phalanx. This particular finger joint position has clearly been associated with finger pulley rupture, which is one of the most common injuries among climbers (Moutet, 2003; Schweizer, 2001). One of the advantages of the crimp grip is that it allows the thumb to act together with the other fingers (also known as 'full' crimp grip). The slope grip corresponds to a major flexion of both the DIP and PIP joints and is typically used for holes or slopers with a depth that is longer than the distal phalanx length (Amca, Vigouroux, Aritan, & Berton, 2012).

Regardless of the grip technique used, hands present anatomical specificities that influence climbing performance. Their most important original characteristic is that the finger muscles are polyarticular, that is, their tendons span multiple joints. In particular, the *flexor digitorum profundus* (FDP) and the *flexor digitorum superficialis* (FDS) are the only two muscles able to flex the distal finger joints. Yet they originate in the forearm and therefore mobilize the fingers through the action of long tendons which span all the finger joints as well as the wrist. This implies that the exertion of fingertip forces generates a complex coordination of all the hand muscles (including extensors) to balance the entire chain of joints from the forearm to the fingertips (Goislard de Monsabert, Rossi, Berton, & Vigouroux, 2012; Snijders, Volkers, Mechelse, & Vleeming, 1987). The second original characteristic of the hand and forearm musculature is to be endowed with a large number of muscles, that is, more than 30 muscles, in a relatively small anatomical volume. These characteristics result in specific physiological functioning with ischemic phenomena appearing in around 40 per cent of maximum voluntary contractions (MVCs) due to the pressure generated by muscle contraction (Pitcher & Miles, 1997). Local fatigue phenomena are thereby generated, which means that studying fatigue in rock climbers requires measuring the physiological status locally rather than using global physiological measurements such as aerobic capacity. Aerobic

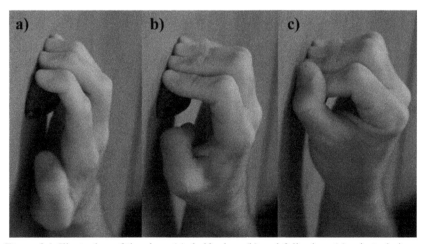

Figure 8.1 Illustration of the slope (a), half crimp (b) and full crimp (c) grip techniques used in rock climbing. The slope grip is characterized by flexion of the finger joints. Half crimp is characterized by hyperextension of the distal joints and the full grip is characterized by addition of the thumb to the other fingers

capacity does not seem to be a limiting factor for climbing performance anyway (Watts, Daggett, Gallagher, & Wilkins, 2004; Watts, Newbury, & Sulentic, 1996). Actually, only 42–67 per cent of the individual running VO_{2max} has been reported to be used during hard rock climbing (Billat, Palleja, Charlaix, Rizzardo, & Janel, 1995; de Geus, Villanueva O'Driscoll, & Meeusen, 2006). Conversely, heart rates have been shown to be disproportionately high compared to the individual VO_2 during climbing (Mermier, Robergs, McMinn, & Heyward, 1997; Sheel, Seddon, Knight, McKenzie, & Warburton, 2003) and blood lactate concentrations after sub-maximum climbing indicated exercise intensities above the individual lactate threshold (Booth, Marino, Hill, & Gwinn, 1999). All these observations suggest that local fatigue phenomena play an important role during climbing.

Methodologies used

To investigate the grip capabilities of climbers, the majority of studies have used a combination of measurements of grip force using instrumented holds and measurements of local physiological parameters. Generally, the researchers used specifically designed hand/finger ergometers as well as tasks unrelated to climbing activities (Watts & Jensen, 2003). This approach was essential to characterize grip capabilities without influence from other factors such as technical skills or psychological aspects (Quaine et al., 2003a). Instrumented holds have been used to obtain one-dimensional (1D) or three-dimensional (3D) force measurements of grip force (Figure 8.2) with, in some studies, a force sensor placed under each finger to identify how the grip force is distributed among the different fingers.

Together with grip force measurements, several studies have also recorded physiological muscle parameters such as electromyography (EMG) or

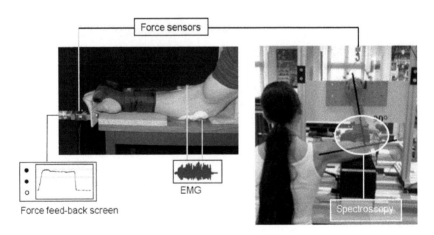

Figure 8.2 Experimental devices used in Vigouroux et al. (2006) and Philippe et al. (2012). In both experiments, fingertip forces were recorded during a fatigue-producing exercise and local physiological parameters were recorded (by electromyography and spectroscopy) to analyse muscle fatigue

spectroscopy parameters. These physiological signals can be used to detect fatigue before the force level is modified and to characterize its physiological nature, for example muscle oxygenation or metabolite accumulation. It has been shown that the frequency content of the EMG signal is a reliable index of muscle fatigue (Basmajian & De Luca, 1985; Petrofsky, 1981). During sustained contractions, the decrease in EMG median frequency is indeed causally related to the decrease in conduction velocity of motor potentials on the sarcolemma and to the decrease in the pH of the interstitial fluid due to the accumulation of lactic acid as well as hydrogen and potassium ions (H+ and K+) (Bigland-Ritchie, Donovan, & Roussos, 1981; Enoka & Stuart, 1992). Near infrared spectroscopy allows the identification of changes in finger flexor muscle oxygenation, which is particularly interesting to study in climbers given the ischemic nature of forearm fatigue (Philippe, Wegst, Müller, Raschner, & Burtscher, 2012; Usaj, 2002).

Maximum grip force: influence of expertise, grip technique and hold size

As expected, numerous studies have reported that climbers are able to exert higher maximum grip force than non-climbers (Cutts & Bollen, 1993; Grant et al., 2003; Quaine et al., 2003a). This conclusion (Table 8.1) has been confirmed by many subsequent studies but was conditioned by the methodology used. Higher differences between climbers and non-climbers were indeed observed with 'finger ergometers' (+ 30 per cent on average) than with 'whole-hand ergometers' (+ 12 per cent on average), which involve many more areas, including the palm of the hand, to exert forces (Cutts & Bollen, 1993). The performance of climbers therefore appears to be highly specific thanks to the particular ability to a produce high fingertip force.

An interesting result according to the literature is that no significant differences in performance have been observed between the crimp and slope grip techniques for a 1-cm depth hold. Contrary to a general belief among climbers, the two different biomechanical configurations actually lead to similar performance when comparing the resultant forces exerted in a one-finger grip and a four-finger grip (Quaine & Vigouroux, 2004; Schweizer, 2001; Vigouroux, Quaine, Labarre-Vila, & Moutet, 2006). However, as expected, the contribution of the thumb in the crimp grip, that is, the full crimp grip, allows a significantly improved performance (Quaine, Vigouroux, Paclet, & Colloud, 2011). Moreover, the involvement of the thumb also modifies the finger force sharing. When using a four-finger crimp grip, the finger force sharing among the fingers is such that: 24 per cent of the resultant force is exerted under the index finger, 32 per cent is exerted under the middle finger, 27 per cent under the ring finger and 17 per cent under the little finger (Table 8.1). The finger sharing with the slope grip position is slightly different and tends towards a more homogenous sharing between fingers (Quaine, Vigouroux, & Martin, 2003b; Vigouroux et al., 2008a). However, when using the thumb, this sharing changes significantly, with a critical drop in the contribution of the little finger, unchanged contributions of the middle and ring fingers and greater action of the index finger on which the thumb exerts an additional force (Quaine et al., 2011). Several neuromuscular studies unrelated to rock climbing

Table 8.1 Examples of results (mean ±SD) reported in the literature (Quaine et al., 2003a; Schweizer, 2001; Vigouroux et al., 2008b; Quaine et al., 2011; Cutts & Bollen, 1993 for each line respectively) for maximum grip exertion in different population during different grip tests

Tested subjects	Type of grip	Force sensor device	Total grip force (N)	Force sharing among the fingers (%, index (I), middle (M), ring (R), little finger (L))
10 Experts	1-cm depth, slope and half crimp, 4-finger grip	1D force sensor, Forearm positioned horizontally	Slope: 434.3 ± 39.06 N (ns) Half crimp: 407.66 ± 26.35 N	Sharing not measured
10 Experts and 10 non-climbers	1-cm depth, Half crimp, 4-finger grip	1D force sensor	Experts: 420 ± 46 N (*) Non-climbers: 342 ±56 N	Sharing not measured
16 climbers	2-cm depth Crimp and slope, 1-finger grip,	1D force sensor, Forearm positioned vertically	Slope: 78 ± 22 N (ns) Half crimp: 82 ± 19 N	Fingers placed in parallel, sharing was not measured
9 climbers	1-cm depth, Full crimp, half crimp and 4-finger grip	3D force sensor, 1 sensor per finger, Forearm positioned vertically	Full crimp: 494.8 ± 68.8 N (*) Half crimp: 422.0 ± 42.9 N	Full crimp: I 39.6%; M 26.7%; R 22.0%; L 11.7% Half crimp: I 24.3%; M 31.6%; R 26.9%; L 17.1%
13 Experts and 12 non-climbers	Whole hand grip and pinch grip	Hand and pinch dynamometer	Whole hand grip (right hand): Climbers, 507 ± 17 N (*) Non-climbers, 445 ± 59 N Pinch-grip (right hand): Climbers, 143 ± 20 N (*) Non-climbers, 101 ± 17 N	Sharing not measured

Notes: (ns) = non-significant difference; (*) = significant difference.

suggest that the force sharing among fingers is determined by the central nervous system and aims at minimizing 'unnecessary' torque along the forearm axis and the wrist radial–ulnar deviation axis (Li, Latash, Newell, & Zatsiorsky, 1998; Vigouroux et al., 2008a). Therefore, the modification of finger force sharing observed in the full crimp grip indicates that the use of the thumb modifies the constraints of wrist equilibrium, probably because of the supplementary action of thumb extrinsic muscles. This influence of the wrist is in agreement with the observations of climbers who sometimes found it more comfortable to modify the wrist joint angle with the full crimp grip when exerting a cross movement for example. Similarly, considering the influence of the wrist equilibrium, it is not surprising to observe that climbers mostly use the combination of ring and middle fingers when gripping a two-finger pocket hold. Compared to other fingers, the middle and ring fingers are indeed the closest to the radial–ulnar deviation axes and therefore probably represent the best option to exert maximum fingertip force while minimizing the disequilibrium of the wrist.

The effect of hold size on grip performance varies and differs according to the grip (Amca et al., 2012; Bourne, Halaki, Vanwanseele, & Clarke, 2011). As shown in Figure 8.3, as grip size increases, maximum performance evolves differently according to the type of grip. Whereas a linear increase is observed with the slope grip, the maximum force decreases beyond a 3-cm depth with the crimp and full crimp grips. The choice of finger technique while climbing thus seems to be more dependent on hold characteristics, such as size or shape, than on any biomechanical advantage. In addition, Amca et al. (2012) also found that the

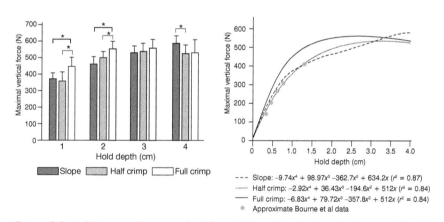

Figure 8.3 A: Mean maximum vertical force (N) and standard deviation according to the hold depth with the slope, half crimp and full crimp grips reported by Amca et al. (2012). Significant differences between grip techniques were observed (* P<0.05) for each hold depth. B: Mean maximum vertical force (N) and fitted polynomial curve used to model the evolution of force according to the hold depth with the three different grips. The approximate mean maximum force results of Bourne et al. (2011) for half crimp technique are presented in the form of a graph

finger techniques are different in terms of force orientation. These authors showed that the crimp grip (with and without the thumb) seems to increase the potential to direct the grip force in the anterio-posterior direction. In other words, the crimp technique could be more suited to 'pulling up the wall' than the slope grip. This point is important given that the entire body balance during climbing movements often requires directing the grip force in the anterio-posterior direction (Noé et al., 2001; Quaine, Martin, Leroux, Blanchi, & Allard, 1996). Consequently, in addition to hold characteristics, the choice of the climber's grip technique also seems to be strongly dependent on the desired climbing movement.

Forearm muscle fatigue

One common way of studying forearm muscle fatigue in climbers is to analyse the evolution of fingertip forces during forearm exercises that mimic climbing movements/tasks, that is, intermittent and static exercise at a high level of sub-maximum grip force applied at the fingertips for several minutes. During this type of exercise, fatigue onset is generally divided into three distinct phases (Figure 8.4) with, first, a plateau phase during which the required level of sub-maximum force is maintained by the participant; second, a sudden drop of the force level; and third, a second plateau where force is maintained at a lower level than the required force. Ferguson and Brown (1997) demonstrated that the force maintained during the first plateau is mainly due to non-aerobic capacities. Using a blood clamp, these authors indeed observed that the characteristics of this first plateau phase remain the same with and without blood flow. However, the subsequent drop in force is limited without a blood clamp whereas the loss of force is drastic and leads to exhaustion with the clamp. The EMG results suggest that during the first plateau and the subsequent drop in force, there is an accumulation of interstitial biochemical by-products due to blood flow obstruction under muscle pressure (Vigouroux & Quaine, 2006). Following the first plateau phase and the drop in force, the physiological indexes indicate that the second plateau phase corresponds to the equilibrium between accumulation of interstitial by-products and re-oxygenation and blood flow between contractions. Spectroscopy studies (Philippe et al., 2012; Usaj, 2002) confirmed that the blood flow between intermittent contractions was crucial to re-oxygenate muscle. It is interesting to note that training and climbing expertise strongly influenced the finger force profile during the entire experimental test. First of all, it was shown that climbers were able to maintain the first plateau phase over a longer period than non-climbers (Quaine et al., 2003a). Secondly, climbers were able to limit the drop of force and showed a higher force level during the second plateau phase (Vigouroux & Quaine, 2006). The EMG and spectroscopy results suggest that this higher performance is due to superior peripheral vascular characteristics and enhanced vasodilator capacity. Hence, the blood flow between two consecutive contractions is increased in expert climbers, thus accelerating the rate at which biochemical by-products are eliminated. Interestingly, the force profile during this type of exercise was also dependent on the climber's individual characteristics. For example, Figure 8.4

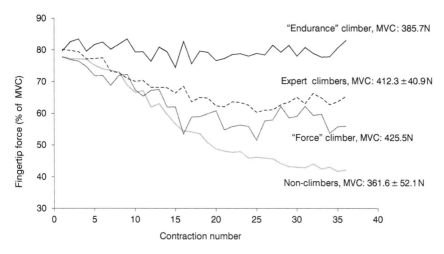

Figure 8.4 Evolution of fingertip forces according to fatigue. Fingertip forces were exerted on a 1-cm depth hold involving 36 contractions with an intermittent rhythm (5 s of contraction followed by 5 s of rest). The instructions were to exert 80 per cent of a maximum voluntary contraction and to keep this level as much as possible. Non-climbers are indicated with black diamonds and climbers with grey diamonds. Two climbers with different profiles: one with an 'endurance' profile (light grey points) and one with a 'force' profile (black points) are also drawn to show the influence of individual characteristics. Results of MVC are indicated on the graph. Source: Data obtained from Vigouroux et al., 2006

shows the fingertip force profile of two elite climbers with similar skill levels. The first produced a higher force level but exhibited a greater drop of the fatigue force profile, the amplitude of which was almost the same as that observed in non-climbers. This climber therefore seems to have developed a 'force' profile that allows exerting a maximum force of limited duration. The second climber exerted a lower level of fingertip force (similar to that of non-climbers) but only exhibited a very small lack of force during the fatigue profile. This climber shows an 'endurance' profile and is able to maintain a prolonged effort. Vigouroux and Quaine (2006) proposed that in addition to vascular capacity, the different climber profiles could be determined based on the muscle type fibres of the forearm muscles. Given these results, it appears crucial for trainers to design specific training programmes for each climber by identifying their forearm fatigue profile in the first place. Investigating such climber characteristics based on fingertip force measurements and/or physiological parameters thus appears to be essential.

When comparing the evolution of fatigue for the crimp and slope grips, Quaine and Vigouroux (2004) did not observe any difference, indicating that the grip technique did not influence the fatigue level. Therefore, fatigue seems to be linked to local physiological phenomena rather than to biomechanical configuration. Further studies should now test if alternating the grip technique could be a way of controlling the onset of fatigue. Another interesting finding of Quaine and Vigouroux (2004) is that, in accordance with the original role of extensor muscles for wrist equilibrium mentioned above, extensor muscles fatigued at the same level and rhythm as flexor muscles. This observation supports the notion that training forearm muscles using only flexion exercises is probably not sufficient to optimize grip capabilities.

Estimation of muscle force during climbing: effect of grip techniques

Although the analysis of maximum grip force performance and fatigue evolution provides important information to characterize climber capabilities, such data is not sufficient to adapt climbing training programmes adequately. Indeed, these values neither inform which muscles are solicited in the climbing grip nor quantify how much force is transmitted through anatomical structures such as muscles, tendons or pulleys. Quantitative information on such internal mechanical efforts is, however, crucial for several reasons: first, identifying the specific muscles solicited in the climbing grip could indicate which development exercises and specific programmes are appropriate; second, measuring internal forces could provide information to help prevent the development of pathology by reinforcing and re-equilibrating forearm musculature as well as make recommendations to avoid risk behaviour, and design rehabilitation procedures.

Biomechanical modelling and experimental setup

To accurately evaluate the internal mechanical efforts, participants have to be equipped with a device by surgery in order to measure over 40 muscles and at least eight pulleys. That direct measurement is technically and ethically hardly possible for healthy participants. The use of biomechanical modelling is an alternative to estimate these forces *in vivo* in each individual. Biomechanical models represent the mechanical behaviour of the hand based on Newton's mechanical principles. These models use experimental data (force measurements, kinematics, EMG) as input (Valero-Cuevas, Zajac, Burgar, 1998; Vigouroux et al., 2006) and generally require mathematical optimization processes (Sancho-Bru, Perez-Gonzalez, Vergara-Monedero, & Giurintan, 2001) in order to estimate the internal forces exerted by muscles, ligaments and joints. Several studies have used musculoskeletal models of the hand to estimate the muscle forces and pulley forces involved in climbing grips. The experiments consisted of testing climbers during various finger/hand tasks such as gripping a hold with the slope grip or crimp grip or exerting joint moments on different joints (i.e. wrist joint, metacarpophalangeal joints and interphalangeal joints). During these experiments, the external forces, the kinematics and EMGs were recorded in order to provide input data for the models.

Forces exerted in the muscles, tendons and pulleys

Vigouroux et al. (2006 and 2008b) were the first to estimate the muscle forces exerted in the crimp and slope grips *in vivo* (Figures 8.5 and 8.6). Two main points were identified in these studies. The first is that high tendon forces were exerted in the FDS and FDP for both slope and crimp grips. Two types of muscle distribution

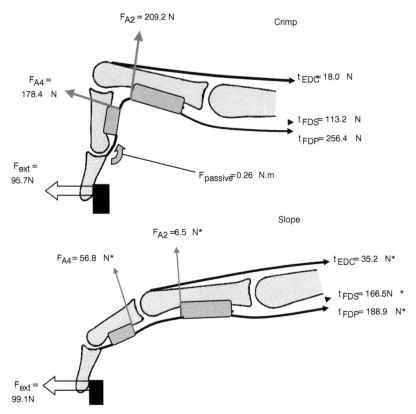

Figure 8.5 Mean estimations of tendon and pulley force computed for the crimp and slope grips in a one-finger grip in six expert climbers. Notes: * means a significant difference between crimp and slope grips. tEDC, tFDS and tFDP represent the tendon forces estimated for the extensor digitorum communis, flexor digiorum superficialis and flexor digitorum profundus respectively. FA2 and FA4 represent the force applied on the A2 and A4 pulleys respectively. Fext represents the external force exerted on a 1-cm depth hold during a MVC and Mpassive represents the passive moment applied on the distal interphalengeal joint in the crimp grip. Source: Vigouroux et al., 2006

were, however, observed according to the grip technique. In the crimp grip, the FDP muscle is mostly involved, whereas in the slope grip, both the FDP and the FDS muscles are recruited to a similar degree. This indicates that climbers should adapt their muscle coordination and improve their muscle strength differentially according to the grip technique used. This conclusion helps to explain the individual differences observed in crimp and slope grip performance according to climber habitus (Quaine & Vigouroux, 2004). Additionally, Schweizer and Hudek (2011) showed that the depth of the hold also influences the pattern of motor unit activations. While increasing the hold depth, higher FDS motor units activation in crimp grip position and higher FDP activation in the slope grip were observed. Training for climbing should thus carefully address to both grip techniques to ensure good performance with each type of grip.

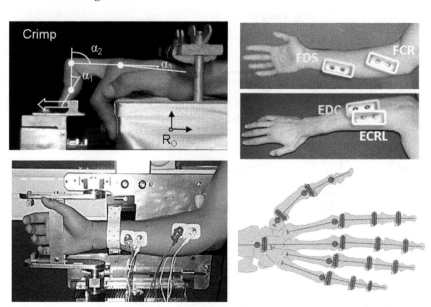

Figure 8.6 Examples of experimental design used to estimate tendon tension in a one-finger crimp grip (upper left-hand panel, Vigouroux et al., 2006) and the muscle maximal strength of the five main hand muscle groups (lower left-hand panel, Vigouroux et al., 2015). Typical placement of EMG electrodes used in hand experiments (upper right-hand panel), FDS: flexor digitorum superficialis, FCR: flexor carpi radialis; EDC: extensor digitorum communis; ECRL: extensor carpi radialis longus. Representation of the hand biomechanical model used to estimate muscle, joint and ligament forces (lower right-hand panel). The rectangles represent flexion/extension degrees of freedom. The circles represent adduction/abduction degrees of freedom

Data on tendon forces have also been used to calculate the intensity of forces exerted on pulleys. In accordance with clinical reports (Bollen & Gunson, 1990; Moutet, 2003), models have estimated that the forces on A4 and A2 pulleys were more than three times higher in the crimp grip than in the slope grip (Vigouroux et al., 2006). Also in accordance with the same clinical reports, Vigouroux et al. (2008b) showed that the middle and ring fingers are more exposed to pulley rupture than the index and little fingers. The pulley forces exerted on these two fingers in the crimp grip are indeed much closer to their rupture thresholds than is the case for the index and little fingers. These quantitative data have been used by surgeons to develop rehabilitation procedures and by researchers to design measurement techniques on cadaver specimens (Schöffl et al., 2009).

Hand and forearm muscle adaptations in climbers

As presented in the preceding paragraph, the finger flexor muscles (FDS and/or FDP) are required to exert forces reaching 250 N during a climbing grip. This force level is much higher than the theoretical maximal strength of these muscles (around 150 N for a single finger flexor tendon), according to the general evaluation from data in the literature (Chao, An, Cooney, & Linscheid, 1989; Valero-Cuevas et al. 1998). To produce such force magnitude, climbers probably increase their maximal muscle strength enormously compared to untrained populations. Conversely, the forces developed in the *extensor digitorum superficialis* (EDC) tendon appear to be equivalent to those developed during other daily tasks such as pinch grip or cylindrical grip (Goislard de Monsabert et al., 2012; Vigouroux, Domalain, Berton, 2011) and are in the range of their theoretical maximal muscle strength (around 60 N for a single finger extensor tendon). From these results, it can be seen that, through training, climbers seem to develop particular adaptations of their maximal muscle strength to generate finger muscle force.

To characterize climbers' muscle adaptation, Vigouroux, Goislard de Monsabert, and Berton (2015) used a biomechanical model of the hand and measurements of the maximum net joint moment to estimate the maximal muscle strength and maximal moment potential of the five main muscle groups of the hand and forearm (Figures 8.6 and 8.7). The main conclusion was that the finger flexor muscles of climbers have a 40 per cent higher strength. As expected, the many years of climbing lead to an increase in finger flexor maximal strength, in accordance with numerous studies in which climbers have been observed to perform significantly better when grasping fingertip holds (Cutts & Bollen, 1993; Grant et al., 2003; Mermier et al., 1997; Philippe et al., 2012; Watts & Drobish, 1998). However, the study of Vigouroux et al. (2015) provided quantitative data on the specific muscle strength profile developed by climbers and on the potential degree of improvement of finger flexor in climbers. In addition to these data on finger flexor muscles, several unexpected results were observed. First, the enhancement of finger flexor maximal strength was not associated with the simultaneous development of finger extensor muscles. Although no significant effect was found, several climbers even presented a lower finger extensor strength than non-climbers. This phenomenon is probably due to an underuse of extensor muscles during training and climbing and may also result from the decrease in antagonist muscle activation, which has been observed in numerous sport/movement expert reports (Fouré, Nordez, & Cornu, 2010; Griffin & Cafarelli, 2005).

The second intriguing finding is that, similarly to finger extensors, wrist muscle strength was not significantly different between climbers and non-climbers. Consequently, it seems that the practice of climbing and current training methods do not result in the uniform improvement in maximal strength of forearm muscle groups since enhancement only occurs in finger flexors and no modifications are observed for other hand and wrist muscles. Because of the greater enhancement of finger flexors, climbers exhibited unfavourable imbalance ratios between flexor and extensor strength around the wrist and MCP joints. In other words, extensor muscles have a low maximal strength compared to flexor muscles. This point is of great importance from a pathological point of view since it is well known from the literature that the co-activation of antagonistic muscles and associated mechanical actions are crucial for the protection of joints from excessive shear forces and excessive involuntary torques by increasing joint rigidity (for a review,

142   *Laurent Vigouroux*

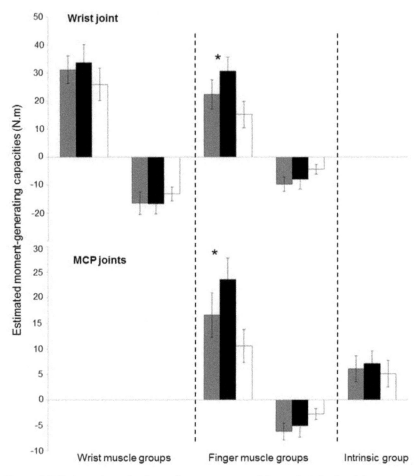

Figure 8.7 Estimated maximal muscle moment potential at wrist joint level (upper panel) and MCP joint level (lower panel) according to Vigouroux et al., (2015). The estimated maximal muscle moment potential was estimated for five main muscle groups: wrist flexors, wrist extensors, finger flexors, finger extensors and intrinsic muscles based on results on maximal muscle strength and muscle moment arms at the respective joints. Non-climbers are indicated in grey, male climbers in black and female climbers in white. Flexion and extension correspond to positive and negative values respectively. No muscle capacity were presented for the intrinsic muscle group at the wrist joint and for the wrist muscle groups at the MCP joints because these muscles do not span these respective joints. Note: * indicates a significant difference between climbers and non-climbers

see Remaud, Guevel, and Cornu, 2007). This conclusion confirms the need for the development of new training tools and new methods in order to improve forearm performance. In particular, these data indicate that finger extensor training would be valuable to re-equilibrate the imbalance ratio of climbers.

Practical applications

Results and data provided by literature could be immediately employed by climbers, trainers and clinicians to prevent injuries and enhance training programmes. First of all, climbers should train their finger capabilities in all the variety of climbing grip techniques in order to be able to adapt to various hold characteristics and various climbing movements. Second, climbers should determine their individual physiological forearm profile in order to adapt their training for optimally improving selected capabilities identified in the literature (i.e. maximal force, maintaining a high level of force intensity, maintaining a long duration of effort). Third, estimated internal forces could be reused by clinicians to optimally adjust injury prevention and the rehabilitation processes. Finally, the results on muscle strengths indicate that a training of forearm and hand muscle groups should be specified to re-equilibrate the climber's muscle capacities for injury prevention and for optimizing hand and finger performances.

Summary

- Compared to non-climbers, climbers exert a high magnitude of fingertip forces on holds and exhibit a 40 per cent enhancement of finger flexor muscle strength compared to non-climbers.
- Climbers limit the effect of fatigue compared to non-climbers mainly due to enhanced peripheral vascular characteristics.
- The choice of the used finger grip technique, for example crimp or slope, depends more on the hold characteristics and on the required climbing movement than on physiological and biomechanical factors.
- Compared to the slope grip, the use of the crimp technique generates high forces in the *flexor digitorum profundus* and on the pulleys, especially for the middle and ring fingers.

References

Amca, A. M., Vigouroux, L., Aritan, S. & Berton, L. (2012). Effect of hold depth and grip technique on maximal finger forces in rock climbing. *Journal of Sports Sciences*, 30(7), 669–677.

Basmajian, J. V., & De Luca, C. J. (1985). *Muscles alive*. Baltimore, MD: Williams & Wilkins.

Bigland-Ritchie, B., Donovan, E. F., & Roussos, C. S. (1981). Conduction velocity and EMG power spectrum changes in fatigue of sustained maximal efforts. *Journal of Applied Physiology*, 51, 1300–1305.

Billat, V., Palleja, P., Charlaix, T., Rizzardo, P., & Janel, N. (1995). Energy specificity of rock climbing and aerobic capacity in competitive sport rock climbers. *Journal of Sports Medicine and Physical Fitness*, 35(1), 20–24.

Bollen, S. R., & Gunson, C. K. (1990). Hand injuries in competition climbers. *British Journal of Sports Medicine*, 24, 16–18.

Booth, J., Marino, F., Hill, C., & Gwinn, T. (1999). Energy cost of sport rock climbing in elite performers. *British Journal of Sports Medicine,* 33(1), 14–18.

144   *Laurent Vigouroux*

Bourne, R., Halaki, M., Vanwanseele, B., & Clarke, J. (2011). Measuring lifting forces in rock climbing: effect of hold size and fingertip structure. *Journal of Applied Biomechanics*, 27, 40–46.

Chao, E. Y., An, K. N., Cooney, W. P., & Linscheid, R. L. (1989). *Biomechanics of the hand.* Singapore: World Scientific.

Cutts, A, & Bollen, S. R. (1993). Grip strength and endurance in rock climbers. *Proceedings of the Institute of Mechanical Engineers*, 207, 87–92.

de Geus, B., Villanueva O'Driscoll, S., & Meeusen, R. (2006). Influence of climbing style on physiological responses during indoor rock climbing on routes with the same difficulty. *European Journal of Applied Physiology*, 98, 489–496.

Enoka, R. M., & Stuart, D. G. (1992). Neurobiology of muscle fatigue. *Journal of Applied Physiology*, 72, 1631–1648.

Ferguson, R. A., & Brown, M. D. (1997). Arterial blood pressure and forearm vascular conductance responses to sustained and rhythmic isometric exercise and arterial occlusion in trained rock climbers and untrained sedentary subjects. *European Journal of Applied Physiology*, 76, 174–180.

Fouré, A., Nordez, A., & Cornu, C. (2010). Pliometric training effects on Achilles tendon stiffness and dissipative properties. *Journal of Applied Physiology*, 109, 849–854.

Goislard de Monsabert, B., Rossi, J., Berton, E., & Vigouroux, L. (2012). Quantification of hand and forearm muscle forces during a maximal power grip task. *Medicine and Science in Sports and Exercise*, 44, 1906–1916.

Grant, S., Shields, C., Fitzpatrick, V., Loh, W. M., Whitaker, A., Watt, I. & Kay, J. W. (2003). Climbing-specific finger endurance: a comparative study of intermediate rock climbers, rowers and aerobically trained individuals. *Journal of Sports Sciences*, 21, 621–630.

Griffin, L., & Cafarelli, E. (2005). Resistance training: cortical, spinal, and motor unit adaptations. *Canadian Journal of Applied Physiology*, 30, 328–340.

Li, Z. M., Latash, M. L., Newell, K. M., & Zatsiorsky, V. M. (1998). Motor redundancy during maximal voluntary contraction in four-finger tasks. *Experimental Brain Research*, 122, 71–78.

Mermier, C. M., Roberts, R. A., McMinn, S. M. & Heyward, V. H. (1997). Energy expenditure and physiological responses during indoor rock climbing. *British Journal of Sports Medicine*, 31, 224–228.

Moutet, F. (2003). Flexor tendon pulley system: anatomy, pathology, treatment. *Chirurgie de la Main*, 22, 1–12.

Noé, F., Quaine, F., & Martin, L. (2001). Influence of steep gradient supporting walls in rock climbing: biomechanical analysis. *Gait and Posture*, 13, 86–94.

Petrofsky, J. S. (1981). Quantification through the surface EMG of muscle fatigue and recovery during successive isometric contractions. *Aviation, Space and Environmental Medicine*, 52, 545–550.

Philippe, M., Wegst, D., Müller, T., Raschner, C., & Burtscher, M. (2012). Climbing-specific finger flexor performance and forearm muscle oxygenation in elite male and female sport climbers. *European Journal of Applied Physiology*, 112, 2839–2847.

Pitcher, J., & Miles, T. (1997). Influence of muscle blood flow on fatigue during intermittent human hand-grip exercise and recovery. *Clinical Experimental Pharmacology and Physiology*, 24, 471–476.

Quaine, F., Martin, L., Leroux, M., Blanchi, J. P., & Allard, P. (1996). Effect of initial posture on biomechanical adjustments associated with a voluntary leg movement in rock climbers. *Archive of Physiology Biochemistry*, 104, 192–199.

Quaine, F., & Vigouroux, L. (2004). Maximal resultant four fingertip force and fatigue of the extrinsic muscles of the hand in different sport climbing finger grips. *International Journal of Sports Medicine*, 25, 634–637.

Quaine, F., Vigouroux, L., & Martin, L. (2003a). Finger flexors fatigue in trained rock climbers and untrained sedentary subjects. *International Journal of Sports Medicine*, 24, 424–427.

Quaine, F., Vigouroux, L., & Martin, L. (2003b). Effect of simulated rock climbing finger postures on force sharing among the fingers. *Clinical Biomechanics*, 18, 78–84.

Quaine, F., Vigouroux, L., Paclet, F., & Colloud, F. (2011). The thumb during the crimp grip. *International Journal of Sport Medicine*, 32, 49–53.

Remaud, A., Guevel, A., & Cornu, C. (2007). Antagonist muscle coactivation and muscle inhibition: effects on external torque regulation and resistance training-induced adaptations. *Neurophysiologie Clinique*, 37, 1–14.

Sancho-Bru, J. L., Perez-Gonzalez, A., Vergara-Monedero, M., & Giurintan, D. J., (2001). A 3-D dynamic model of human finger for studying free movements. *Journal of Biomechanics*, 34, 1491–1500.

Schöffl, I., Oppelt, K., Jungert, J., Schweizer, A., Neuhuber, W., & Schöffl, V. (2009). The influence of the crimp and slope grip position on the finger pulley system. *Journal of Biomechanics*, 42, 2183–2187.

Schweizer, A. (2001). Biomechanical properties of the crimp grip position in rock climbers. *Journal of Biomechanics*, 34, 217–223.

Schweizer, A., & Hudek, R. (2011). Kinetics of crimp and slope grip in rock climbing. *Journal of Applied Biomechanics*, 27, 116–121.

Shea, K. G., Shea, O. F., & Meals, R. A. (1992). Manual demands and consequences of rock climbing. *Journal of Hand Surgery*, 17, 200–205.

Sheel, A. W., Seddon, N., Knight, A., McKenzie, D. C. R., & Warburton, D. E. (2003). Physiological responses to indoor rock climbing and their relationship to maximal cycle ergometry. *Medicine and Science in Sports and Exercise*, 35, 1225–1231.

Snijders, C. J, Volkers, A. C., Mechelse, K., & Vleeming, A. (1987) Provocation of epicondylalgia lateralis (tennis elbow) by power grip or pinching. *Medicine and Science in Sports and Exercise*, 19, 518–523.

Usaj, A. (2002). Differences in the oxygenation of the forearm muscle during isometric contractions in trained and untrained subjects. *Cellular and Molecular Biology Letters*, 7, 375–377.

Valero-Cuevas F. J., Zajac F. E., & Burgar, C. G. (1998). Large index-fingertip forces are produced by subject-independent patterns of muscle excitation. *Journal of Biomechanics*, 31, 693–703.

Vigouroux, L., Domalain, M., & Berton, E., (2011). Effect of object width on muscle and joint forces during thumb/index fingers grasping. *Journal of Applied Biomechanics*, 27, 173–180.

Vigouroux, L., Ferry, M., Colloud, F., Paclet, F., Cahouet, V., & Quaine, F. (2008a). Is the principle of minimization of secondary moment validated during various fingertip force production conditions? *Human Movement Science*, 27, 396–407.

Vigouroux, L., Goislard de Monsabert, B., & Berton, E. (2015). Estimation of hand and wrist muscle capacities in rock-climbers. *European Journal of Applied Physiology*, 115(5), 947–957.

Vigouroux, L., & Quaine, F. (2006). Fingertip force and electromyography of finger flexor muscles during a prolonged intermittent exercise in elite climbers and sedentary individuals. *Journal of Sports Sciences*, 24, 181–186.

Vigouroux, L., Quaine, F., Colloud, F., Paclet, F., & Moutet, F. (2008b). Middle and ring fingers are more exposed to pulley rupture than index and little during sport-climbing: a biomechanical explanation. *Clinical Biomechanics*, 23, 562–570.

Vigouroux, L., Quaine, F., Labarre-Vila, A., & Moutet, F. (2006). Estimation of finger muscle tendon tensions and pulley forces during specific sport-climbing grip techniques. *Journal of Biomechanics*, 39, 2583–2592.

Watts, P., & Drobish, K. M. (1998). Physiological responses to simulated rock climbing at different angles. *Medicine and Science in Sports and Exercise*, 30, 1118–1122.

Watts, P., & Jensen, R. (2003). Reliability of peak forces during a finger curl motion common in rock climbing. *Measurement in Physical Education and Exercise Science*, 74(4), 263–267.

Watts, P., Newbury, V., & Sulentic, J. (1996). Acute changes in handgrip strength, endurance, and blood lactate with sustained sport rock climbing. *Journal of Sports and Medicine and Physiological Fitness*, 36(4), 255–260.

Watts, P. B., Daggett, M., Gallagher, P., & Wilkins, B. (2004). Metabolic response during sport rock climbing and the effects of active versus passive recovery. *International Journal of Sports Medicine*, 21(3), 185–190.

9   Muscular strength and endurance in climbers

Jiří Baláš

This chapter discusses the role of, and explores what should be understood by, the terms muscular strength, power and endurance – attributes that are considered amongst the most important predictors of climbing performance. It also describes climbing specific tests that correspond to the loading, movement and body positions typically found whilst climbing. Test specificity requires similar motor unit recruitment, type of contraction, speed of contraction, position of body segments and time characteristics of contraction to be considered. Climbing specific tests may be divided into four areas. 1) Finger flexors strength, involving isometric contraction of the finger flexors on a hold 2–3 cm deep with an open or crimp grip, with the tested arm above the head. 2) Finger flexors endurance, with either a) intermittent test until exhaustion with the 5–12 second (s) contraction and 2–4 s relief at 30–80 per cent maximal voluntary contraction (MVC), or b) continuous finger hang with both hands on a 2–3 cm deep rung. 3) Shoulder girdle power with either a one- or two-arm explosive upward movement. 4) Shoulder girdle strength and endurance, bent-arm hang on one or both arms. Supporting normative data is provided for a large range of climbing specific tests, and for a broad spectrum of climbing abilities.

Introduction

The sport climbing is a multifaceted activity, requiring a combination of strength, endurance and power. Training climbers in these qualities is challenging, as they represent diverse physiological functions. It is possible to differentiate between muscular strength, endurance and power based on the physiological responses to exercise; these will briefly be defined. Strength, or more precisely muscular strength, is the ability to generate maximal external force (Zatsiorsky & Kraemer, 2006). Muscular endurance is the ability to produce submaximal force for longer periods of time (Heyward & Gibson, 2014). According to the type of contraction, strength may be either static or dynamic. During static or isometric contractions, the distance between the start and the end of a muscle fibre does not change. During dynamic contractions, when the length of muscle fibre shortens, we speak of a concentric contraction; conversely, when the fibre absorbs external energy and lengthens, we speak of an eccentric contraction. Muscles have a greater capacity to generate muscular strength during an isometric contraction, whilst strength is always lower during a concentric movement. The amount of strength is dictated by the number of actin myosin cross-bridge cycles, which is also inversely related to speed of contraction. Maximal muscular power describes the highest level of power (work/time) achieved during a muscular contraction (Cormie, McGuigan, & Newton, 2011).

In climbing, the greatest demands are placed on maximal isometric strength and endurance of the forearm muscles, the isometric strength, endurance and power of shoulder girdle muscles and the strength of the core muscles (Baláš, Pecha, Martin, & Cochrane, 2012; Mermier, Janot, Parker, & Swan, 2000; Michailov, 2014; Michailov, Mladenov, & Schöffl, 2009; Nachbauer, Fetz, & Burtscher, 1987). Enhanced ability in these areas is likely to represent climbing specific adaptations. Whether assessing or training, consideration should be given to how representative the movements are of actual climbing performance. In order to ensure specificity, several factors should be considered, including the type of contraction, speed of contraction, motor units involved, position of body segments, and the temporal characteristics of the work–relief ratio during prolonged contractions.

Finger flexor strength

Assessments of finger flexor strength and endurance have received the most attention from climbers and scientists. Finger strength is dependent on many factors, which are considered in the following text. Discussion of the development of tools for the assessment of finger strength and endurance helps us to understand the physiological and biomechanical basis of ability in these areas.

Handgrip dynamometry

The earliest research assessing climbing specific strength used handgrip dynamometry (Figure 9.1a) (Cutts & Bollen, 1993; Watts, Martin, & Durtschi, 1993). Dynamometry has several advantages over more recent measures as it is easy to perform, requires limited equipment, comparisons may easily be made between studies and reliability has been confirmed with a variety of devices in large populations (España-Romero et al., 2010; Peolsson, Hedlund, & Oberg, 2001). However, the criterion validity of grip dynamometry, in relation to climbing performance, remains controversial, as it has been shown that absolute values of grip strength are not directly related to climbing ability. Although when grip strength is related to body mass, the differences are significant (Watts, 2004). Despite this, the use of strength to body mass ratio has been criticised as it disadvantages subjects with higher body mass (Vanderburgh, Mahar, & Chou, 1995). Baláš et al. (2014) demonstrated significant differences of handgrip strength to body mass ratio in climbers of differing climbing abilities; although when strength was normalised to body mass by linear regression the differences were not significant. Aside from the normalisation of mass to grip strength, other issues have been raised. Watts et al. (2008) reported that electromyographic activity (EMG) of the forearm flexors was lowest during handgrip dynamometry, when compared to six common climbing grips, leading the authors to question the specificity of handgrip dynamometry. On the other hand, hand dynamometry represents one of several common grips found in climbing, with the thumb in opposition, and all elite climbers demonstrate a high level of strength when normalised to body mass (Baláš et al., 2012). It is suggested that high levels of handgrip strength are necessary in order to achieve high levels of climbing performance, although increases in handgrip strength do not necessarily guarantee high levels of climbing ability.

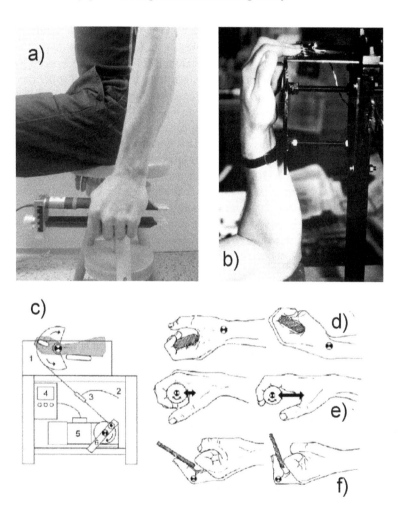

Figure 9.1 a) Handgrip dynamometry; b) finger flexor strength testing proposed by Grant et al. (1996, 2001) and lately used by MacLeod et al. (2007), Philippe et al. (2012) and Fryer et al. (2015b). The testing may be conducted in either a standing or seated position, with the shoulder and elbow flexed at 90 degrees. c–f) Isokinetic device proposed by Schweizer and Furrer (2007) to assess concentric and eccentric flexion of the wrist (d), basis of fingers (e) and proximal interphalangeal joint (f)

Climbing specific dynamometry

In an effort to develop more specific measures of finger strength, devices have been constructed that mimic the arm and hand positions typically found within climbing. One of the first attempts to assess finger flexor strength in this way was presented by Grant et al. (1996, 2001) using a custom-built apparatus (Figure 9.1b). Using the new climbing specific dynamometer advanced climbers were found to have significantly greater isometric strength than lower grade climbers and non-climbers, when normalised to body mass by linear regression (right hand, male: 446 N, 359 N, 309 N, respectively). Similar differences were found in females (right hand: 321 N, 251 N, 256 N, respectively). The reliability of maximal strength testing using similar hand and arm positions was later determined by Watts and Jensen (2003); the internal consistency of two attempts ranged from R = 0.90 to R = 0.95 for the right and left hand, respectively. R in this case represents intraclass coefficient of reliability and values greater than 0.9 indicate high reliability.

In an attempt to further improve the specificity of tests and testing devices, Schweizer and Furrer (2007) assessed dynamic finger strength. The authors used an isokinetic device to assess both the eccentric and concentric strength of the forearm flexors (Figure 9.1c). Eccentric strength of the forearm flexors is, as Schweizer and Furrer suggested, more relevant to actual climbing than concentric strength since the hold is loaded by the climber's body mass and the finger flexors absorb gravitational forces. The study in question found significant correlation between climbers red-point performance and both concentric and eccentric strength, relative to body mass, in three tests: wrist flexion, R = 0.50 and R = 0.57 (concentric and eccentric contraction, respectively); flexion on the basis of fingers, R = 0.47 and R = 0.48; and flexion of the proximal interphalangeal (PIP) joint, R = 0.32 and R = 0.32 (Figure 9.1d–f). Interestingly, the greatest relationship with performance was found in the least specific movement – concentric wrist flexion. The authors postulate that this is due to a fear of executing a movement involving the PIP joint, as this movement induces an extreme load on pulleys A2, A3 and A4 with a high risk of inducing a pulley rupture. It is also speculated by the authors that the high correlation between wrist flexion and climbing performance was due to the biomechanics of wrist flexion; 58 per cent of wrist flexion is provided by the finger flexors (m. digitorum profundus (FDP), m. digitorum superficialis (FDS)) and 42 per cent by the wrist flexors (flexor carpi ulnaris, flexor carpi radialis). As such, high levels of wrist strength are reflected by a high degree of finger flexor strength.

Finger strength difference in boulderers and lead climbers

Wall, Starek, Fleck, and Byrnes (2004) asked both boulderers and lead climbers to apply external force to a hold two distal joints deep, placed directly above the shoulder, with the climber in a kneeling position with their arm flexed 180° at the shoulder and completely extended at the elbow. The levels of strength recorded were associated with bouldering performance to a greater degree (R = 0.67) than lead routes (R = 0.50), confirming the greater importance of finger flexor strength in bouldering. Similarly, the finger strength of competitive boulderers has been evaluated using a two finger grip on a 10 mm deep hold (Michailov et al., 2009). Values of strength correlated with highest red point (RP) boulder ascent outside (R = 0.63) to a greater degree than placement in a World Cup competition (R = 0.50). In a development over previous finger strength research, Fanchini et al. (2013) highlighted the importance of neuromuscular activation speed in bouldering – the ability to develop high forces on a small hold in as shorter time as possible. The authors found that whilst maximal strength was slightly higher in boulderers than in lead climbers (~14 per cent), the rate of force development was substantially greater (~36 per cent). Further research suggests that bouldering may also be distinguished from lead climbing by shorter duration of ascents (~30 s versus ~2–7 min), greater number of route attempts, shorter time spent in static contractions (25 per cent versus 37 per cent of total climb time) and more powerful movements (Billat, Palleja, Charlaix, Rizzardo, & Janel, 1995; White & Olsen, 2010).

The role of arm position on finger flexor strength development

The moderate relationships found between finger strength and climbing performance, in the aforementioned studies, indicates that the tests were either not sufficiently specific, or that they are also influenced by other important factors, such as power, flexibility, technique, tactics or psychological factors. In the previously discussed studies, several different custom-made devices were used, with varying grips and body positions, inevitably requiring different types of contractions and/or muscle activation. The following section describes the role of arm and body position and the effect of grip when assessing finger flexor strength.

During sport climbing typically the arm is placed in a position where the shoulder is at greater than 90° abduction or flexion when applying force to a hold. Consequently, arm position should be taken into consideration when testing the finger flexors, as non-specific positions may lead to results with lower validity to climbing performance. The effect of arm position on maximal finger flexor strength has been evaluated in four positions (Baláš, Panáčková, et al., 2014), handgrip with arm near the body extended at the elbow (Figure 9.2c), 90/90 position (Figure 9.2d, e), 130/50 position (Figure 9.2f), 180/0 position (Figure 9.2g). The highest variability explained by climbing ability in finger strength was found in the 180/0 ($\eta_p^2 = 0.25$) and 130/50 positions ($\eta_p^2 = 0.25$), whilst the variability in the 90/90 position was slightly lower ($\eta_p^2 = 0.16$). The handgrip test had the lowest validity to reported climbing ability ($\eta_p^2 = 0.05$). It was concluded that positions 180/0 and 130/50 are most suitable for the assessment of finger flexor strength in climbers. The results are in agreement with Watts et al.'s (2008) earlier findings, who recorded greater EMG activity in common climbing movements in comparison to maximal voluntary handgrip dynamometry (Figure 9.2c). It was suggested that the force for contact with most holds in rock climbing is generated by the effect of body mass along the gravitational line. Thus, the external force pulls the hand onto the hold and muscular force must maintain the specific hand position against the external force.

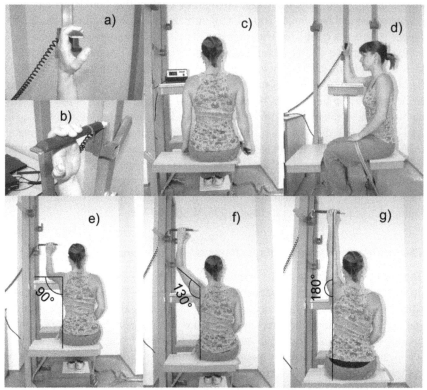

Figure 9.2 a, b) Finger position on the gauge; c) handgrip – grip strength measurement with shoulder at 0° and elbow fully extended; d, e) 90/90 position – measurement with the shoulder at 90° flexion and externally rotated at 45° on a shelf with the elbow flexed at 90°; f) 130/50 position – measurement with the shoulder abducted at 130° and elbow flexed at 50°; g) 180/0 position – measurement with the shoulder 180° flexed and elbow fully extended

Source: Baláš, Mrskoč, Panáčková, & Draper, 2014.

The role of different hand grips

The most common grips used in climbing are the open hand (Figure 9.3a), half crimp, full crimp (Figure 9.3b), pinch grip, and one or two fingers grips (Figure 9.3c, d). The way in which a hold is grasped substantially changes the muscle activation of the forearm flexors (Watts et al., 2008). The most commonly analysed grips are the full crimp and open handed grips (Schöffl et al., 2009; Schweizer, 2001; Schweizer & Hudek, 2011). Climbers, when gripping small holds, often prefer the full crimp grip; however, it induces greater load on finger pulleys (Schweizer, 2001; Vigouroux, Quaine, Labarre-Vila, & Moutet, 2006). To learn more about the biomechanical principles of grip positions, the reader is referred to Chapter 8. Finger flexion is enabled by the activity of the FDP and FDS. The degree of activation of the finger flexors depends on the hold size (Schweizer & Hudek, 2011). In the open

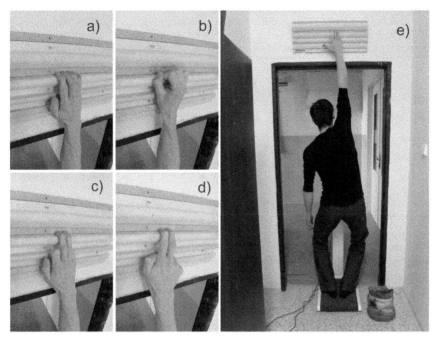

Figure 9.3 The four different grips and the position on the scale: a) open grip; b) crimp grip; c) middle and ring fingers; d) index and middle fingers; e) the basic position on the scale

Source: Baláš, Mrskoč, et al., 2014.

grip and crimp grip on very small holds there is greater activation of FDP than the FDS. The FDS demonstrates greater recruitment when using the crimp grip on larger holds. The effect of hold depth (1, 2, 3, 4 cm) and grip (full crimp, half-crimp, open) on vertical force production has been analysed by Amca et al. (2012). The authors reported greater vertical forces with increased hold depth with an open grip. However, a plateau of maximal vertical force production with the crimp grip was attained on small holds (2 cm) with small decline in vertical force on large holds (>3 cm). To summarise, when testing both open and crimp grips, the hold should be between ~2 and ~3 cm deep to facilitate the production of maximal contractions.

When testing maximal finger strength, grip preferences should also be taken into consideration, as testing an open grip may not necessarily assess maximal specific finger strength if the preferred grip is a crimp grip. Moreover, depending on the flexor being assessed the size of the hold should be taken into consideration as a small hold does not provide the opportunity for high levels of activation in the FDS. It is also worth considering that in the crimp grip, the thumb is frequently used over the index finger. The use of the may increase the strength by another 17–20 per cent without any negative increase in pulley load (Amca et al., 2012; Quaine, Vigouroux, Paclet, & Colloud, 2011).

The validity of four different grips during maximal finger strength testing has been assessed using electronic scales (Figure 9.3e) (Baláš, Mrskoč, et al., 2014).

Table 9.1 Bivariate (in italic) and partial correlations (bold) among climbing abilities (RP, OS) and finger strength in four different grip positions – open grip, crimp grip, index + middle finger (II+III), middle + ring (III + IV) finger. The partial correlation is used to control for the effect of body mass

	RP	OS	Open grip	Crimp grip	II+III	III+IV	Body mass
RP	1	0.968	0.628	0.625	0.521	0.636	–0.131
On sight	**0.968**	1	0.638	0.648	0.541	0.647	–0.121
Open grip	**0.806**	**0.811**	1	0.908	0.871	0.847	0.498
Crimp grip	**0.788**	**0.808**	**0.880**	1	0.823	0.856	0.476
II+III	**0.677**	**0.694**	**0.830**	**0.770**	1	0.860	0.490
III+IV	**0.746**	**0.753**	**0.821**	**0.831**	**0.836**	1	0.375

Source: Baláš, Mrskoč, et al., 2014.

The open grip, crimp grip, index and middle fingers, and middle and ring fingers were tested on a 2.3 cm deep wooden rung. Testing scores showed high internal consistency (R = 0.88–0.97) and test–retest reliability (R = 0.88–0.94) with standard error of measurement ranging between 22 N and 53 N. Table 9.1 shows bivariate and partial correlations between maximal strength in the four grips and climbing ability. A high association of absolute strength and strength to body mass ratio were found for all grips. The highest association was reported for the four fingers positions and lowest association for index and ring finger grip. The relationship for crimp ($R^2 = 0.62$) and open grip ($R^2 = 0.66$) positions to climbing performance is the highest recorded value found in relation to all previous studies concerning finger strength; this may be explained by the use of a suitable grip size and arm position during the testing and large heterogeneous sample size, with climbing abilities ranging from IV to X (International Climbing and Mountaineering Federation; UIAA). Normative values for the different abilities are provided in Table 9.3.

Finger flexor endurance

One of the first studies to assess finger flexor endurance came from Nachbauer et al. (1987). The authors assessed a two-arm, four-finger hang on a 1 cm deep wooden rung and a one-arm finger hang on a 5 cm deep wooden rung. The reliability for the two-arm hang was satisfactorily high (R = 0.96), although lower for the one-arm hang (R = 0.82–0.89). Climbers with an ability greater than VI UIAA demonstrated significantly longer hang time on a 1 cm rung than lower grade climbers of < VI UIAA (34.1 ± 17.7 s versus 19.3 ± 15.7 s). Smaller differences were stated for the one-arm hang (right hand 22.9 ± 15.1 s; 14.0 ± 13.7 s; left hand 19.0 ± 16.7 s; 11.6 ± 10.0 s). The two-arm hang appeared more specific for the testing of finger flexor endurance. However, the use of a 1 cm deep hold, as previously discussed, is unlikely to assess the muscular endurance of FDS, major activation of which is demonstrated only on holds bigger than the length of distal finger part (Schweizer & Hudek, 2011). A finger hang on a 3 cm (2.5 cm + 0.5 cm radius) rung was found to be more suitable to test finger flexors endurance in larger samples, as it enables lower grade climbers to also hang for a short while (Baláš et al., 2012). The authors of the study stated high correlation to the climbing ability in males (R = 0.87) and females (R = 0.81). However, short hang times in lower grade climbers are likely to indicate maximal strength rather than muscular endurance. Normative values are provided in Table 9.3.

Assessing endurance Cutts and Bollen (1993) used continuous testing at 80 per cent of climbers' MVC using a hand dynamometer. Results were calculated as a force–time integral, and climbers were shown to outperform non-climbers; the force–time integral describes the amount of muscular work completed during the test. Ferguson and Brown (1997) compared continuous and intermittent testing (5 s contraction – 2 s relief) at 40 per cent MVC in climbers and non-climbers. During the continuous test, time to exhaustion was similar between the groups; however, during the intermittent tests climbers endured two times longer than non-climbers did. This was explained by greater vasodilatation capacity of the forearm muscles and therefore greater blood flow. Conversely, Grant et al. (2003) did not find any differences between climbers, rowers and aerobically trained subjects in either a continuous or intermittent test (6–4 s; 18–12 s). Testing was undertaken on the device simulating climbing grip (Figure 9.1b). Climbers showed greater MVC, and, despite similar time until failure, climbers completed the test with higher absolute levels of strength (see Table 9.2). Therefore, it is suggested that it is not only important to record time to failure, but also the level of MVC to evaluate local muscular endurance. In fact, high values of MVC were found to be negatively correlated with time of contraction (Carlson & McCraw, 1971), that is, the strongest subjects demonstrated the worst endurance time and vice versa.

The same climbing specific device was used in a similar study comparing climbers and non-climbers during continuous (40 per cent MVC) and intermittent (40 per cent MVC, 10–3 s) testing (MacLeod et al., 2007). The times to failure for both tests were similar between climbers and non-climbers; however, the force–time integral was significantly different. Moreover, a significant relationship was stated for blood re-oxygenation during 3 s relief and force–time integral ($R^2 =$ 0.41). In a similar study, Philippe et al. (2012) stated that not only were there greater values of force–time integral in the intermittent and continual tests in climbers, but also longer time until exhaustion in the intermittent test than the previous study. This might be explained by higher climbing ability in climbers from Philippe et al. (2012; OS VIII+ to X+) than MacLeod et al. (2007; OS VII+/VIII- to IX). It is, therefore, suggested that elite sport climbers have higher specific adaptation for local intermittent contraction than advanced climbers do. Recently, it has been demonstrated that these specific adaptations encompass 1) significantly higher de-oxygenation with increasing climbing ability; 2) parameters of relative re-oxygenation which are in close relationship to muscular endurance (force–time integral); 3) higher blood flow and higher heart rate in the relief period in advanced and elite climbers, indicating lower blood occlusion; 4) recovery after testing which is significantly faster in elite and advanced climbers despite reaching lower values of O_2 saturation during the contractions (Fryer, Stoner, Dickson, et al., 2015; Fryer, Stoner, Lucero, et al., 2015).

Table S Maximal voluntary contraction (MVC), continual and intermittent tests on "climbing specific" devices in males (M) and females (F) of different climbing abilities

Study	Dynamometer		MVC (N)	MVC/body mass (N·kg⁻¹)	Continuous test (s)	Intermittent test (s)	Force–time integral in the continuous test (N·s)	Force–time integral in the intermittent test (N·s)
Cutts & Bollen (1993)							80 % MVC	
Non-climbers (N=12, M)	Hand dynamometry		445 ± 59	6.3 ± 1.0			9300 ± 4000	
	Pince[a]		101 ± 17	1.4 ± 0.2			3800 ± 1400	
Climbers (N=13, M)	Hand dynamometry		507 ± 17	7.2 ± 1.2			11900 ± 4600	
	Pince[a]		143 ± 20	2.0 ± 0.3			6400 ± 2000	
Ferguson & Brown (1997)						40 % MVC		
Non-climbers (N=10, M)	Modified dynamometry		635 ± 55/660 ± 65		122 ± 14	420 ± 69[b]		
Climbers (N=5, M)			715 ± 34/730 ± 7		140 ± 11	853 ± 76[b]		
Grant et al. (2003)						40 % MVC		
Rowers (N=9, M)	'Grant' dynamometry		321 ± 50	4.1 ± 0.6	153 ± 40	1433 ± 1210[c]		
Aerobically trained (N=9, M)			288 ± 61	4.0 ± 0.8	189 ± 76	1242 ± 812[c]		
Climbers (N=9, M)			383 ± 36	5.3 ± 0.5	150 ± 54	1454 ± 1083[c]		
MacLeod et al. (2007)						40 % MVC	40 % MVC	40 % MVC
Non-climbers (N=9, M)	'Grant' dynamometry		375 ± 91	5.0 ± 1.2	105 ± 29	252 ± 107[d]	15816 ± 6263	35325 ± 9724
Climbers (N=11, M)			485 ± 65	7.4 ± 1.2	111 ± 28	278 ± 83[d]	21043 ± 4474	51769 ± 12229

					40 % MVC	40 % MVC	40 % MVC
Philippe et al. (2012)							
Non-climbers (N=6, M)	'Grant' dynamometry	402 ± 74	5.4 ± 0.6	101 ± 26	194 ± 84[d]	15929 ± 3737	30688 ± 13628
Non-climbers (N=6, F)		228 ± 32	3.6 ± 0.6	117 ± 16	205 ± 98[d]	10523 ± 7009	18042 ± 7459
Elite climbers (N=6, M)		491 ± 77	7.0 ± 1.3	93 ± 31	295 ± 244[d]	17433 ± 2879	52760 ± 33731
Elite climbers (N=6, F)		312 ± 57	5.8 ± 1.3	132 ± 54	453 ± 241[d]	15609 ± 4819	53023 ± 25048
Fryer et al. (2015a, b)					40 % MVC	40 % MVC	40 % MVC
Non-climbers (N=9, MF)	'Grant' dynamometry	245 ± 60	3.2 ± 1.1	107 ± 43	246 ± 132[d]	10799 ± 5882	25524 ± 16007
Intermediate (N=9, MF)		273 ± 72	3.4 ± 0.6	175 ± 105	332 ± 128[d]	17391 ± 5933	33717 ± 7646
Advanced (N=10, MF)		299 ± 57	4.2 ± 0.6	141 ± 56	264 ± 60[d]	16826 ± 7435	31990 ± 11463
Elite (N=10, MF)		412 ± 141	5.9 ± 1.8	102 ± 39	365 ± 267[d]	15605 ± 4830	53252 ± 29984

Notes:
a Pince grip: index and middle finger in opposition to thumb using hand dynamometer
b 5 s contraction, 2 s relief
c 6 s contraction, 4 s relief
d 10 s contraction, 3 s relief

The optimal contraction–relief ratio and percentage of MVC for intermittent testing is still under debate; however, it is clear that it should be informed by actual climbing performance. During lead climbing, the time of contact between fingers and hold is typically ~10–12 s and the contraction–relief ratio was found to be between 3:1 and 7:1 (Donath, Roesner, Schöffl, & Gabriel, 2013; Schädle-Schardt, 1998). Therefore, it is suggested that the optimal relief ratio should last from ~2 to 4 s.

To conclude, testing finger flexor endurance should involve both continuous and intermittent testing. A continuous finger hang on a 2.5–3 cm rung satisfactorily differentiates climbers of differing climbing ability. However, intermittent contractions seem to provide a more valid score of local endurance and better reflect unique climbing specific physiological adaptations.

Shoulder girdle strength and power

Describing the muscular activity of the shoulder girdle in climbing represents even more of a challenge than that of the finger flexors. The shoulder girdle in conjunction with the core provide stability for the body in almost all moves and positions. The strength and power of the shoulder girdle, for example, are important when completing moves with poor foot support, whilst shoulder endurance is indispensable on long overhanging routes.

Pull-ups were one of the first tests used to assess dynamic strength in climbers (Grant et al., 1996, 2001). Advanced climbers achieved better results (males on average 16.2, SD 7.2, and females on average 2.1, SD 3.0) than lower grade climbers and non-climbers (males ~four and females ~zero pull-ups). The study identified the important role of dynamic shoulder girdle strength; however, the high number repetitions indicated that this test might not assess muscular strength, but rather muscular endurance in advanced climbers. Similarly, shoulder girdle isometric strength testing, for which the climbers were ask to pull down a handle attached to a load gauge, showed high association with lead climbing performance (R = 0.66) and bouldering (R = 0.62) (Wall et al., 2004). Isokinetic strength in flexion–extension and external–internal rotation of the shoulder has also been found to be greater in climbers than in non-climbers (Wong & Ng, 2008, 2009). Climbers demonstrated a lower ratio of flexors/extensors and external/internal rotators of shoulder. This ratio may be used as an indicator of unilateral asymmetry in sport training or rehabilitation. Unilateral muscular asymmetries are often associated with higher injury incidences, training interruptions and/or reduced capacity to produce maximal performance.

Traditional campus-board exercises have been used as a test of shoulder girdle power (Draper et al., 2011). The climber starts hanging on big holds (either shoulder width, or a wider position), then the climber initiates an explosive pull up movement subsequently releasing one hand to slap as high as possible on the scaled board above (Figure 9.4). The authors found that the score achieved was closely related to climbing ability for both variations (R = ~0.7). Based on a slightly higher correlation with climbing ability, the authors recommended a narrow variant to test the power of the shoulder girdle.

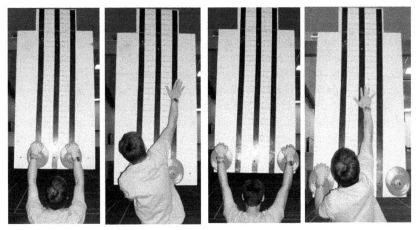

Figure 9.4 The starting and finishing position for the narrow and wide grip power tests of shoulder girdle muscles

Source: Draper et al., 2011.

A second similar test to that of Draper et al. (2011) was presented by Laffaye et al. (2014). The test starts in the same position as the previous test, hanging, with hands placed 55 cm apart. The climber then performs an explosive pull up movement releasing both hands to slap the scaled board as high as possible. The distance of the lower hand from the starting hold represents the test score. In addition to height, an accelerometer was used to record the time–force parameters. The achieved distance distinguished not only climbing ability groups but also boulderers (77.0 ± 11.3 cm) from lead climbers (61.3 ± 10.4 cm). Further, boulderers outperform lead climbers in the following areas: higher velocity 1.81 ± 0.28 versus 1.63 ± 0.59 m·s⁻¹; power related to body mass 28.4 ± 7.6 versus 23.4 ± 3.7 W·kg⁻¹; and time 743 ± 12 versus 788 ± 13 ms. The distance achieved explained only 49 per cent of the relative power (W·kg⁻¹); this was explained by the four different climbers' typology which were identified as: a) weak and slow; b) powerful and slow; c) weak and quick; d) powerful and quick. Bouldering specialists were characterised as powerful and quick, whilst lead climbers were described as either as weak and slow or weak and quick. The use of an accelerometer shows that a typical power test may not only assess the power component. Consequently, the speed of the movement is an important parameter for strength diagnostics, especially in bouldering.

Shoulder girdle endurance

The most commonly used test of shoulder girdle endurance is the bent-arm hang. Using this test, Grant et al. (1996, 2001) only found greater time to failure in advanced climbers (53.1 ± 13.2 s males and 27.5 ± 19.4 s females), whilst lower grade climbers and non-climbers displayed similar performances (~32 s males and ~14 s females). Baláš et al. (2012) found a closer relationship between this test and climbing ability in females ($R^2 = 0.64$) in comparison to males ($R^2 = 0.49$). In male climbers, the relationship was weakened by the high variability in bent-arm hang time. Differences between performances in males and females were especially apparent in lower grade climbers, which were explained by the work and leisure activities of the males. The level of muscular endurance of the shoulder girdle is similar in both sexes for higher climbing abilities. Therefore, it is suggested that training shoulder girdle muscular endurance in beginner females represents one of the main factors that would improve their climbing performance and to a lesser degree in advanced females, and male climbers. Elite climbers are able to perform very long two-arm hangs; as such a one-arm hang might be more suitable. Normative values are presented in Table 9.3.

Table 9.3 Normative values for simple strength and endurance tests related to climbing ability RP in lead climbing. Norms are based on the published data (Baláš, Mrskoč, et al., 2014; Baláš et al., 2012) with supplementary measurements

UIAA	Handgrip (kg•kg⁻¹)	Open grip (kg•kg⁻¹)	Crimp grip (kg•kg⁻¹)	III + IV (kg•kg⁻¹)	Bent-arm hang(s)	Finger hang(s)
Male climbers						
	$n = 238$	$n = 69$	$n = 69$	$n = 69$	$n = 256$	$n = 253$
4	0.56	0.43	0.44	0.37	19	0
5	0.60	0.52	0.53	0.42	29	14
6	0.64	0.61	0.62	0.48	39	28
7	0.68	0.70	0.71	0.53	49	42
8	0.72	0.79	0.80	0.59	59	56
9	0.76	0.89	0.89	0.65	68	70
10	0.79	0.98	0.98	0.70	78	84
11	0.83	1.07	1.07	0.76	88	98
12	0.87	1.16	1.16	0.81	98	112
13	0.91	1.25	1.25	0.87	108	126
Female climbers						
	$n = 147$	$n = 53$	$n = 53$	$n = 53$	$n = 172$	$n = 172$
4	0.45	0.39	0.44	0.31	12	0
5	0.50	0.47	0.52	0.38	21	13
6	0.55	0.55	0.60	0.45	31	28
7	0.60	0.63	0.68	0.52	40	43
8	0.65	0.71	0.76	0.59	50	58
9	0.70	0.79	0.84	0.66	60	73
10	0.75	0.87	0.92	0.73	69	88
11	0.80	0.95	1.00	0.80	79	103
12	0.85	1.03	1.08	0.87	89	118

Summary

- Isometric finger strength and endurance, and shoulder girdle power, strength and endurance increase with climbing ability level.
- Testing climbing specific strength and endurance should correspond to actual climbing positions and movements.
- Handgrip dynamometry is not a suitable test for finger strength assessment in climbers.
- Four finger positions, hold depth 2–3 cm and arm position in shoulder flexion are recommended when testing finger strength and endurance.
- Boulderers outperform lead climbers in finger strength and shoulder girdle power.

Acknowledgements

Special thanks to David Giles for his valuable comments and help with the English translation.

References

Amca, A. M., Vigouroux, L., Aritan, S., & Berton, E. (2012). Effect of hold depth and grip technique on maximal finger forces in rock climbing. *Journal of Sports Sciences, 30*(7), 669–677.

Baláš, J., Mrskoč, J., Panáčková, M., & Draper, N. (2014). Sport-specific finger flexor strength assessment using electronic scales in sport climbers. *Sports Technology, 7*(3–4), 151–158.

Baláš, J., Panáčková, M., Kodejška, J., Cochrane, D., & Martin, A. J. (2014). The role of arm position during finger flexor strength measurement in sport climbers. *International Journal of Performance Analysis in Sport, 14*(2), 345–354.

Baláš, J., Pecha, O., Martin, A. J., & Cochrane, D. (2012). Hand-arm strength and endurance as predictors of climbing performance. *European Journal of Sport Science, 12*(1), 16–25.

Billat, V., Palleja, P., Charlaix, T., Rizzardo, P., & Janel, N. (1995). Energy specificity of rock climbing and aerobic capacity in competitive sport rock climbers. *Journal of Sports Medicine and Physical Fitness, 35*(1), 20–24.

Carlson, B. R., & McCraw, L. W. (1971). Isometric strength and relative isometric endurance. *Research Quarterly, 42*(3), 244–250.

Cormie, P., McGuigan, M. R., & Newton, R. U. (2011). Developing maximal neuromuscular power: part 1 – biological basis of maximal power production. *Sports Medicine, 41*(1), 17–38.

Cutts, A., & Bollen, S. R. (1993). Grip strength and endurance in rock climbers. *Proceedings of the Institution of Mechanical Engineers, Part H: Journal of Engineering in Medicine, 207*(2), 87–92.

Donath, L., Roesner, K., Schöffl, V., & Gabriel, H. H. W. (2013). Work-relief ratios and imbalances of load application in sport climbing: another link to overuse-induced injuries? *Scandinavian Journal of Medicine & Science in Sports, 23*(4), 406–414.

Draper, N., Dickson, T., Blackwell, G., Priestley, S., Fryer, S., Marshall, H., … Ellis, G. (2011). Sport-specific power assessment for rock climbing. *Journal of Sports Medicine and Physical Fitness, 51*(3), 417–425.

España-Romero, V., Ortega, F. B., Vicente-Rodriguez, G., Artero, E. G., Rey, J. P., & Ruiz, J. R. (2010). Elbow position affects handgrip strength in adolescents: validity and reliability of jamar, dynex, and TKK dynamometers. *Journal of Strength and Conditioning Research, 24*(1), 272–277.

Fanchini, M., Violette, F., Impellizzeri, F. M., & Maffiuletti, N. A. (2013). Differences in climbing-specific strength between boulder and lead rock climbers. *Journal of Strength and Conditioning Research, 27*(2), 310–314.

Ferguson, R. A., & Brown, M. D. (1997). Arterial blood pressure and forearm vascular conductance responses to sustained and rhythmic isometric exercise and arterial occlusion in trained rock climbers and untrained sedentary subjects. *European Journal of Applied Physiology & Occupational Physiology, 76*(2), 174–180.

Fryer, S., Stoner, L., Dickson, T., Draper, S. B., McCluskey, M. J., Hughes, J. D., ... Draper, N. (2015a). Oxygen recovery kinetics in the forearm flexors of multiple ability groups of rock climbers. *Journal of Strength and Conditioning Research, 29*(6), 1633–1639.

Fryer, S., Stoner, L., Lucero, A., Witter, T., Scarrott, C., Dickson, T., ... Draper, N. (2015b). Haemodynamic kinetics and intermittent finger flexor performance in rock climbers. *International Journal of Sports Medicine, 36*(2), 137–142.

Grant, S., Hasler, T., Davies, C., Aitchison, T. C., Wilson, J., & Whittaker, A. (2001). A comparison of the anthropometric, strength, endurance and flexibility characteristics of female elite and recreational climbers and non-climbers. *Journal of Sports Sciences, 19*(7), 499–505.

Grant, S., Hynes, V., Whittaker, A., & Aitchison, T. (1996). Anthropometric, strength, endurance and flexibility characteristics of elite and recreational climbers. *Journal of Sports Sciences, 14*(4), 301–309.

Grant, S., Shields, C., Fitzpatrick, V., Ming Loh, W., Whitaker, A., Watt, I., & Kay, J. W. (2003). Climbing-specific finger endurance: a comparative study of intermediate rock climbers, rowers and aerobically trained individuals. *Journal of Sports Sciences, 21*(8), 621–630.

Heyward, V. H., & Gibson, A. L. (2014). *Advanced fitness assessment and exercise prescription* (7 ed.). Champaign, IL: Human Kinetics.

Laffaye, G., Collin, J. M., Levernier, G., & Padulo, J. (2014). Upper-limb power test in rock-climbing. *International Journal of Sports Medicine, 35*(8), 670–675.

MacLeod, D., Sutherland, D. L., Buntin, L., Whitaker, A., Aitchison, T., Watt, I., ... Grant, S. (2007). Physiological determinants of climbing-specific finger endurance and sport rock climbing performance. *Journal of Sports Sciences, 25*(12), 1433–1443.

Mermier, C. M., Janot, J. M., Parker, D. L., & Swan, J. G. (2000). Physiological and anthropometric determinants of sport climbing performance. *British Journal of Sports Medicine, 34*, 359–366.

Michailov, M. (2014). Workload characteristics, performance limiting factors and methods for strength and endurance training in rock climbing. *Medicina Sportiva, 18*(3), 97–106.

Michailov, M., Mladenov, L., & Schöffl, V. (2009). Anthropometric and strength characteristics of world-class boulderers. *Medicina Sportiva, 13*(4), 231–238.

Nachbauer, W., Fetz, F., & Burtscher, M. (1987). Testprofil zur Erfassung spezieller sportmotorischer Eigenschaften der Felskletterer. / A testprofile for gathering specific sport-motor characteristics of rock climbers. *Sportwissenschaft, 17*(4), 423–438.

Peolsson, A., Hedlund, R., & Oberg, B. (2001). Intra- and inter-tester reliability and reference values for hand strength. *Journal of Rehabilitation Medicine, 33*(1), 36–41.

Philippe, M., Wegst, D., Muller, T., Raschner, C., & Burtscher, M. (2012). Climbing-specific finger flexor performance and forearm muscle oxygenation in elite male and female sport climbers. *European Journal of Applied Physiology, 112*(8), 2839–2847.

Quaine, F., Vigouroux, L., Paclet, F., & Colloud, F. (2011). The thumb during the crimp grip. *International Journal of Sports Medicine, 32*(1), 49–53.

Schädle-Schardt, W. (1998). Die zeitliche Gestaltung von Belastung und Entlastung im Wettkampfklettern als Element der Trainingssteuerung [The temporal organization of loading and unloading in competitive climbing as an attribute of training]. *Leistungssport, 28*(1), 23–28.

Schöffl, I., Oppelt, K., Juengert, J., Schweizer, A., Neuhuber, W., & Schöffl, V. (2009). The influence of the crimp and slope grip position on the finger pulley system. *Journal of Biomechanics, 42*(13), 2183–2187.

Schweizer, A. (2001). Biomechanical properties of the crimp grip position in rock climbers. *Journal of Biomechanics, 34*(2), 217–223.

Schweizer, A., & Furrer, M. (2007). Correlation of forearm strength and sport climbing performance. *Isokinetics and Exercise Science, 15*(3), 211–216.

Schweizer, A., & Hudek, R. (2011). Kinetics of crimp and slope grip in rock climbing. *Journal of Applied Biomechanics, 27*(2), 116–121.

Vanderburgh, P. M., Mahar, M. T., & Chou, C. H. (1995). Allometric scaling of grip strength by body mass in college-age men and women. *Research Quarterly for Exercise and Sport, 66*(1), 80–84.

Vigouroux, L., Quaine, F., Labarre-Vila, A., & Moutet, F. (2006). Estimation of finger muscle tendon tensions and pulley forces during specific sport-climbing grip techniques. *Journal of Biomechanics, 39*(14), 2583–2592.

Wall, C. B., Starek, J. E., Fleck, S. J., & Byrnes, W. C. (2004). Prediction of indoor climbing performance in women rock climbers. *Journal of Strength and Conditioning Research, 18*(1), 77–83.

Watts, P. B. (2004). Physiology of difficult rock climbing. *European Journal of Applied Physiology, 91*, 361–372.

Watts, P. B., & Jensen, R. L. (2003). Reliability of peak forces during a finger curl motion common in rock climbing. *Measurement in Physical Education and Exercise Science, 7*(4), 263–267.

Watts, P. B., Jensen, R. L., Gannon, E., Kobeinia, R., Maynard, J., & Sansom, J. (2008). Forearm EMG during rock climbing differs from EMG during handgrip dynamometry. *International Journal of Exercise Science, 1*(1), 4–13.

Watts, P. B., Martin, D. T., & Durtschi, S. (1993). Anthropometric profiles of elite male and female competitive sport rock climbers. *Journal of Sports Sciences, 11*, 113–117.

White, D. J., & Olsen, P. D. (2010). A time motion analysis of bouldering style competitive rock climbing. *Journal of Strength and Conditioning Research, 24*(5), 1356–1360.

Wong, E. K. L., & Ng, G. Y. F. (2008). Isokinetic work profile of shoulder flexors and extensors in sport climbers and nonclimbers. *Journal of Orthopaedic & Sports Physical Therapy, 38*(9), 572–577.

Wong, E. K. L., & Ng, G. Y. F. (2009). Strength profiles of shoulder rotators in healthy sport climbers and nonclimbers. *Journal of Athletic Training, 44*(5), 527–530.

Zatsiorsky, V. M., & Kraemer, W. J. (2006). *Science and practice of strength training* (2nd edition). Champaign, IL: Human Kinetics.

10 Biomechanics of ice tool swinging movement

*Annie Rouard, Thomas Robert and
Ludovic Seifert*

Ice climbing has recently been introduced as a competitive practice and involves quadruped locomotion with ice tools in each hand and crampons on each foot. Progression results in contradictory actions: the climber has to determine the best target, followed by a swinging motion to anchor the axe, combining accuracy and strength, so that the climber can pull on the axe to climb up the cliff. Finally, the axe is unanchored by the climber. These successive actions are frequently repeated during progression resulting in fatigue conditions. Analyses of competitions indicates that performance is related to shorter times either for anchor or swing. Low expertise climbers spend more time in static conditions to find the target, using symmetric location of four supports resulting in greater fatigue. Biomechanical data suggests that experts adjust their movement to the kind of ice axe. They are characterized by highly controlled coordination of the upper limb joints. The cocking phase appeared with a proximo-distal coordination associated to lower muscular co-activations, the movement successively involving shoulder, elbow and wrist. The strike phase is characterised by high joint moments with peak co-activations just before the impact, the upper limb stiffening in order to transmit maximal force and velocity to the pick. The distal wrist joint controls the accuracy of the impact. The high co-activations of the digitorum muscles allowed a strong hanging that was very important to transmit force, velocity and accuracy from the upper limb to the axis. Fatigue affects the grasping muscles more than the muscles involved in the ballistic movement.

Introduction

As highlighted in Chapter 1, mountain climbing has changed tremendously since the mid-18th century. This transformation is reflected both in the variety of types of climbing that can be adopted to ascend a rock face or mountain, and in the corresponding technologies (e.g. ropes, camming devices, bolts, synthetic fibre boots, ice tools and crampons) available to individuals who attempt to achieve such heights. Although ice climbing is a recent type of practice that appeared in the 1970s, it's a good example of such transformation, because it now varies from 'pure' ice climbing to dry-tooling (i.e. ice tools and crampons are used for mixed route where rock alternates with ice) (Duez, 2009). As emphasized by Blanc-Gras and Ibarra (2012) and Duez (2009) the shape of ice tools and crampons changed through the decades and as did the types of practice (e.g. mountaineering, ice climbing, dry-tooling); for instance, the shaft of the ice tool can be more or less curved and its blade can be more or less inclined (~60° between blade and nail of shaft for ice climbing tool), which modify the centre of mass of the ice tool (Blanc-Gras & Ibarra, 2012) (see later in the chapter for further discussion about inertial parameters of the various ice tools).

Moreover, ice climbing is one of very few physical activities recently introduced either as competitive sport, or recreational pursuit, and/or complementary practice of rock climbing. Indeed, World Cup and World championship competitions in ice climbing started in 2002 with two types of competition – speed and lead difficulty climbing – regulated by the International Climbing and Mountaineering Federation (UIAA) (http://www.iceclimbingworldcup.org/rules-and-regulations.html). These competitions take place on artificial ice structure presenting ice and rock parts with fixed holds. Although the icy part of the climbing structure is cleaned by the organizers, competitive ice climbing mainly corresponds to hook existing hole on the ice structure or hold on the rocky structure. Ice climbing in natural environment mostly requires cleaning the icefall when the climber performs the first ascent and following by a mix of swinging an hooking actions of the ice tools (Seifert et al., 2014). As ice climbing is very new competitive practice, the scientific literature is scarce and does not focus on the ice tool swinging movement. Therefore, the first section of this chapter presents an overview of ice tool swinging by providing the characteristics of ice climbing both in competition and in traditional practice. The second section presents a biomechanical analysis of the swinging movement. The third section studies the effect of isometric fatigue on the swinging movement. The fourth section investigates the effect of the stick shape of the ice tool (by comparing three types of ice tools) on the swinging movement, reporting biomechanical and subjective experience analyses. The final section addresses practical applications for climbers.

Overview of the activity

Ice climbing involves quadruped locomotion as climbers ascend a vertical frozen waterfall surface with ice tools in each hand and crampons on each foot. Only the extremities of these tools are anchored in the frozen waterfall surface. Moreover, although ice climbers attempt to determine their own climbing paths during traditional practice, skilled coordination of upper and lower limbs emerges from the interaction of each climber with the specific properties of the icefall during ascent. This is because specific patterns of coordination and the quality of the ice could not be totally identified before starting to climb. Indeed, key properties of the icefall (e.g. shape, steepness, temperature, thickness and ice density) vary stochastically through the ascent, dependent on specific weather patterns, the ambient temperature throughout the climb (when a part of the icefall switches from shadow to sun) and the altitude of the location. These environmental properties are not completely under the control of the climber, and probe the skills of each individual to interact and to actualize with his environment. As explained in Chapter 11, expert ice climbers are able to exploit a larger range of coordination patterns (horizontal, diagonal, vertical and crossed located angular positions between right and left support) and types of action (e.g. swinging and hooking) than beginners (Seifert et al., 2014). Indeed, beginners principally swing their ice tools to create their own holes and rarely hook existing holes in the icefall (Seifert et al., 2014). Second, experts are able to detect various sources of regulating information (e.g. size, depth and shape of the holes in the icefall), specifying a range of functional actions (e.g. swinging versus hooking), whereas beginners would tend to perceive global, structural icefall characteristics (e.g. existing steps in icefall), which may not specify actions and would explain the lower climbing fluency of beginners (Seifert et al., 2014). Third, analysis of the subjective experience of expert ice climbers shows that the ice tools are not external components in the actions/cognitions of experts (Adé, Gal-Petitfaux, Seifert, & Poizat, 2016). In action, ice tools amplify and make manifest what might have remained vague or even unnoticed in their absence. For example, the sounds of the blade striking the ice and the vibrations felt in the forearm via the axe shaft provides climbers with vital information about the quality of the ice and the adequacy of the anchor sites, thereby letting them make appropriate adaptations (Adé et al., 2016). On this basis, expertise in ice climbing also means an 'expert coupling' between the climber, the ice tools and the environment. These characteristics of expertise may be also observed during ice climbing competitions. However, no published studies exist about skills used during ice climbing competitions. Therefore, we have analysed the world cup that occurred at Champagny (France) in 2014 (http://www.iceclimbingworldcup.org/events-15-UIAA-Ice-Climbing-World-Cup-Champagny-en-Vanoise-France-2014.html).

Our analysis was based on 21 women who competed in the lead ice climbing competition. They climbed an artificial icefall of 24 m that could be divided in three sections: a vertical icy section, an overhang icy section and a dry-tooling section. Among these 21 climbers, 10 of them fell, 6 of them did not complete the route before the time limit and 5 of them completed the whole route. The mean time for the non-finishers was 240 seconds (s) to complete the vertical icy section while the finishers took 120 s. The longer ascent durations of the non-finishers might come from the longer anchor time of the ice tools (8 s versus 5 s for the finishers) and of the crampons (6 s versus 4 s for the finishers), reflecting more isometric efforts. The longer ascent durations of the non-finishers were also characterized by a higher number of ice tool swinging actions (32 versus 23 actions for the finishers). In sum, the analysis of the world cup emphasized that to be successful, the finishers switch more quickly to the next support (i.e. using dynamic moves and anticipatory strategies) whereas the non-finishers spent more time isometric to secure their anchorage, which would reflect a strategy to control body equilibrium. Our observation confirmed previous studies showing that the lack of expertise is highly related to too much time spent in static conditions using symmetric location of hands and feet supports (Seifert, Coeurjolly, Hérault, Wattebled, & Davids,

2013; Seifert et al., 2014). Security reasons might explain this need to maintain controlled body equilibrium because, as observed in those previous studies (Seifert et al., 2013; Seifert et al., 2014), the non-finishers performed numerous swinging actions of the ice tools before the definitive anchorage and the pulling action of the arms. The criteria of a safe anchorage are an optimum depth of the blade and a stable position (i.e. immobility) of the blade during anchorage.

Biomechanical approach of the swinging movement

One of the critical aspects of the ice climbing activity is the swinging movement that leads to securely and efficiently placing the axe into the ice. The strike motion must fulfil several objectives that may be contradictory:

- It is a ballistic motion that must be accurate, as the targeted area may be small.
- It must lead to a safe and secured axe placement, so that the climber can pull on the axe to climb up the cliff, but the axe should not be too strongly anchored as it has to be unanchored by the climber as he moves up.
- It must be energetically efficient in order to limit the amount of fatigue induced.

In addition, this motion is repeated several times during a climb, alternating with a pulling motion (to move up) and unanchoring the ice tools in critical conditions:

- non-standardized environment, often in extreme conditions (cold, humidity);
- precarious and unusual balance;
- tiring overhead arm posture and limited toe stance.

The strike motion in ice climbing thus has to combine strength, balance and accuracy. Because of these different constraints, the nature of the motion is not obvious: is it an accuracy motion, a hammering task or a throwing type of motion? How does the climber manage to compromise strength versus accuracy? What are the effects of fatigue?

In order to answer these questions, an experiment was designed to observe and quantify the strike motion of expert ice climbers. Participants were asked to perform series of 30 strike motions, whose objective was to securely anchor their axe in 'dry ice' (designed by Entre-prises©, http://www.entre-prises.fr) on self-defined targets (Figure 10.1, left panel). The only constraint was to secure the axe placement. Three different ice tools were used (Petzl©: Quark, Nomic and Ergo; Figure 10.2).

A motion capture system (Vicon MX T20; Vicon Motion Systems, 100 Hz) was used to record the three dimensional (3D) trajectories of the reflective markers placed on specific anatomical points on the climber, and point on the handle, shaft and blade of the ice axes (Figure 10.1). Joint angles were computed using a global optimization inverse kinematic procedure (Wang et al., 2005). This automated procedure consists of positioning a kinematic model of the upper body at each time frame, initially personalized to the subject being studied, so that markers located on this model best matched their measured 3D positions. The corresponding net

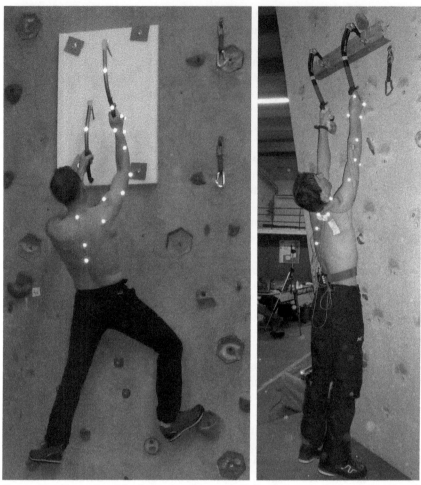

Figure 10.1 Example of the ice tool striking task (left panel) and of the exhaustion task (right panel)

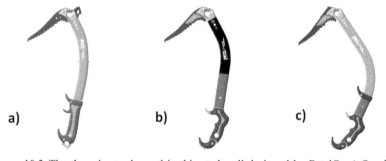

Figure 10.2 The three ice tools used in this study, all designed by Petzl©: a) Quark, b) Nomic and c) Ergo

joint torques were estimated using an inverse dynamic procedure (Robert et al., 2013). At the same time, muscular activation was recorded with surface electrodes on the main muscles of the hand, elbow and shoulder (model P3X8, Biometrics Ltd, UK, 100 Hz). To evaluate the effectiveness of the strike, the characteristics of the ice/axe impact were also analysed: accuracy (distance between the self-selected target and the hit point), orientation at impact (angle between the pick tip/head line and the perpendicular to the wall) and the pick tip's impact velocity.

Results indicated that the striking motion of expert climbers was characterized by an accurate location of impact with a mean distance between the impacted point and the targeted point of less than 2 cm (Robert et al., 2013). Interestingly, the mean velocity of the pick's tip at the time of impact was very consistent (8.03 ± 0.55 m.s^1) although the velocity was not an explicit constraint. Haake et al. (1997) reported similar values (9 m.s^{-1}) for a typical strike on ice suggesting that such magnitude of impact velocity is required to anchor and thus characterizes expert ice climbers.

Another very repeatable impact characteristic is the angle of the pick at the time of impact for all the subjects and the repetitions. The value of the angle formed by the pick's tip and the axe head depended on the type of axe (Figure 10.3). This invariant angle across climbers and the capacity to adapt it to the pick's geometry may reflect that the tool configuration determines the spatial component of the strike.

Similar to throwing motions (Rash and Shapiro, 1995), the strike motion consists of two phases: the cocking phase, that is, the movement of the ice axe away from the ice until its maximal backward position, happens during the first two thirds of the total movement duration; and the striking phase, from the maximal backward position of the ice axe's head to the impact on the ice, takes place during the last third of the motion.

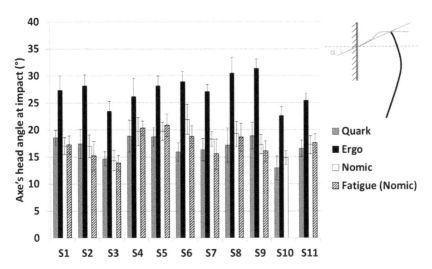

Figure 10.3 Angle (average ± SD across trials) between the horizontal and the line joining the axe's tip and axe's head for the 11 subjects (S1 to S11) and in four different conditions: before fatigue with the three different axes and after fatigue with one of them (Nomic)

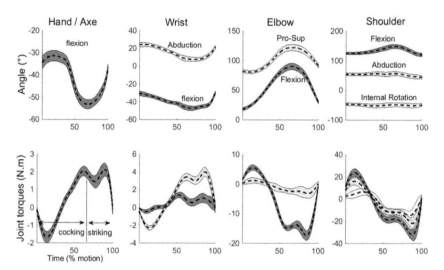

Figure 10.4 Example of joint angles for a typical subject (average ± SD across trials) related to the time (in percentage of the total time of the swing)

Apart the fact that the striking phase is about two times faster, kinematics during both phases appear very similar, with joint angles showing almost the same patterns (Figure 10.4). In other words, backward ice axe motion (cocking) resembles a slower inverse striking motion.

Although the similar kinematic patterns, muscular activations differed for both phases with lower activations and a proximo-distal coordination for the long cocking phase and a "block" one during the strike (i.e. all muscles strongly activated simultaneously) (Figure 10.5).

The cocking was initiated by the deltoidus anterior activation with co-activations of the teres major to stabilize the scapula. The elbow flexion during this phase was performed with low activations of the biceps brachii that could reflect the possible use of gravity to flex the elbow. Activation of the extensor carpi reflected the wrist extension during this cocking swing when moderate co-activation of extensor and flexor digitorum indicated the muscular cost to hang the axe.

These muscular activations led to movements outside the classical functional axes, characterized, for the cocking phase, by extension *and* abduction of the wrist, and flexion *and* supination of the elbow, with opposite motions for the striking phase.

The joints extension during the striking phase started by the activation of the main elbow extensor (triceps brachii) following by simultaneous peak activities for all the studied muscles of all the joints just before the impact. The simultaneous activations of all the upper limb muscles could be related to task accuracy as observed in pointing movements by Laursen et al. (1998), Gribble et al. (2003), and Itaguchi and Fukuzawa (2012). Mainly this result suggests a stiffening of the joints, the upper limb being like a mono-articular structure to transmit the high joint torques produced during the striking phase to the pick (Robert et al., 2013). Similar peak torques about 50 to 70 per cent of the averaged male static force capacity (Chaffin et al., 2006)

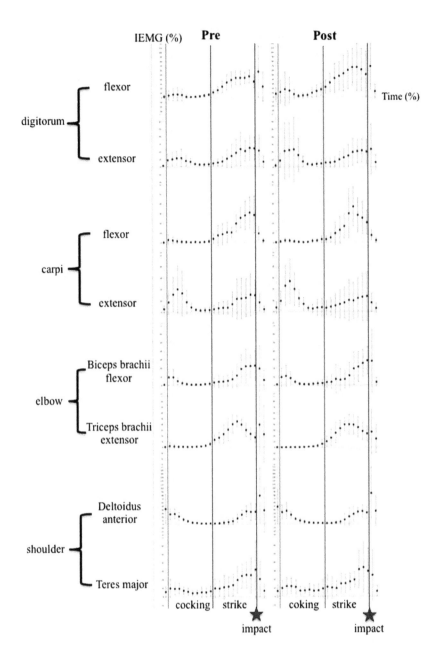

Figure 10.5 Normalized integrated electro-myographic signal (IEMG) (%) for the two phases (cocking/strike) for upper limb muscles: digitorum (flexor and extensor), carpi (flexor and extensor), elbow (biceps and triceps brachii) and shoulder (deltoidus anterior and teres major), before (Pre) and after fatigue (Post)

were reported for other striking activities (Elliot et al., 2003). They were nonetheless lower than those observed in elite American football quarterback throwers (e.g. Rash & Shapiro, 1995).

Looking at ranges of motion, we can first observe that the shoulder is relatively weakly mobilized compared to other joints, in particular to the elbow (Figure 10.6). This should be mitigated by the fact that, because of a longer level arm, shoulder rotations induce larger motions in the axe head.

Also interesting is the motion between the ice tool and the hand's palm: we observed quite a large rotation (about 30°) of the tool relative to the hand in the axe's plane. The small standard deviations either for kinematics or wrist electromyographic signal (EMG) reflected a consistent and repeatable motion (Figure 10.5). These results clearly indicated a controlled movement of the distal wrist joint. The compliance of the distal joint allowed controlling the accuracy of the impact.

Nonetheless, the striking motion appears to be distributed among all the arm joints, starting from the shoulder. These results were in accordance with the leading joint hypothesis (LJH) (Dounskaia, 2010) suggesting that joints of a multi-articular limb play different roles in movement production according to their mechanical subordination in the joint linkage. There is one leading joint (shoulder) that conditions the other joints' actions (elbow and wrist). The movement of the upper arm joints were performed in the same planar motion of the axe's head. This relation of motions along individual degrees of freedom had already been observed and reported in several motions such as hammering (Schoenmarklin and

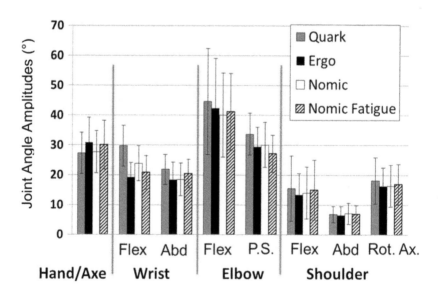

Figure 10.6 Joint angles amplitude (average ± SD across subjects and trials) for the different arm's degrees of freedom in four different conditions: before fatigue with the three different axes and after fatigue with one of them (Nomic).Flex: flexion; Abd: abduction; P.S.: prono-supination; Rot. Ax.: axial rotation

Marras, 1989) or throwing (Moritomo et al., 2007). This strategy seems indeed interesting to induce a higher pick impact velocity by summing the angular velocities and joint torques of shoulder–elbow and wrist joints.

At the opposite, higher co-activation was observed for digitorum muscles to stiff the hanging axe. The fingers' stiffness allowed velocity and accuracy to be transmitted to the axe producing better anchoring. This result indicated the main contribution of the gripping task in the ice climbing striking movement.

Finally, kinematics results indicate strong continuity of the joint angles between both phases indicating the importance of the cocking phrase for the performance of the striking phase. From the muscular point of view, the cocking phase allows the muscles responsible for the striking movement to be stretched. These stretch-shortening successive actions probably increase muscular efficiency as observed in other sports such as vertical jump (van Ingen Schenau et al., 1997).

Effect of fatigue

Fatigue in ice climbing can result from the different kinds of actions: grasping of the axe handle, anchoring the axe and remaining suspended on it, that is, alternative kinds of isometric and dynamical repetitive actions. In this way, we simulated the fatigue through a hanging ecological task in which each climber gripped with both ice axes and hung to exhaustion (Figure 10.1, right panel). The effects of fatigue were evaluated by comparing the swing and a 5 s grip strength test before and after the fatigue test.

In fatigued conditions, no changes were observed in terms of accuracy, the axe's angle or impact velocity (Figures 10.3 and 10.6) from the phase durations (cocking swing, strike, impact). Although the impact characteristics remained the same, results indicated a high decrease of the grip strength (44 per cent) after the fatiguing test indicating a strong alteration of the grasping function. Muscle coordination remained the same in fatigue and fresh conditions (Figure 10.5). Nevertheless, the distal flexor muscles of the digitorum and carpi appear most affected by fatigue, with an increase of amplitude and a decrease of frequency activation indicating a kind of submaximal fatigue (Figure 10.7). Other muscles appear less affected by fatigue in the movement with amplitude increase during the cocking phase for the biceps brachii, and frequency decrease for the extensor digitorum and duration increase for deltoidus during the strike phase. The extensor muscles presented any indicator of muscular fatigue.

All these results suggest that a hanging fatigue task marginally altered the kinematics of the strike and conversely strongly affected the grasping task as observed in rock climbing (Quaine et al., 2003) and in handgrip tasks (Soo et al., 2010).

Influence of the type of ice tool

In this study, we investigated three different types of ice tools used in ice climbing designed by Petzl© (Quark, Nomic and Ergo (Figure 10.2)): mountaineering (e.g. snowy and icy gully), ice climbing and dry-tooling. These tools presented very

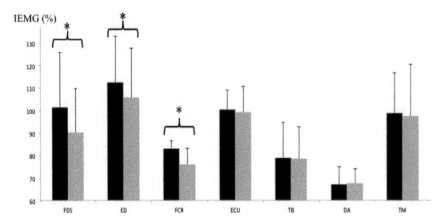

Figure 10.7 Burst mean power frequency during strike phase for muscles. Note: FDS: flexor digitorum superficialis, ED: extensor digitorum, FCR: flexor carpi radialis, ECU: extensor carpi ulnaris, TB: triceps brachii, DA: deltoidus anterior, TM: teres major. Light grey: Pre-fatigue condition; dark gray: Post-fatigue condition. *: significant difference, $p < 0.05$

different geometries, and also different mass distribution. The different designs may have influenced the muscle force required to perform the strike motion.

Few differences could be observed in accuracy, velocity impact and motion kinematics (similar joint angle patterns and amplitudes) (Figure 10.6). These results suggest that experts are able to adapt to the different tools.

The main effect can be observed on the angle between the line formed by the pick's tip and the axe head and the horizontal with greater values for the Ergo compared to the other tools. Nerveless, for each tool, the angle remained relatively invariant among the different subjects (Figure 10.3). This result suggested that the axe's or pick's geometry strongly determined the swing kinematic. This hypothesis was confirmed by the analysis of the subjective experience of the climbers.

The subjective experience of three types of ice tool was examined from the enactive perspective, using the theoretical and methodological framework of course of action (Theureau, 2003). Two types of data were collected: (a) video recordings and (b) verbalisations during post-protocol interviews. The data were processed in two steps: (a) a reconstruction of each climber's course of action and (b) identification and comparison of their typical concerns. The main results indicated that the Quark was experienced as the most *accurate* because the blade keeps a straight trajectory (i.e. without any lateral disturbance) during the striking motion (Pouponneau, 2015). Moreover, the climbers experienced the striking motion as perpendicular to the ice surface, with a close relationship to a hammer striking motion. The striking motion of the Nomic was experienced as efficient, corresponding to a good blend between accuracy and force generation. Climbers mentioned that they did not need to perform a striking motion with great amplitude to get a deep and accurate anchorage of the blade (Pouponneau, 2015). In other words, the striking motion of the Nomic was felt as a forearm movement initiated by the elbow rather than an arm movement initiated by the shoulder. Finally, for the Ergo, the climbers mentioned a relative disturbance regarding the inertia of the ice tools during the striking motion, as well as a lack of lateral stability, which led the subjects to feel a lack of accuracy (Pouponneau, 2015). Moreover, the climbers reported the need for guiding and controlling the striking motion in order to guarantee the anchorage. In fact, many times the climbers experienced a bounce of the blade instead of an anchorage. In comparison to the Quark where the striking motion was experienced as perpendicular to the ice surface, the Ergo required a curved striking motion to get a successful anchorage of the blade (Pouponneau, 2015). Put together, the analyses of the subjective experience of various types of ice tools were very informative in understanding the climber–ice tool coupling. In particular, the climbers often referred to ice tools as being extensions of their bodies, allowing them to act, perceive and feel the structure of the ice. The ice tools became a constituent of the climbers' bodies in action, reconfigured perceptual modalities, opened and 'capacitated' possibilities for action, and thereby participated in their expertise. This process, called 'appropriation' (Havelange, 2010), concentrates the process of integrating the ice tool with the climber's own body, individuating its usage, and more or less transforming the ice tool over time (e.g. as done by Bruno Sourzac who added metallic wings on each side of the blade to ensure anchorage in the soft and ventilated ice of Cerro Torre in Patagonia). Integration as the idea of incorporating the ice tool is often associated with the notion of the ice tool becoming transparent in action (Havelange, 2010; Lenay, 2006) in the sense that it is so deeply incorporated into the physical body that the climber is no longer aware of it.

Conclusion and practical applications

This first biomechanical study on ice climbing suggested that experts adjust their movement according to the kind of ice axe. They were characterized by highly controlled coordination of the upper limb joints. The cocking phase appeared with a proximo-distal coordination associated to lower muscular co-activations, the movement successively involving shoulder, elbow and wrist. The strike phase presented high joint moment. Muscles simultaneously developed peak activation just before the impact. These co-activations stiffened the upper limb allowing maximal force and velocity to be transmitted to the pick. The accuracy of the impact seems to be controlled by the distal wrist joint. Finally, the high co-activations of the digitorum muscles to hang from the axe appeared to be a determinant for the transmission of the force–velocity–accuracy actions of the upper limb joints. These results suggest the development of some specific exercises to improve muscular control, that is, a succession of relax dissociated contractions and flexion during the cocking following by extension with all joints stiffened. A strong hanging appeared very important to transmit the force from the upper limb to the pike at the impact. As fatigue appeared to affect the grasping muscles more than the muscles involved in the ballistic movement, specific training fatigue programmes have to be designed both for the hang/grasp and the ballistic movement.

Summary

- Short time to anchor and swing for the best experts in competitions.
- Low muscular activations in the cocking phase followed by strong co-activation during the striking phase.
- Stiff the upper limb and strong hanging to transmit force and accuracy to the pike.
- Adaptation of the strike motion to the type of ice axe.
- Accuracy of the axe controlled by the wrist in the sagittal plane.

Acknowledgements

This project received funding from the National Institute of Sport and Expert Performance (ID: 11-R-012) and the support of the French Federation of Alpine Clubs (FFCAM) and the National School of Skiing and Alpinism (ENSA of Chamonix, France). We also thank Fanny Bertrand, Mathieu Brun and Clément Pouponneau for their contributions in the data collection and analysis.

References

Adé, D., Gal-Petitfaux, N., Seifert, L., & Poizat, G. (2016). Artefacts and expertise in sport : an empirical study of ice climbing. *International Journal of Sport Psychology*, in press.

Blanc-Gras, J., & Ibarra, M. (2012). *The Art of Ice Climbing*. Chamonix, France: Blue Ice Edition.

Chaffin, D. B., Andersson, G. B., & Martin, B. J. (2006). *Occupational Biomechanics* (4th Edition), New York: Wiley-Interscience.

Dounskaia, N. (2010). Control of human limb movements: the leading joint hypothesis and its practical applications. *Exercise and Sport Science Review, 38(4)*, 201–208.

Duez, J. (2009). Les instruments de l'alpiniste [The climber's tools]. *Technique et Culture, 52(2)*, 330–351.

Elliot, B., Fleisig, G., Nicholls, R., & Escamilia, R. (2003). Technique effects on upper limb loading in the tennis serve. *Journal of Science and Medicine in Sport, 6 (1)*, 76–87.

Gribble, P. L., Mullin, L. I., Cothros, N. & Mattar, A. (2003). Role of cocontraction in arm movement accuracy. *Journal of Neurophysiology, 89*, 2396–2405.

Haake, S. J., Blackwood, W. D., & Yoxall, A. (1997). Photoelastic analysis of ice axe impacts. In *Proceedings of the International Society of Optical Engineering*, 482–489.

Havelange, V. (2010). The ontological constitution of cognition and the epistemological constitution of cognitive science: phenomenology, enaction and technology. In J. Stewart, O. Gapenne, & E. Di Paolo (Eds), *Enaction: Toward a New Paradigm for Cognitive Science* (pp. 335–359). Cambridge, MA: MIT Press.

Itaguchi, Y., & Fukuzawa, K. (2012). Effects of arm stiffness and muscle effort on position reproduction error in the horizontal plane. *Perceptual and Motor Skill, 114(3)*, 757–773.

Laursen, B., Jensen, B. R., & Sjøgaard, G. (1998). Effect of speed and accuracy demands on human shoulder muscle electromyography during a repetitive task. *European Journal of Applied Physiology and Occupational Physiology, 78(6)*, 544–548.

Lenay, C. (2006). Énaction, externalisme et suppléance perceptive [Enaction, externalism and perceptive substitution]. *Intellectica, 43*, 27–52.

Moritomo, H., Apergis, E. P., Herzberg, G., Werner, F. W., Wolfe, S. W., & Garcia-Elias, M. (2007). IFSSH committee report of wrist biomechanics committee: biomechanics of the so-called dart-throwing motion of the wrist. *The Journal of Hand Surgery, 32(9)*, 1447–1453.

Pouponneau, C. (2015). *Analyse de l'activité de glaciéristes dans une perspective de conception de matériel de progression pour l'escalade et la montagne : contribution à l'élaboration d'un programme de recherche technologique en ergonomie du sport [Analysis of ice climbers activity in order to design ice tools in climbing and mountaineering].* PhD Thesis. University of Bourgogne – Franche Comté, Dijon, France.

Quaine, F., Vigouroux, L. & Martin, L. (2003). Finger flexors fatigue in trained rock climbers and untrained sedentary subjects. *International Journal of Sports Medicine, 24*, 424-427.

Rash, G. S., & Shapiro, R. (1995). A three-dimensional dynamic analysis of the quarterback's throwing motion in American football. *Journal of Applied Biomechanics, 11(4)*, 443–459.

Robert, T., Rouard, A., & Seifert, L. (2013). Biomechanical analysis of the strike motion in ice-climbing activity. *Computer Methods in Biomechanics and Biomedical Engineering. Suppl 1*, 90–92.

Schoenmarklin, R. W., & Marras, W. S. (1989). Effects of handle angle and work orientation on hammering: I. wrist motion and hammering performance. *Human Factors, 31*, 397–411.

Seifert, L., Coeurjolly, J. F., Hérault, R., Wattebled, L., & Davids, K. (2013). Temporal dynamics of inter-limb coordination in ice climbing revealed through change-point analysis of the geodesic mean of circular data. *Journal of Applied Statistics, 40(11)*, 2317–2331.

Seifert, L., Wattebled, L., Herault, R., Poizat, G., Adé, D., Gal-Petitfaux, N., & Davids, K. (2014). Neurobiological degeneracy and affordance perception support functional intra-individual variability of inter-limb coordination during ice climbing. *PloS One, 9(2)*, e89865.

Soo, Y., Sugi, M., Yokoi, H., Arai, T., Nishino, M., Kato, R., Nakamura, T. & Ota, J. (2010). Estimation of handgrip force using frequency-band technique during fatiguing muscle contraction. *Journal of Electromyography and Kinesiology, 20*, 888–895.

Theureau, J. (2003). Course of action analysis & course of action centered design. In E. Hollnagel (Ed.), *Handbook of Cognitive Task Design* (pp. 55–81). Mahwah, NJ: Lawrence Erlbaum Associates.

Van Ingen Schenau, G., Bobbert, M., & De Haan, A. (1997). Does elastic energy enhance work and efficiency shortening cycle? *Journal of Applied Biomechanics, 13*, 389–415.

Wang, X., Chevalot, N., Monnier, G., Ausejo, S., Suescun, A., & Celigueta, J. (2005). Validation of a model-based motion reconstruction method developed in the Realman Project. *SAE Transactions Journal of Passenger Cars – Electronic and Electrical Systems, 114*, 873–879.

Wilk, K. E., Meister, K., Fleisig, G., & Andrews, J. (2010). Biomechanics of the overhead throwing motion. *Sports Medicine and Arthroscopy Review, 8(2)*, 124–134.

Part IV
Motor control and learning

11 How expert climbers use perception and action during successful climbing performance

Ludovic Seifert, Dominic Orth, Chris Button and Keith Davids

Climbing in various performance environments, from indoor walls to rock and ice surfaces to mountains, provides considerable psycho-emotional and physiological demands, which challenge the organisation of action in climbers. This chapter addresses key properties (*speed, accuracy, form* and *adaptability*) of the organisation of action when climbing in different environments (indoors, rock, ice climbing and mountaineering). We highlight how climbers use perception and action to organise their behaviours and enhance their expertise in climbing through the continuous and active exploration of environmental properties by climbers. From this perspective, adaptability is the foundation of expertise because it underpins the ongoing co-adaptation of each climber's behaviours to a set changing and interacting constraints, which are individually perceived and acted upon. Finally, we consider how skills are transferred between different surfaces to support climbers who achieve or maintain high performance levels in a variety of performance contexts.

Introduction

Research on expert sport performance has been traditionally explained in cognitivist, computational and hierarchical models of motor control (Abernethy, Poolton, Masters, & Patil, 2008; Schmidt & Lee, 2011) and performance (Ericsson, Krampe, & Tesch-Römer, 1993; Ericsson & Lehmann, 1996). Within these models, experts display greater: (i) *perceptual* (i.e. anticipation, discrimination, recognition and recall of information), (ii) *attentional* (i.e. reproduction and automatisation of actions when multitasking), (iii) *cognitive* (i.e. problem representation: superior knowledge constructs organised in a comprehensive and structured manner and improved problem-solving), and (iv) *motor* (i.e. automaticity of movement patterns) skills than non-experts (Abernethy et al., 2008). Ericsson and Lehmann (1996) defined an expert as an individual with at least ten years or 10000 hours of deliberate and intense practice, on average. These traditional conceptions of expertise are limited because they do not consider the ongoing coupling of an individual with a performance environment (Davids, Glazier, Araújo, & Bartlett, 2003; Seifert, Button, & Davids, 2013) that underpins expert performance.

Climbing is practised in many performance environments, including: indoors and outdoors, differing heights, short (e.g. up to a maximum of 7–8m height in 'bouldering') or long ascents (e.g. from one pitch to multi-pitches averaging 20–30m each), at low or high altitudes, on rocky, snowy, icy or mixed surfaces, with or without tools for support (e.g. ice tools, crampons or even ropes), in sport format (with bolts) or traditional (without bolts), and with more or less engagement with other climbers (e.g. solo, top-rope or on-sight) (Lockwood & Sparks, 2013). During performance a climber needs to assess the quality of ice or rock properties, risks of avalanches, weather forecasts, and possibility of a fall back option or an escape route. This degree of environmental uncertainty, coupled with the ensuing psycho-emotional and physiological demands involve ongoing adaptations that distinguish expert and non-expert climbers. Thus, expertise assessment cannot only look at the performance outcome (e.g. ability to climb 9a in rock climbing). This chapter presents the key properties of expertise (i.e., speed, accuracy, form and adaptability of actions) when climbing in different, with a special focus on *adaptability*. *Adaptability* is a key focus because it provides insights into the ongoing co-adaptation of each climber to a set of changing and interacting constraints, which are individually perceived and acted upon. We also consider how skills are transferred between different surfaces to support climbers who achieve or maintain high performance levels in a variety of performance contexts. We conclude with ideas on practical applications to promote exploratory behaviours and adaptive behaviours, to enhance expertise in climbing.

Performance and key properties of skills in climbing

As discussed in Chapter 14, various scales assess climbing grade of difficulty, and the maximal grade of difficulty reached by a climber cannot be synonymous with his performance level. The grade of difficulty and the level of engagement, such as lead-climbing (securing ascent with existing bolts), top-roping or seconding (removing bolts), free soloing (without any rope), climbing an existing route or not (i.e. an ascent of a route described in a guide book) (see Chapters 15 and 16 about psychological factors), constrain performance and should be taken in account when climbing skills are studied. Consequently, a double grade scale has been developed in mountaineering, traditional rock climbing and ice climbing: route difficulty (graded from E–easy to ABO–abominable) and route engagement (graded from I to VII, rated on possibility of dangers like falling stones or ice, avalanche risks, and opportunities for escapee, fall back and rescue) (Batoux & Seifert, 2007; Blanc-Gras & Ibarra, 2012). These scales do not provide a means of assessing how climbing skill can be related to route difficulty. According to Johnson (1961) skill can be defined as the combination of *speed*, *accuracy*, *form* and *adaptability*, which probably interact to different degrees during climbing to influence performance outcomes (Figure 11.1).

Speed

Speed is a criterion for success and survival because the faster one climbs, the shorter the length of exposure to danger, especially in places like the high altitude

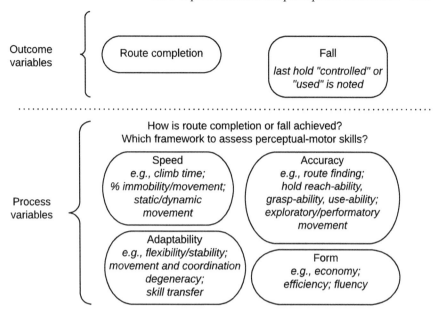

Figure 11.1 Framework to intertwine the outcome variables (climbing performance outcome) and process variables (key components of skill)

summits of the Himalayas where weather conditions can alter rapidly. The professional Swiss mountaineer, Ueli Steck, considered the fastest climber in the world, exemplifies this rule. In his book, *Speed*, Ueli Steck (2014) explains how he broke the speed record during a soloing ascent of three north faces in the Alps: the Eiger (in 2h47 by the Heckmair route in 2008), the Grandes Jorasses (in 2h21 by the Colton-McIntyre route in on-sight climbing in 2008) and the Cervin (in 1h56 by the Schmid route in on-sight climbing in 2009). Speed climbing is a real challenge for some climbers because another popular Swiss climber, Dani Arnold, has recently beaten the speed record of the Schmid route of the Cervin in 1h46 (22 April 2015). Speed climbing is also attempted in constraining environments. For instance, Ueli Steck has speed climbed in the Himalayas on summits up to 8000m, on the south face ascent of the Shisha Pangma (8013m in 10h30 in 2011) and a soloing ascent of the south face of the Annapurna (8091m in 28h in 2013). The first summiteers of these mountains took four days to climb the north face in 1938.

On indoor walls, 'speed' climbing is one of the three types of competitive constraints along with 'lead' and 'bouldering'. Speed climbing competitions started in 2012 and involve climbing, as quickly as possible, routes of 3m width and 10 or 15m height, with a negative incline of 5° in a top-rope condition without falling. The design of such routes is regulated by the International Federation of Sport Climbing (https://www.ifsc-climbing.org/index.php/world-competition/event-regulation) and is the same across the world with a grade difficulty estimated around 6b. There are two types of route: 10m height with 24 handholds and 16 additional footholds or 15m height with 40 handholds and 22 additional footholds. In 2014, the 10m route was climbed in 4.2s, and the 15m route in 5.6s (world record at that time).

In 'lead' climbing, speed cannot be the absolute criteria of expertise because climbers need to alternate climbing with route finding and resting. Instead, expertise could reflect the ability to climb fast the hard sections and to recover during the easy sections, suggesting that climbing is a sequential task, which should be performed fluently to be efficient. It means that a non-fluent and inefficient ascent could be characterised by too many phases of immobility. Previous studies have shown that longer immobility is often observed in non-experts compared to experts, for different reasons:

- Non-expert climbers exhibit more static than dynamic movements assessed by hip displacement during performance (Billat, Palleja, Charlaix, Rizzardo, & Janel, 1995; Fryer et al., 2012; Nieuwenhuys, Pijpers, Oudejans, & Bakker, 2008; Pijpers, Oudejans, Bakker, & Beek, 2006). In one study, Billat et al. (1995) reported that advanced climbers spent 63 per cent of a route duration immobile and 37 per cent ascending, and non-experts were immobile for even longer.
- Non-experts also exhibit more exploratory movements (touched and grasped holds) than performatory movements (holds used to move the body upward) (Nieuwenhuys et al., 2008; Pijpers et al., 2006).
- Non-experts take longer route climb times (Draper et al., 2011; Sanchez, Boschker, & Llewellyn, 2010; Seifert et al., 2013b).
- Non-experts spend greater time in three-hold support (Sibella, Frosio, Schena, & Borghese, 2007).
- Non-experts show greater response times (Pijpers et al., 2006).

Obviously, temporal aspects of performance must be understood in context, because periods of immobility may not be inappropriate stops, but rather could reflect active resting (Sanchez, Lambert, Jones, & Llewellyn, 2012). For instance, Fryer et al. (2012) showed that expert climbers spent a greater proportion of their climbing time in static states, and more of the static time actively resting (i.e. limb shaking), compared to climbers of intermediate skill levels. That is, time spent actively recovering en route might prevent fatigue (Fryer et al., 2012). In ice climbing, Seifert et al. (2013b, 2014b) showed that expert ice climbers exhibited a greater number of stops, but for shorter average time durations. The fact that these climbers also exhibited shorter total climb times suggest that such behaviours can play a functional role in climbing (e.g. route finding, active resting, postural regulation). However, rather than assessing duration and frequency of stops en route, it could be valuable to utilise more advanced temporal measurement analyses (such as harmonic analysis of the acceleration of the hips; Cordier, Dietrich, & Pailhous, 1996) and to add spatial indicators of performance. Using Fourier transformation, Cordier et al. (1996), using a harmonic analysis, revealed that expert climbing performance could be characterised by an oscillating pendulum acting as a mass-spring system that works like a dissipative system, that is, a system where dissipation of energy is minimised by harmonic movements. Finally, speed analysis (i) only makes sense according to the context of performance, (ii) requests cautions with the interpretation of immobility phases, and (iii) invite to link speed with form analyses (e.g., through space/time fluency analysis).

Accuracy

Performance *accuracy* usually relates to the minimisation of errors. Errors in climbing can involve hold stand-ability, reach-ability, grasp-ability and use-ability. Accuracy can be examined at global (i.e. 'route finding' to detect easy and difficult sections, such as 'crux points') and local levels (i.e. limb movements to fully exploit environmental properties). Experts generally display better perceptual attunement to and calibration of informational variables (Fajen, Riley, & Turvey, 2009), because they tend to rely on a range of perceptual variables that enable the reach, grasp and use of holds with accuracy. Thus, using correct grasping patterns for a given hold to move the body upward reveals great perceptual attunement and calibration of informational variables specifying accurate actions. Assuming that accuracy can be assessed through the ability to perceive affordances (opportunities for action) in a performance environment (Gibson, 1979), analysis of relations between *exploratory* and *performatory* movements could explain how climbers perceive 'climb-ability' of a surface and exploit environmental properties to act (Boschker & Bakker, 2002; Boschker, Bakker, & Michaels, 2002b; Pijpers et al., 2006). During indoor wall climbing, Pijpers et al. (2006) distinguished exploratory and performatory touching movements of potential holds on a rock surface, with or without them being used as support during ascent. Therefore, calculating the ratio between 'touched-grasped' and "used" holds to move upward could indicate the accuracy of a climber's perception and action systems. According to the 'three-holds rule', skilled climbers negotiate a surface by touching fewer than three surface holds before grasping a functional one (Sibella, Frosio, Schena, & Borghese, 2007). This distinction between touched, grasped and used holds is also present in 'lead' climbing competitions when a competitor falls before the top. In particular the IFSC rules indicate that

> a hold shall be considered as 'controlled' where a competitor has made use of the hold to achieve a stable or controlled position, whereas a hold from which a competitor has made a controlled climbing movement in the interest of progressing along the route shall be considered as 'used'.

To help the judges to make their decision, the IFSC rules indicate that

> a controlled climbing movement may be either 'static' or 'dynamic' in nature and in general will be evidenced by (i) a significant positive change in position of the competitor's centre of mass; and (ii) the movement of at least one hand in order to reach either the next hold along the line of the route.

These rules reinforce the idea that repetitive exploratory movements may lead to early fatiguing and falling. Thus, computing the ratio between exploratory and performatory movements is an ideal candidate to assess climbing accuracy. Previous studies have already revealed how *route* and *hold designs* induce more or less exploratory behaviours (Seifert, Boulanger, Orth, & Davids, 2015) and accuracy in performatory movements (Nougier, Orliaguet, & Martin, 1993). For instance, grasping horizontal edge holds can lead to adoption of a 'face-to-the-wall' body orientation, whereas vertical edge hold grasping can induce a 'side-to-the-wall' body orientation (Seifert et al., 2015). Designing complex climbing routes, with holds offering dual edge orientations, affords (invites climbers to explore) two types of grasping patterns and body orientations (Seifert et al., 2015). In fact, moving between a right-orientated vertical edge hold to a left-orientated vertical edge hold would lead the body to rotate as if on the hinges of a door. Hold design has been found to influence climbers' movement patterns and especially movement time during hold grasping (Nougier et al., 1993). Complexity of manual grips (2cm versus 1cm depth) and posture difficulty (low versus high angle of inclination of footholds) result in shorter movement times for grasping (Nougier et al., 1993), with less time spent exploring. Moreover, hold design may impact on the force–time pattern and the force orientation exhibited by the climber (further details in Chapters 7 and 8), meaning that climbing requires accuracy both at kinematical and kinetic levels.

The exploratory/performatory movements ratio could be adapted to assess performance accuracy in ice climbing by analysing the proportion of repetitive swings of ice tools to the number of completed anchorages (Seifert, Wattebled, et al., 2013, 2014). The swinging/anchoring ratio of ice tool behaviours could reveal the attunement of each climber to icefall properties (e.g. thickness, density, shape and steepness) for accurate exploitation. For instance, when the ice is soft or ventilated, climbers can anchor their ice tools in one swing, whereas when ice is dense and thick, climbers often need to repeat numerous swings to a acquire deep anchorage. Expert climbers can typically detect variations in icefall thickness in order to reduce action frequency needed to acquire definitive anchorages. In fact, expert ice climbers exhibit greater perceptual attunement to visual, acoustic and haptic sources of information specifying action, which allow climbers to detect the 'use-ability' of existing holes in an icefall. Conversely, beginners seem mostly attuned to visual characteristics of an icefall, focusing on size and depth of holes and steps. Beginners exhibit a global perception of icefall shape for which big and deep holes are synonymous with deep and stable anchorages (Seifert et al., 2014b). They tend to mechanically repeat the same actions to create a deep hole anchorage. Finally, low levels of accuracy may lead to more exploratory movements and errors (in which a movement does not completely fit with environmental properties), leading to falls.

Form

As developed in Chapter 3, *form* relates to effort, economy and efficiency, with the latter defined as the ratio of external work performed relative to energy expended during task performance. Due to the complexity of outdoor climbing terrains and climber movements, valid measurement of external work remains elusive and determination of economy during climbing is not possible. Computer models have been developed to estimate the mechanical costs of climbing. For instance, Russell, Zirker, and Blemker (2012) used an inverse dynamic model to investigate joint angles and torques, to quantify total mechanical work. They showed that experts used kinematic motions of climbing that corresponded to muscle fibres operating much closer to their optimum length than non-experts. These biomechanical and physiological aspects of *form* have been well summarised in Chapters 2, 6, and 7. Another attempt was to assess the perceptive and cognitive aspects of *form* (e.g. route finding) through climbing *fluency* that indicates efficiency of the path taken through the route (Cordier, Mendès-France, Bolon, & Pailhous, 1993; Cordier, Mendès-France, Pailhous, & Bolon, 1994). Perceptive and cognitive aspects of *form* are particularly meaningful for on-sight climbing. In that case, exhibiting continuous climbing using a straightforward path through a route can be qualitatively described as 'fluent climbing' and globally captures skilled climbing performance. Relevant analyses include climb distance (Green & Helton, 2011; Seifert, Orth, et al., 2014; Seifert, Wattebled, et al., 2014), hand movement distance (Nieuwenhuys et al., 2008), centre of mass to wall distance (Sibella et al., 2007; Zampagni, Brigadoi, Schena, Tosi, & Ivanenko, 2011), inter-limb relative positions (Seifert et al., 2013c, 2014b; Seifert, Coeurjolly, Hérault, Wattebled, & Davids, 2013), but the most prominent computation is of the geometric entropy index value from the hip displacement (Boschker & Bakker, 2002; Boschker, Bakker, & Michaels, 2002a; Cordier et al., 1993, 1994; Sanchez et al., 2012; Sibella et al., 2007).

The geometric index of entropy (H) has been calculated by recording the path distance covered by the hips (L) and the perimeter of the convex hull around that path (c), according to the following equation (Cordier et al., 1993, 1994): $H = \log n2L/c$. The geometric entropy measures reveal the amount of fluency/curvature of a curve: the higher the entropy, the higher the disorder of the system (Cordier et al., 1993, 1994). A low entropy value is associated with low energy expenditure and greater climbing fluency, characteristic of experts. The geometric entropy index remains a spatial measure of body motion that does not consider the displacement of the hips over time, only the projection of the path. Entropy measures do not consider the way that a trajectory is achieved and when a climber pauses for the purposes of route finding or for postural regulation, it is not taken into consideration by the geometric entropy index. Thus, it is necessary to get an index of climbing fluency that integrates both *spatial* and *temporal* measurements into a single outcome, such as velocity and acceleration (Cordier et al., 1996) and jerk (Ladha, Hammerla, Olivier, & Plötz, 2013; Pansiot, King, McIlwraith, Lo, & Yang, 2008; Seifert, Orth, et al., 2014). Analyses of the jerk coefficient of hip trajectory and orientation, that is, third time derivative of position or the rate of change of acceleration, indicating trajectory smoothness (e.g. Seifert et al., 2014a), have revealed decreases of jerk coefficients with practice, providing a useful indicator of climbing fluency. However, and to conclude, climbing fluency remains an indirect measure of efficiency and more broadly of form, which is mostly adapted for on-sight climbing and complex climbing tasks demanding high adaptability. Moreover, capturing climbing fluency from a single point (i.e. hip) is limited because the same hip path can be obtained from various limb movements and coordination patterns when kinematic, kinetic and muscular levels are considered. Concerning kinematics, the computation of the centre of mass and full body analysis would be more appropriate. For instance, Boulanger, Seifert, Hérault, and Coeurjolly (2016) have presented an application of a machine learning method to automatically detect and classify climbing activities using inertial measurement units (IMUs) attached to the wrists, feet and pelvis of the climber. This full-body activity detection/classification is based on the following decision tree:

- *Immobility* when all limbs are immobile and the pelvis is immobile.
- *Postural regulation* when all limbs are immobile and the pelvis is moving.
- *Hold interaction* when at least one limb is moving and the pelvis is immobile.
- *Traction* when at least one limb is moving and the pelvis is moving (Boulanger et al., 2016).

However, hold interaction could correspond to a change in the hold used before the next traction, a change in the position and orientation of the hand/foot on a hold, or successive limb movements to determine which hold is the most appropriate for the next traction. Thus, a second layer of detection has been performed at the limb level, which distinguishes 'when a limb is immobile', 'using hold', 'changing to the next hold' or 'exploring the hold' (Boulanger et al., 2016). Applied to 94 trails performed by climbers of various skill levels, the automatic detection showed a higher number of exploratory movements and longer immobility duration in beginners than in more experienced climbers (Boulanger et al., 2016).

Adaptability

Adaptability implies that performance remains proficient in varying and even unpredictable environmental contexts. Expert behaviour is characterised by stable and reproducible movement patterns, which are consistent over time, resistant to perturbations and reproducible in that a similar movement pattern may recur under different task and environmental constraints. However, it is not stereotyped and rigid but flexible and adaptive. Adaptability relates to a functional relationship between *stability* (i.e. persistent behaviours) and *flexibility* (i.e. variable behaviours) during performance (Davids et al., 2003; Warren, 2006). Skilled climbers are able to exhibit stable patterns of behaviour when needed, but can vary actions depending on dynamic performance conditions (Seifert, Button, et al., 2013). Although humans become more stable and economical with experience and practice, stability and flexibility are not opposing characteristics of performance. Notably, flexibility is not a loss of stability, but a sign of adaptability (van Emmerik & van Wegen, 2000; Warren, 2006). Even if movement patterns display regularities and similarities in their structural components, an individual is not locked into performing a rigidly stable solution, but can adapt an emergent movement pattern in order to maintain behavioural functionality. The capacity for an individual to adapt to environmental changes by exploiting different coordination patterns reflects neurobiological system *degeneracy*. Edelman and Gally (2001) defined degeneracy as 'the ability of elements that are structurally different to perform the same function or yield the same output' (p. 13763). Degeneracy allows an individual to vary motor behaviours (e.g. type of action, movement and coordination patterns) without compromising function at different levels of organisation. System degeneracy in climbing is revealed as a large range of hand grasping patterns and body positions regularly used to exploit a specific hold (e.g. crimp, gaston, jug, mono, pinch, pocket, sloper and undercling grasping patterns; bridge, campus, crossover, deadpoint, flag, heel hook, knee bar and mantle body positions; Phillips, Sassaman, & Smoliga, 2012). For instance, experienced climbers can exhibit three different hand grasping positions for different hold depths (from 1 to 4cm): slope, half crimp (crimp without thumb) and full crimp (crimp with thumb) (Amca, Vigouroux, Aritan, & Berton, 2012). Their data indicated that maximal vertical and antero-posterior forces increased according to hold depth but the form of this increase differed depending on grasping patterns. They concluded that choosing one or other grasping pattern is not primarily due to internal biomechanical factors (e.g. muscle length, moment arms, joint angle) but rather to optimise finger-hold contacts/interactions (Amca et al., 2012). This study exemplifies that a range of grasping patterns is available to achieve a task-goal, with more or less functional equivalence between patterns depending on task constraints (e.g. hold depth).

Since environmental constraints are neither predictable nor controllable, ice climbing also illustrates nicely how experts have to use numerous types of actions and patterns of inter-limb coordination during performance by exploiting system degeneracy (Seifert et al., 2014b). For instance, experts tend to alternate exploitation of horizontal, diagonal, vertical and crossed angular support positions on an icefall surface (Figure 11.2a). Indeed, expert climbers sometimes move their right and left supports across the vertical mid-line of their bodies to exploit surface properties and hook existing holes in an icefall (Seifert et al., 2014b) (Figure 11.2b. Conversely, beginners show a more constricted range of movement and coordination patterns as they adopt a basic quadruped climbing pattern that resembles climbing a ladder (Figure 11.2c). In particular, support anchorages employed by beginners remain the same with both arms (or legs) extended (or flexed), corresponding to simultaneous muscular activation of arms (or legs), because they prioritise stability and security of posture rather than taking risks to climb quickly (Seifert, Wattebled, et al., 2013).

Multi-stable patterns of coordination in expert ice climbers reflect a functional adaptation to dynamic environmental properties, with different types of actions emerging (i.e. swinging, kicking, stepping, hooking) depending on icefall shape. In dense ice without any holes, climbers usually swing their ice tools and kick their crampons, and in hollow ice, they hook holes with ice tools and crampons. Multi-stability of coordination patterns and a large repertoire have been revealed by observing the efficient coupling of a skilled climber with the properties of a

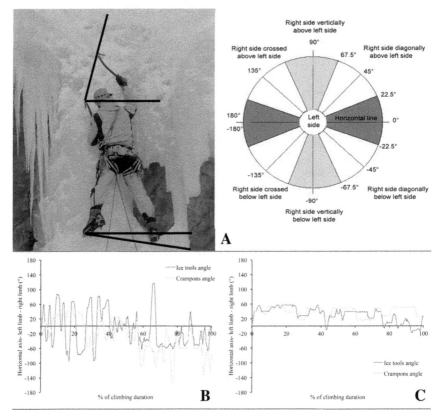

Figure 11.2 Inter-limb coordination in ice climbing. Panel A shows how climbers coordinate the angle formed between the two ice tools in the horizontal plane. In this example the angle (formed by the two thick black lines) would be assigned a specific value around 80° (the same procedure was done for crampons). Panel B shows example raw data of ice tools and crampons couplings over time (upper graph) for an expert in comparison panel C that shows the beginner coordination over the same period of time (300s). Note the presence of plateaus in the beginner in contrast to the relatively continuous changes in the expert climber

performance environment, likely predicated on inherent neurobiological system degeneracy (Davids & Glazier, 2010; Edelman & Gally, 2001). High levels of adaptability may facilitate *skills transfer*, helping climbers to switch from rock to ice, or vice versa, helping them to remain fluent on a mixed route during mountaineering.

Expertise and transfer in climbing

How well does an indoor climbing wall simulate the performance environments of rock or ice climbing? This is an important issue of skill transfer since some climbers may choose not to train on cliffs or mountains, because of fear or a lack of confidence in their ability to correctly assess altitude effects, weather conditions and unmarked routes, or they may simply live too far from the mountains. Moreover, some expert climbers deliberately use indoor climbing walls for fitness training because weather conditions and route conditions do not allow daily practice. As such, it is imperative that there are effective ways of designing representative training sessions that afford uncertainties and the psychological requirements of outdoor climbing in indoor climbing wall contexts. The question of skill transfer also concerns the relationships between lead climbing and bouldering, so that performers and practitioners typically seek to train transferrable (or generalisable) skills (Collins & Collins, 2012). For instance, Adam Ondra is able to climb among the most difficult routes around the world (e.g. *Change*, 9b+, at Flatanger Cave in Norway, in 2012: http://www. adamondra.com/adam-ondra-climbs-change-9b) and to win the IFSC World Cup 2015 (ranked first in lead climbing and third in bouldering) at Kranj in Slovenia. Numerous other examples can exemplify how skill transfer emerges from the influence of prior experiences under a particular set of interacting constraints on performance under a different set of constraints compared to those where the skills were acquired (Newell, 1996). Seifert et al. (2013) evaluated the role of experience in skill transfer from indoor climbing to ice climbing outdoors, showing that *specificity–generality* of transfer might influence efficiency for climbing in various environments. *Specificity* of transfer emerges when the existing skill repertoire of an individual *cooperates* with the new task to be learned, facilitating positive transfer (i.e. performance improvement) (Issurin, 2013; Rosalie & Müller, 2012). Here specificity is predicated on the specificity of information that can be used to organise climbing actions. *General* transfer occurs when the existing skill repertoire and task dynamics do *not cooperate closely or compete*, and non-specifying information is used to organise actions. In one study, Seifert et al. (2013) showed that experienced climbers, who had previously acquired multiple movement patterns, were able to transfer climbing fluency to the novel task constraints of ice climbing.

Three main properties supported *general* transfer of climbing experience between the task constraints of indoor and ice climbing (Seifert, Wattebled, et al., 2013):

- Unpredictability of performance environments requiring the continuous coupling of perception and action.
- Alternation between maintaining body equilibrium (stability) and climbing quickly up a vertical surface (transitioning).
- Use of quadruped locomotion patterns involving the extremities of each limb to negotiate an ascent.

The task constraints of ice climbing reveal at least three, information-based particularities in comparison to rock climbing which might induce *specificity* of transfer between each discipline (Seifert, Wattebled, et al., 2013):

- Tools, such as ice tools for the hands and crampons for the feet, form parts of the landscape of available affordances used by an ice climber to interact with the surface properties of an icefall.

- Icefall properties tend to be stochastically distributed throughout a particular frozen waterfall surface (for instance, icefall texture can vary greatly, presenting more or fewer holes, inviting climbers to hook available holes or create holes by swinging their ice tools).
- Climbers can discover specific climbing paths by creating their own more or less stable anchorages with tools and secure an ascent by inserting ice screws into specific icefall locations.

These findings demonstrated how individuals solve different motor problems, exploiting positive *general* transfer processes, but design of *specific* task constraints enabled participants to pick up specifying information for tool use in climbing an icefall.

Conclusions

Analysis of organisation of action, such as hip movements and performatory and exploratory actions of upper/lower limbs, provide a precise way of understanding the relationship between skilled behaviour and expertise in climbing. This chapter reviewed studies observing climbing skill in hip and limb organisation, to highlight skilled adaptations to various climbing contexts. Expertise was associated with spatially efficient route progression and lower levels of immobility. Whilst higher ability levels are associated with better strength and conditioning performance, these measures do not successfully predict performance amongst individuals of similar ability levels, and perception–action relations and psychological processes also contribute. Improved performance on new routes or in new environments (skill transfer) is supported by exploratory actions, predicated on system degeneracy and an individual's skill repertoire. These findings imply how training contexts should be designed for improving performance on new routes.

Practical applications

Achieving expertise can be directed at the grade level of the individual performer and his/her environment by encouraging *exploratory* movements, which become *performatory* movements, linking *speed, accuracy, efficiency* and *adaptability*. Inducing exploration of system degeneracy during emergent performer interactions can promote *skill transfer*. The challenge is how to set up opportunities for efficient exploration that manages the dangers of performing in unpredictable contexts. Representing uncertainty within the relative safety of indoor settings may prepare climbers for performance in more demanding contexts, through the design of informational constraints in the training context.

Highlights

- Expertise is the product of speed, accuracy, form and adaptability.
- Adaptability is the most challenging component of expertise to be developed.

- Skill transfer can be enabled through exploratory behaviour.
- Exploration can lead to exploitation of inherent system degeneracy.

Acknowledgements

This project received the support of the CPER/GRR 1880 Logistic, Mobility and Numeric and FEDER RISC (ID: 33172). This project also received funding from the French National Agency of Research (ID: ANR-13-JSH2-0004 DynaMov).

References

Abernethy, B., Poolton, J. M., Masters, R. S. W., & Patil, N. G. (2008). Implications of an expertise model for surgical skills training. *ANZ Journal of Surgery*, 78(12), 1092–1095. doi:10.1111/j.1445-2197.2008.04756.x

Amca, A., Vigouroux, L., Aritan, S., & Berton, E. (2012). Effect of hold depth and grip technique on maximal finger forces in rock climbing. *Journal of Sports Sciences*, 30(7), 669–677.

Batoux, P., & Seifert, L. (2007). *Ice climbing and dry-tooling: from Mont Blanc to Leman.* Chamonix, FR: JMEditions.

Billat, V. L., Palleja, P., Charlaix, T., Rizzardo, P., & Janel, N. (1995). Energy specificity of rock climbing and aerobic capacity in competitive sport rock climbers. *The Journal of Sports Medicine and Physical Fitness*, 35(1), 20–24.

Blanc-Gras, J., & Ibarra, M. (2012). *The art of ice climbing.* Chamonix, FR: Blue Ice Edition.

Boschker, M. S. J., & Bakker, F. C. (2002). Inexperienced sport climbers might perceive and utilize new opportunities for action by merely observing a model. *Perceptual and Motor Skills*, 95(1), 3–9.

Boschker, M. S. J., Bakker, F. C., & Michaels, C. F. (2002a). Effect of mental imagery on realizing affordances. *The Quarterly Journal of Experimental Psychology. A Human Experimental Psychology*, 55(3), 775–792.

Boschker, M. S. J., Bakker, F. C., & Michaels, C. F. (2002b). Memory for the functional characteristics of climbing walls: perceiving affordances. *Journal of Motor Behavior*, 34(1), 25–36.

Boulanger, J., Seifert, L., Hérault, R., & Coeurjolly, J. (2016). Automatic sensor-based detection and classification of climbing activities. *IEEE Sensors*, 16(3), 742–749. doi:10.1109/JSEN.2015.2481511

Collins, L., & Collins, D. (2012). Conceptualizing the adventure-sports coach. *Journal of Adventure Education and Outdoor Learning*, 12(1), 81–93.

Cordier, P., Dietrich, G., & Pailhous, J. (1996). Harmonic analysis of a complex motor behaviour. *Human Movement Science*, 15(6), 789–807.

Cordier, P., Mendès-France, M., Bolon, P., & Pailhous, J. (1993). Entropy, degrees of freedom, and free climbing: a thermodynamic study of a complex behavior based on trajectory analysis. *International Journal of Sport Psychology*, 24, 370–378.

Cordier, P., Mendès-France, M., Pailhous, J., & Bolon, P. (1994). Entropy as a global variable of the learning process. *Human Movement Science*, 13, 745–763.

Davids, K., & Glazier, P. S. (2010). Deconstructing neurobiological coordination: the role of the biomechanics-motor control nexus. *Exercise and Sport Science Reviews*, 38(2), 86–90. doi:10.1097/JES.0b013e3181d4968b

Davids, K., Glazier, P. S., Araújo, D., & Bartlett, R. M. (2003). Movement systems as dynamical systems: the functional role of variability and its implications for sports medicine. *Sports Medicine*, 33(4), 245–260.

Draper, N., Dickson, T., Blackwell, G., Fryer, S., Priestley S., Winter, D., & Ellis, G. (2011). Self-reported ability assessment in rock climbing. *Journal of Sports Sciences*, 29(8), 851–858.

Edelman, G. M., & Gally, J. A. (2001). Degeneracy and complexity in biological systems. *Proceedings of the National Academy of Sciences of the United States of America*, 98(24), 13763–13768. doi:10.1073/pnas.231499798

Ericsson, K. A., Krampe, R. T., & Tesch-Römer, C. (1993). The role of deliberate practice in the acquisition of expert performance. *Psychological Review*, 3, 363–406.

Ericsson, K. A., & Lehmann, A. C. (1996). Expert and exceptional performance: evidence of maximal adaptation to task constraints. *Annual Review of Psychology*, 47, 273–305.

Fajen, B. R., Riley, M. R., & Turvey, M. T. (2009). Information, affordances, and the control of action in sport. *International Journal of Sports Psychology*, 40(1), 79–107.

Fryer, S., Dickson, T., Draper, N., Eltom, M., Stoner, L., & Blackwell, G. (2012). The effect of technique and ability on the VO2–heart rate relationship in rock climbing. *Sports Technology*, 5(3–4), 143–150.

Gibson, J. (1979). *The ecological approach to visual perception.* Boston, MA: Houghton Mifflin.

Green, A., & Helton, W. (2011). Dual-task performance during a climbing traverse. *Experimental Brain Research*, 215, 307–313.

Issurin, V. (2013). Training transfer: scientific background and insights for practical application. *Sports Medicine*, 43(8), 675–694.

Johnson, H. W. (1961). Skill = speed × accuracy × form × adaptability. *Perceptual and Motor Skills*, 13, 163–170.

Ladha, C., Hammerla, N., Olivier, P., & Plötz, T. (2013). ClimbAX: skill assessment for climbing enthusiasts. In J. Häkkila, K. Whitehouse, A. Krüger, Y. Tobe, O. Hilliges, K. Yatani, … F. Mattern (Eds), *ACM Conference on Ubiquitous Computing, UbiComp'13 Adjunct* (pp. 235–244). Zurich, Switzerland: ACM Press.

Lockwood, N., & Sparks, P. (2013). When is risk relevant? An assessment of the characteristics mountain climbers associate with eight types of climbing. *Journal of Applied Social Psychology*, 43(5), 992–1001. doi:10.1111/jasp.12063

Newell, K. M. (1996). Change in movement and skill: learning, rentention and transfer. In M. L. Latash, & M. T. Turvey (Eds), *Dexterity and its development* (pp. 393–430). Mahwah, NJ: Erlbaum.

Nieuwenhuys, A., Pijpers, J., Oudejans, R., & Bakker, F. (2008). The influence of anxiety on visual attention in climbing. *Journal of Sport & Exercise Psychology*, 30, 171–185.

Nougier, V., Orliaguet, J.-P., & Martin, O. (1993). Kinematic modifications of the manual reaching in climbing: effects of environmental and corporal constraints. *International Journal of Sport Psychology*, 24, 379–390.

Pansiot, J., King, R., McIlwraith, D., Lo, B., & Yang, G. (2008). ClimBSN: climber performance monitoring with BSN. In *IEEE Proceedings of the 5th International Workshop on Wearable and Implantable Body Sensor Networks* (pp. 33–36). The Chinese University of Hong Kong: IEEE.

Phillips, K., Sassaman, J., & Smoliga, J. (2012). Optimizing rock climbing performance through sport-specific strength and conditioning. *Strength and Conditioning Journal*, 34(3), 1–18.

Pijpers, J. R., Oudejans, R. D., Bakker, F. C., & Beek, P. J. (2006). The role of anxiety in perceiving and realizing affordances. *Ecological Psychology*, 18(3), 131–161.

Rosalie, S., & Müller, S. (2012). A model for the transfer of perceptual-motor skill learning in human behaviors. *Research Quarterly for Exercise and Sport*, 83(3), 413–421.

Russell, S., Zirker, C., & Blemker, S. (2012). Computer models offer new insights into the mechanics of rock climbing. *Sports Technology*, 5(3–4), 120–131.

Sanchez, X., Boschker, M. J. S., & Llewellyn, D. J. (2010). Pre-performance psychological states and performance in an elite climbing competition. *Scandinavian Journal of Medicine & Science in Sports*, 20(2), 356–363.

Sanchez, X., Lambert, P., Jones, G., & Llewellyn, D. J. (2012). Efficacy of pre-ascent climbing route visual inspection in indoor sport climbing. *Scandinavian Journal of Medicine & Science in Sports*, 22(1), 67–72.

Schmidt, R. A., & Lee, T. D. (2011). *Motor control and learning: a behavioral emphasis* (5th Edition). New York: Human Kinetics Publisher.

Seifert, L., Boulanger, J., Orth, D., & Davids, K. (2015). Environmental design shapes perceptual-motor exploration, learning, and transfer in climbing. *Frontiers in Psychology*, 6, 1819. doi:10.3389/fpsyg.2015.01819

Seifert, L., Button, C., & Davids, K. (2013a). Key properties of expert movement systems in sport: an ecological dynamics perspective. *Sports Medicine*, 43(3), 167–178.

Seifert, L., Coeurjolly, J. F., Hérault, R., Wattebled, L., & Davids, K. (2013b). Temporal dynamics of inter-limb coordination in ice climbing revealed through change-point analysis of the geodesic mean of circular data. *Journal of Applied Statistics*, 40(11), 2317–2331.

Seifert, L., Orth, D., Boulanger, J., Dovgalecs, V., Hérault, R., & Davids, K. (2014a). Climbing skill and complexity of climbing wall design: assessment of jerk as a novel indicator of performance fluency. *Journal of Applied Biomechanics*, 30(5), 619–625.

Seifert, L., Wattebled, L., Herault, R., Poizat, G., Adé, D., Gal-Petitfaux, N., & Davids, K. (2014b). Neurobiological degeneracy and affordance perception support functional intra-individual variability of inter-limb coordination during ice climbing. *PloS One*, 9(2), e89865.

Seifert, L., Wattebled, L., L'Hermette, M., Bideault, G., Herault, R., & Davids, K. (2013c). Skill transfer, affordances and dexterity in different climbing environments. *Human Movement Science*, 32(6), 1339–1352.

Sibella, F., Frosio, I., Schena, F., & Borghese, N. A. (2007). 3D analysis of the body center of mass in rock climbing. *Human Movement Science*, 26(6), 841–852.

Steck, U. (2014). *Speed*. Chamonix, France: Guérin.

van Emmerik, R. E. A., & van Wegen, E. E. H. (2000). On variability and stability in human movement. *Journal of Applied Biomechanics*, 16, 394–406.

Warren, W. H. (2006). The dynamics of perception and action. *Psychological Review*, 113(2), 358–389. doi:10.1037/0033-295X.113.2.358

Zampagni, M. L., Brigadoi, S., Schena, F., Tosi, P., & Ivanenko, Y. P. (2011). Idiosyncratic control of the center of mass in expert climbers. *Scandinavian Journal of Medicine & Science in Sports*, 21(5), 688–699.

12 What current research tells us about skill acquisition in climbing

Dominic Orth, Chris Button, Keith Davids and Ludovic Seifert

Skilled movement has been defined as a refined organization of behaviours to optimize the ratio of mechanical work to energy expenditure in satisfying the interacting environmental, task and individual constraints (Newell, 1996). This chapter discusses how current research on learning in climbing can be used to support improvement in skill performance by managing practice task constraints during training. The aims of this chapter are twofold: first, to review the effects of practice constraints on skilled behaviour in climbing, and second, to develop a theoretical framework for guiding perceptual-motor learning in route climbing through learning design.

Introduction

Climbing requires an individual to adapt to a more or less vertical and ever-changing structure of a climbing surface with the task of completing a route without falling (Orth, Davids, & Seifert, 2015). Skilled behaviour in climbing is predicated on how an individual dynamically adapts actions to varied climbing surface properties (variations in shape, texture and relative distancing of features; Davids, Brymer, Seifert, & Orth, 2014). Due to the extreme postural constraints imposed by the small protrusive/sunken edges embedded into a sloped surface, climbers need to continuously regulate their use of the environment relative to their internal state during performance. For example, muscular fatigue reduces the ability to produce the required friction force at the fingertips (Vigouroux & Quaine, 2006) and can be intensified if an individual becomes 'blocked' (i.e. cannot perceive how to use holds to continue climbing; White & Olsen, 2010), uses inefficient movements (de Geus, O'Driscoll, & Meeusen, 2006), or does not perceive and exploit opportunities to rest (Fryer et al., 2012). Hence, improving climbing skill, in tasks requiring route finding (such as bouldering, sport and traditional climbing), can be facilitated by helping learners to detect and use relevant information sources during climbing to support successful performance and energy efficient actions (Orth et al., 2015).

In the emergence of skilled behaviour, three timescales of change (slow, moderately fast and fast) appear to exist. According to Cordier et al. (1993), 'fast' variables account for the dynamics of motor *performance*. Changes in the fast timescale, typically expressed in seconds, are observed as the temporary (re)organization of behaviours in a discrete performance trial. 'Moderately fast' variables account for *learning*, refer to the relatively persistent adaptation of the individual to the environment, in a timescale perhaps expressed over several hours (Cordier, Mendès-France, Bolon, & Pailhous, 1993). The effects of learning can be observed over many performance repetitions (referred to as learning dynamics) and under retention and transfer conditions (Davids, Button, & Bennett, 2008). Finally, Cordier et al. (1993) defined 'slow' variables to account for the dynamics underlying the emergence of highly skilled behaviours. This timescale may be expressed across many months or years, and can be reflected in the structural/ functional adaptations developed through progressive training (e.g. Bläsing, Güldenpenning, Koester, & Schack, 2014; Vigouroux & Quaine, 2006).

This chapter considers how skilled climbing is improved through learning, summarizing behavioural data observed as individuals negotiate climbing environments over repeated trials of practice and pre- and post-test interventions. Relatively few studies have reported learning effects during route climbing tasks and the aims of this chapter are twofold: to review effects of practice task constraints on skilled behaviours in climbing, and to propose a theoretical framework for enhancing perceptual-motor learning in route climbing. The chapter is organized into four sections. The first section considers the effects of skill on learning dynamics in climbing, considering potential mechanisms. Next we consider the perceptual-motor basis of skilled behaviour in climbing, leading to a framework for conceptualizing progressive improvement on the basis of skilled affordance perception in the third section. Finally, we discuss interventions that exemplify how the theoretical framework developed in earlier sections can be applied to a specific learning problem in climbing.

The effect of skill on the rate and level of learning in climbing

In a series of innovative studies, Cordier and colleagues (Cordier, Dietrich, & Pailhous, 1996; Cordier et al., 1993; Cordier, Mendès-France, Bolon, & Pailhous, 1994; Cordier, Mendès-France, Pailhous, & Bolon, 1994) evaluated the effects of practice during ten trials on the same route (set at a French Rating Scale of difficulty [F-RSD] of 6a). Skill level effects were assessed by contrasting the performance of an advanced group (F-RSD between 7a and 7b), with an intermediate group (F-RSD between 6b and 6c). Each climber's position on the wall was analysed by digitizing the movement of a light-emitting diode (LED), attached to the back at the waist, and video recorded with a camera during climbing. Digitized trajectories were projected onto the climbing wall plane, and spatial and temporal characteristics of performance were analysed. From the positional data several variables were calculated to characterize overall stability including: the geometric index of entropy (Cordier et al., 1993; Cordier, Mendès-France, Bolon, et al., 1994; Cordier, Mendès-France, Pailhous, et al., 1994); spectral (Cordier et al., 1996); fractal (Cordier et al., 1993); harmonic (Cordier et al., 1996); and phase portrait analyses (Cordier et al., 1996).

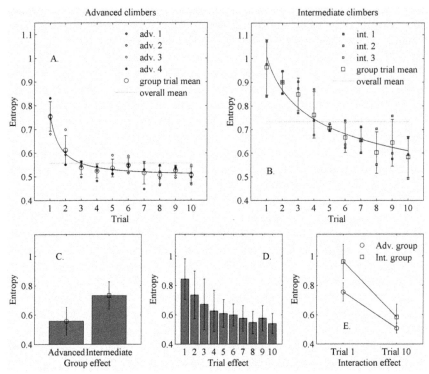

Figure 12.1 Data adapted from Cordier et al. (1993, p. 373) showing practice and skill effects as indexed by entropy of the hip trajectory when climbing the same route over ten trials. Int. = Intermediate climber, Adv. = Advanced climber. Error bars = ±1 standard deviation

Cordier and colleagues showed how the existing skill level of learners affected their subsequent level and rate of performance improvement. Figure 12.1 summarizes the results of analyses undertaken by Cordier et al. (1993), displaying skill differences (Figure 12.1 Panels A, B and C); learning rates (Figure 12.1 Panels A, B and D), and level of learning (reflected in magnitude of change over ten trials; Figure 12.1 Panel E). The advanced group (Panel A) reached a stable state (a plateau in the rate of improvement) earlier (identified in Trial 3 in Cordier et al., 1993) than the intermediate group (Panel B) (identified in Trial 8 in Cordier et al., 1993). Both groups achieved a similar level of performance in terms of movement efficiency (captured by geometric index entropy) by the tenth trial of practice (see Figure 12.1, Panel E).

Cordier et al. (1996) emphasized that the advanced group typically used regular lifting movements (every 3 seconds [s] on average), whereas the intermediate group showed no clear tendency for displacements to recur at any particular frequency. Furthermore, phase portrait analyses of each group revealed that advanced individuals displayed more regular movement characteristics (stable dynamics), whereas intermediate climbers exhibited less predictable dynamics.

These findings suggest how advanced climbers achieve a stable 'coupling' between their repertoires of existing capabilities and changing environmental features (changing as function of the climbers' movements). In contrast, the relative difficulty of the route for the intermediate climbers meant that these less skilled individuals were less 'coupled' to the climbing surface throughout practice (Cordier et al., 1996, p. 805). The more sensitive temporal movement analyses placed into perspective the large learning effect along the spatial dimension shown by the intermediate climbers who achieved similar levels of movement efficiency (as indexed by entropy) relative to the advanced group (refer to Figure 12.1, Panel E), but still required practice to improve efficient temporal dynamics.

The practical implications of these findings suggests that once an individual finds a globally effective route pathway, a key constraint on improving performance on a given practice route, it should influence the temporal structuring of actions. For example, once an effective route path has been determined, a climber may further improve performance by linking movements in a more periodic fashion. For climbers where the gap between the route difficulty and their current ability is too small, as was the case with the advanced group, the learning effect may be limited, with subsequent trial-to-trial dynamics likely to follow a power law function (such as discussed in Guadagnoli & Lee, 2004; Newell, Mayer-Kress, Hong, & Liu, 2009). Emphasizing training at an easy relative difficulty may, therefore, be inefficient for progression of the individual's red-point (highest performance grade achieved with physical practice) or on-sight (highest performance without prior physical practice) ability level. On the other hand, for individuals learning on a route that is close to the limit of their ability level it may be expected that a learning effect can continue to be meaningful over multiple days of practice.

The role of perception-action coupling and climbing affordances in learning

Perception-action coupling refers to the patterned relationships that are formed between human movements and perceived information in a performance environment. It is a concept that underpins the design of practice contexts (Handford, Davids, Bennett, & Button, 1997). The suggestion is that internal and external sources of information can be detected by the individual's sensory system and perceived directly, providing affordances for action. Affordances are defined as opportunities for action in a performance environment with reference to a particular individual (Gibson, 1979). A major difference between individuals of varying experience levels is in the information attended to, and, therefore, the possible opportunities (affordances) available to be utilized.

The relationship between skill and affordance perception was examined in detail by Boschker et al. (2002). One experiment involved three groups of climbers: an advanced group (F-RSD from 7a to 7c+), a lower grade/intermediate group (F-RSD from 4c to 5c), and an inexperienced group (no climbing experience whatsoever). Participants were required to visually inspect a route of 23 holds (set between 5c to 6a F-RSD) for a defined period of time, and the task-goal was to recall the position and orientation of the holds needed to complete the route. In the first trial, an inspection period of 2.5 minutes was given; in subsequent trials participants were then given a 5 second view period. The average accuracy group values for successive trials are shown in Figure 12.2, Panel A (see also Boschker et al., 2002, p. 29). In another experiment, an inexperienced group and an advanced group undertook the same recall task as the first experiment, but participants were instructed to 'think aloud during the reproduction task, verbally

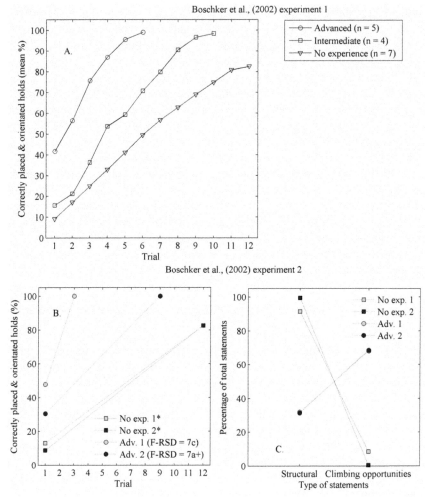

Figure 12.2 Recall performance and verbal reports during a route recall task reported in Boschker et al. (2002). The task involved a climbing route set between 5c to 6a F-RSD. Participants repeatedly attempted to reconstruct the route until it was fully and accurately reproduced or until the end of Trial 12. Adv. = advanced climber, No exp. = no experience in climbing, F-RSD = French rating scale of difficulty. * = actual values at Trial 12 were not reported. Trial 12 data for both inexperienced climbers in Panel B is instead taken from the estimated mean percentage of the no experienced group at Trial 12 from Experiment 1

reporting everything they thought about, especially what was perceived when looking at the climbing wall and why they reproduced the holds in the way they did' (Boschker et al. 2002, p. 32). Verbal reports were divided into statements referring to 'structural features' or 'climbing opportunities' (for details refer to Boschker et al., 2002, pp. 32–33) (Figure 12.2, Panels B and C).

These results of Boschker et al. (2002) showed that the advanced climbers had more accurate recall than both intermediate and less experienced climbers after 2.5 minutes of preview (Figure 12.2, Panel A, Trial 1 data). Additionally, general experience in climbing tasks supported a higher rate of recall over repeated trials (Figure 12.2, Panels A and B). According to Boschker et al. (2002) the same mechanism underpinned superior Trial 1 performance and superior trial-by-trial performance. They proposed that individuals had picked up 'clustered'[1] information if they recalled more than nine items after the 5 s viewing period, thus exceeding short-term memory capacity (but see Wagman & Morgan, 2010). Specifically, to overcome inherent limitations on short-term memory, climbers must use different types of information allowing them to draw on experience (i.e. long-term memory) rather than storing more information in short-term memory.

In climbing, information can be nested in the form of climbing opportunities that reflect the functional properties of holds, which refer to their reachability, graspability, and stand on-ability, as well as opportunities for specific climbing moves (Boschker et al., 2002). For example, various climbing techniques require specific bodily configurations with respect to orientation and relative positions of numerous holds (Seifert et al., 2015). This allows multiple holds to be collectively perceived as a single, nested, climbing opportunity (Boschker et al., 2002, p. 31). Data reported in Experiment 2 (Figure 12.2, Panels B and C) support this contention, indicating that as individuals gain climbing experience, they perceive affordances of hold properties (i.e. functional properties). Inexperienced individuals almost exclusively attend to the structural details of a surface (Figure 12.2, Panel C; see also Seifert, Wattebled, et al., 2014). This invites speculation that, should climbers perceive movements in series (as nesting of climbing actions in sequence), this skill might facilitate recall of more holds and may be one of the reasons recall performance increases with skill level (Boschker et al., 2002).

Practically, these findings imply that skilled behaviour is underpinned by perception of affordances that support effective and efficient climbing. An individual's attention during practice of a climbing route should, therefore, be guided toward the functional properties of the climbing surface that support skilled behaviour. Understanding what prevents holds from being perceived as climbing opportunities may help to improve skilled affordance perception. Fundamentally, this would emphasize designing route properties (such as the architecture of holds or wall slope) during training based on the individual's unalterable (such as anthropometrics) and trainable capabilities (such as strength) in order to ensure that climbing affordances are designed within the effectivities (i.e. capacities) of each individual. Indeed, even inexperienced climbers can perform recall tasks at the same level as advanced climbers as long as the route is within their current climbing ability, whilst advanced climbers lose their recall performance advantage over inexperienced climbers when tested on an 'impossible to climb' route (Pezzulo et al., 2010). Following this line of reasoning, interventions that improve action capabilities, such as finger and hand grip strength and endurance (Vigouroux & Quaine, 2006) or upper-limb power and endurance (Laffaye, Collin, Levernier, & Padulo, 2014), may support training transfer (such as climbing unfamiliar routes in competition) on the basis of the behavioural opportunities made available this way. Indeed, this expectation suggests that certain exercises can enable positive transfer based on motor system adaptation; however, these expectations are not always reasonable, particularly in more advanced individuals (Issurin, 2013).

Improving skilled perception of affordances though constraints manipulations

Temporary constraints manipulation can be used to affect affordance perception and potentially lead to meaningful qualitative changes in behaviour. According to Gibson (1979), 'The observer may or may not perceive or attend to the affordance, according to their needs, but the affordance, being invariant, is always there to be perceived' (cited in Pijpers, Oudejans, & Bakker, 2007, p. 108). Pijpers et al. (2007) argued that, since an environment can contain many affordances (e.g. a hold can be grasped in different ways), many factors, such as an individual's internal states, influences their selection. Design factors, such as climbing height (Pijpers, Oudejans, Bakker, & Beek, 2006) or top-rope versus leading conditions (Hardy & Hutchinson, 2007), reflect environmental and task constraints that do not change the available affordances, but that can interact with an individual's intentions, constraining affordance perception based on altered needs. For example, increased anxiety may lead an individual to focus their intention toward remaining fixed to a surface, with attention directed toward perceiving affordances that support stability. This can be observed in behaviours like reduced distance between grasped holds or a more proximal (closer to the body) attentional focus (Pijpers et al., 2006).

Figure 12.3 represents an integration of the concepts raised so far, placing into perspective the evolution of learning with respect to factors that affect skilled affordance perception. The model makes initial assumptions that affordance perception is qualitatively distinct based on actions supported, and that skilled affordance perception correlates with skilled climbing. Early in learning, fundamental affordance perception supports baseline needs such as avoiding falling. With more advanced performers, or through practice, affordances are perceived in terms of improving performance, such as periodically chaining movements. The model in Figure 12.3 is layered into concentric circles to indicate how affordances are nested atop relative to each other, where the perception of more advanced affordances entails the, perhaps, implicit perception of fundamental concerns. For example, perceiving hold usability can support remaining fixed to a surface although this may not be the intention of an individual, which may be instead efficient progression. The model also indicates that beginners can perceive skilled affordances, as a function of relative route difficulty. For example, a beginner inspecting a route with numerous and very large easy to grasp holds can

Perception of climbing affordances as a function of the individual's intentions, attention, relative route difficulty and practice

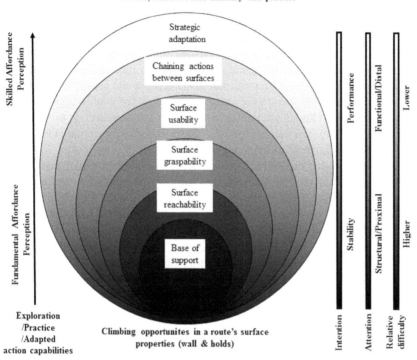

Figure 12.3 Affordance perception and skill in climbing

still perceive hold usability. However, as task difficulty increases (e.g. holds get smaller), a beginner's action capabilities may require their needs to shift towards affordances for seeking out characteristics of holds that support stability.

Implementation: effect of constraints manipulation on learning dynamics and the transfer of skill in climbing

Learning design is based on the structuring of practice and provision of learning opportunities by managing interactions at the level of the individual learner and their training constraints (Renshaw, Chow, Davids, & Hammond, 2010). Practically, simple constraints manipulation, such as providing instructions (Boschker et al., 2002) or modifying hand hold properties (Orth, Davids, & Seifert, 2014), can directly impact upon whether climbing affordances are utilized. Thus, effective learning design involves managing the interaction between constraints that facilitate progression toward skilled affordance perception during training. In this final section, we exemplify a learning intervention regarding a specific training problem.

Orth et al. (2014) assessed the impact of practice under three different conditions on climbing entropy. Routes were designed assuming that participants would use pre-existing experience to perceive affordances for supporting efficient traversal. Six individuals (with a self-reported red-point F-RSD = 6a) were observed over four separate days practising on three routes. On each day, participants climbed the three routes once each in counterbalanced order. Routes were each set at 5c F-RSD, but were different in terms of handhold orientation set into each route, including: handholds with horizontally aligned edges graspable with the knuckles running parallel to the ground; handholds with vertically aligned edges graspable with the knuckles running perpendicular to the ground; and handholds with both a horizontally aligned edge and a vertically aligned edge. The double-edged route was designed to allow climbers to explore a variety of grasping actions by presenting a choice at each hold. A transfer test was also included using a combination of the hold types from the three different learning conditions (Figure 12.4).

Data suggests that experienced climbers only displayed a learning effect on the double-edged route (Figure 12.4). Additionally, positive transfer can be inferred from the clear difference between Trial 1 (on-sight) on the double-edged route and the on-sight transfer test performance. Implications of these findings are twofold. First, in experienced climbers, an existing platform of expertise can support rapid adaptation to a route, even if unfamiliar. On the other hand, introduction of choice into handhold properties affords adaptation and problem solving at the level of route finding. Orth et al. (2014) suggested that successful transfer was induced because of the experience of climbers on the double-edged route. Specifically, the capacity to use existing experience to adapt rapidly to the multiple hold choices found in the new climbing route underpinned the positive transfer of skill. In a follow up study, Seifert et al. (2015) used the same experimental procedure as Orth et al. (2014), but considered potential mechanisms underpinning positive transfer by assessing the number of exploratory actions in relationship to entropy. A key finding was that whilst Trial 1 conditions showed both high levels of entropy and exploratory behaviour, on the transfer test, more efficient performance was associated with higher amounts of exploratory behaviour. According to Seifert et al. (2015), these findings indicate that climbers can learn to explore efficiently. Thus, a potential behavioural mechanism underpinning positive transfer might be effective exploratory behaviours.

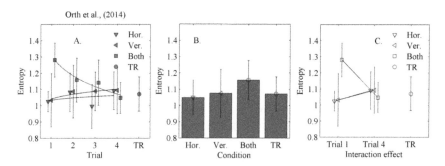

Figure 12.4 Geometric index of entropy for each trial (A), for each condition (B) and for the interaction between trial and condition (C). Hor. = horizontal edge condition, Ver.=vertical edge condition, Both = double-edged condition, TR= transfer test.

Source: Data adapted from Orth et al. (2014).

Practically speaking, any on-sight climb might be conceptualized as a skill transfer problem, requiring adaptations during performance with unfamiliar surface properties and in contexts with dynamic environments (such as outdoors). Assuming positive transfer is supported by skilled affordance perception, helping individuals to explore and learn how to find information specifying efficient climbing opportunities is one approach that might improve on-sight climbing ability. Similarly, motor adaptions, such as improving a beginner's ability to explore balance for longer periods of time, are likely to assist with the transfer of skill or learning (improved rate of learning in new contexts due to experience), because motor adaptations can support longer periods of remaining in contact with holds.

Future research and perspective: the role of exploratory behaviour in understanding the relationship between learning and affordances

Many of the ideas discussed imply that exploration during practice is a potential mechanism that can help learners to improve performance over time. In climbing, exploratory behaviour has been observed with respect to qualitatively different climbing affordances (Table 12.1). For example, exploratory behaviours related to the functional properties of holds can reveal opportunities for movement at the hips without subsequent displacement (Boulanger, Seifert, Hérault, & Coeurjolly,

Table 12.1 Specific forms of exploration directed toward qualitatively distinct affordance

Affordance layer	Movement pattern	Intention	Information foci	Example
Base of support	'X' shaped, COM (centre of mass) immobile	Maintain contact with the surface	Holds for hands and feet	Seifert et al., 2011
Surface reachability	Touching not grasping, COM immobile	Explore reachability	Individual– surface distance	Pijpers et al., 2006
Surface graspability	Grasping actions without subsequent usage, COM immobile	Explore graspability	Surface geometric properties (structure)	Fuss et al., 2013
Surface usability	Performatory actions with progression, COM mobile	Use surfaces to prepare or achieve route progression	Movement opportunities (function)	Boschker et al., 2002
Chaining	Spatial-temporal efficiency of linked actions	Use upcoming surface to regulate current positioning	Distant surfaces, movements in series	Cordier et al., 1993
Strategic adaptations	Within route active recovery/ exploration	Use of surfaces to rest or plan	Distant surfaces, internal state	Fryer et al., 2012; Sanchez et al., 2012

2015). Exploration in postural regulation during periods of immobility suggest that prolonged pauses during climbing may still be useful to the learner. Postural exploration seems particularly relevant for beginners considering this may allow the individual to determine more efficient positions and new body–wall orientations that may be important for more advanced movements. On the other hand, the more advanced individual may benefit from immobility for different reasons. For example, one possibility is that static states can afford resting and recovery and should be distinguished from exploration as a performatory behaviour (Fryer et al., 2012). Another possibility is that the individual may benefit from immobility by visually exploring upcoming holds, perhaps indicated by the amount of fixations made and their relative distance to the individual during immobility (Sanchez, Lambert, Jones, & Llewellyn, 2012).

Another form of exploration includes reaching to touch a hold but not grasping it or using it to support the body weight (Seifert et al., 2015). This form of exploration is believed important for achieving an accurate body-scaling to the environment (Pijpers et al., 2007) and, perhaps, as different techniques, such as dynamic moves, become part of an individual's action capabilities this boundary of reachability may distinguish individuals of different abilities. Making adjustments in how a hold is grasped prior to using it to support displacement is also a form of exploration perhaps in terms of graspability or usability. For example, prior to applying force to a hold climbers can be seen, in some cases, to make adjustments to how they position their hand on a hold. Such exploratory behaviour may be important to improve the amount of friction that can be applied to the hold (Fuss, Weizman, Burr, & Niegl, 2013), or enable a qualitatively different way of using the hold, such as in cases where multiple edge orientations are available (Seifert, Orth, et al., 2014).

It has also been speculated that exploration can support perception of opportunities for new climbing moves (Seifert, Orth, Herault, & Davids, 2013). This may be observed by examining how climbing actions are different over practice. For example, from one trial to the next, different route pathways, body orientations or grasping patterns might be used, reflecting exploration emerging during the dynamics of learning. Thus, during intervention the nature of learning behaviour may be better understood by evaluating the level at which exploration emerges. A substantial challenge, therefore, for future of learning research in climbing is in measuring exploration at different levels of analysis with respect to performance, both in technically manageable and theoretically consistent ways.

Conclusion

Here we discussed how skill acquisition in climbing can be understood, revealed through temporary interactions between the individual learner and the performance environment throughout practice. Pedagogical practice in climbing should focus on helping individuals to skilfully interact with climbing environments, where even inexperienced individuals bring to the task a unique set of adaptations that can form the basis from which to design a learning environment. Such a learning process entails a progression in the individual's capacity to efficiently adapt to new climbing routes, a process facilitated by skilled affordance perception.

Practical implications

- Observing performance over repeated trials of practice allows the evolution toward skilled behaviour to be assessed. Additionally, through pre- and post-test measures of performance, and testing the transfer of skill and learning, the relative importance of an intervention can be interpreted.
- The transition toward skilled behaviour involves developing exploratory behaviour across different levels (i.e. hands/feet, limb and hip orientations), which support each learner's current needs (such as stability or improved performance).
- The practitioner can influence affordance perception though manipulating constraints during training to influence each individual's intentions, needs and action capabilities. For example, a task or environment can be modified to encourage the individual to actively explore.

Summary

- Learners in climbing appear to first improve performance through route finding by determining an efficient spatial pathway, followed by improved temporal linking of movements by reducing stationary periods during ascent. A high degree of spatial-temporal efficiency enhances climbing performance.
- Dynamic internal (e.g. strength or confidence) and external (e.g. handhold positions and postural orientations) factors directly influence climbing opportunities (affordances) perceived and used by learners during practice.
- Skilled perception of climbing opportunities is essential for climbing efficiency. Early in learning, affordance perception provides a means of remaining fixed to a surface. Later in learning, a climber perceives affordances for linking movements in a more periodic manner, supporting efficient and effective performance.

Acknowledgements

The authors would like to thank Frederic Noé and Peter Wolf for their comments and ideas that improved the chapter. This project received the support of the CPER/GRR 1880 Logistic, Mobility and Numeric and FEDER RISC (ID: 33172). This project also received funding from the French National Agency of Research (ID: ANR-13-JSH2-0004 DynaMov).

Note

1 The term 'nested' is preferred here because the term 'clustered' implies that only spatial information has been perceived, thus it does not effectively capture the possibility that perceiving affordances also includes temporal properties.

References

Bläsing, B. E., Güldenpenning, I., Koester, D., & Schack, T. (2014). Expertise affects representation structure and categorical activation of grasp postures in climbing. *Frontiers in Psychology*, 5(1008), 1–11.

Boschker, M. S., Bakker, F. C., & Michaels, C. F. (2002). Memory for the functional characteristics of climbing walls: perceiving affordances. *Journal of Motor Behavior, 34*(1), 25–36.

Boulanger, J., Seifert, L., Hérault, R., & Coeurjolly, J. F. (2015). Automatic sensor-based detection and classification of climbing activities. *Sensors Journal, IEEE*, 16(3), 742–749.

Cordier, P., Dietrich, G., & Pailhous, J. (1996). Harmonic analysis of a complex motor behavior. *Human Movement Science, 15*(6), 789–807.

Cordier, P., Mendès-France, M., Bolon, P., & Pailhous, J. (1993). Entropy, degrees of freedom, and free climbing: a thermodynamic study of a complex behavior based on trajectory analysis. *International Journal of Sport Psychology, 24*, 370–378.

Cordier, P., Mendès-France, M., Bolon, P., & Pailhous, J. (1994). Thermodynamic study of motor behaviour optimization. *Acta Biotheoretica, 42*(2–3), 187–201.

Cordier, P., Mendès-France, M., Pailhous, J., & Bolon, P. (1994). Entropy as a global variable of the learning process. *Human Movement Science, 13*(6), 745–763.

Davids, K., Brymer, E., Seifert, L., & Orth, D. (2014). A constraints-based approach to the acquisition of expertise in outdoor adventure sports. In K. Davids, R. Hristovski, D. Araújo, N. B. Serre, C. Button, & P. Passos (Eds), *Complex systems in sport* (pp. 277–292). New York: Routledge.

Davids, K., Button, C., & Bennett, S. (2008). *Dynamics of skill acquisition: a constraints-led approach*. Champaign, IL: Human Kinetics.

de Geus, B., O'Driscoll, S. V., & Meeusen, R. (2006). Influence of climbing style on physiological responses during indoor rock climbing on routes with the same difficulty. *European Journal of Applied Physiology, 98*(5), 489–496.

Fryer, S., Dickson, T., Draper, N., Eltom, M., Stoner, L., & Blackwell, G. (2012). The effect of technique and ability on the VO2–heart rate relationship in rock climbing. *Sports Technology, 5*(3–4), 143–150.

Fuss, F. K., Weizman, Y., Burr, L., & Niegl, G. (2013). Assessment of grip difficulty of a smart climbing hold with increasing slope and decreasing depth. *Sports Technology, 6*(3), 122–129.

Gibson, J. J. (1979). *The ecological approach to visual perception*. Boston, MA: Houghton Mifflin.

Guadagnoli, M. A., & Lee, T. D. (2004). Challenge point: a framework for conceptualizing the effects of various practice conditions in motor learning. *Journal of Motor Behavior, 36*(2), 212–224.

Handford, C., Davids, K., Bennett, S., & Button, C. (1997). Skill acquisition in sport: some applications of an evolving practice ecology. *Journal of Sports Sciences, 15*(6), 621–640.

Hardy, L., & Hutchinson, A. (2007). Effects of performance anxiety on effort and performance in rock climbing: a test of processing efficiency theory. *Anxiety, Stress, and Coping, 20*(2), 147–161.

Issurin, V. B. (2013). Training transfer: scientific background and insights for practical application. *Sports Medicine, 43*(8), 675–694.

Laffaye, G., Collin, J. M., Levernier, G., & Padulo, J. (2014). Upper-limb power test in rock-climbing. *International Journal of Sports Medicine, 35*(8), 670–675.

Newell, K. M. (1996). Change in movement and skill: learning, retention, and transfer. In M. L. Latash & M. T. Turvey (Eds), *Dexterity and its development* (pp. 393–429). NJ: Psychology Press.

Newell, K. M., Mayer-Kress, G., Hong, S. L., & Liu, Y. T. (2009). Adaptation and learning: characteristic time scales of performance dynamics. *Human Movement Science, 28*(6), 655–687.

Orth, D., Davids, K., & Seifert, L. (2014). Hold design supports learning and transfer of climbing fluency. *Sports Technology, 7*(3–4), 159–165.

Orth, D., Davids, K., & Seifert, L. (2015). Coordination in climbing: effect of skill, practice and constraints manipulation. *Sports Medicine, 46*(2), 255–268.

Pezzulo, G., Barca, L., Bocconi, A. L., & Borghi, A. M. (2010). When affordances climb into your mind: advantages of motor simulation in a memory task performed by novice and expert rock climbers. *Brain and Cognition, 73*(1), 68–73.

Pijpers, J. R., Oudejans, R. R., & Bakker, F. C. (2007). Changes in the perception of action possibilities while climbing to fatigue on a climbing wall. *Journal of Sports Sciences, 25*(1), 97–110.

Pijpers, J. R., Oudejans, R. R., Bakker, F. C., & Beek, P. J. (2006). The role of anxiety in perceiving and realizing affordances. *Ecological Psychology, 18*(3), 131–161.

Renshaw, I., Chow, J. Y., Davids, K., & Hammond, J. (2010). A constraints-led perspective to understanding skill acquisition and game play: a basis for integration of motor learning theory and physical education praxis? *Physical Education and Sport Pedagogy, 15*(2), 117–137.

Sanchez, X., Lambert, P., Jones, G., & Llewellyn, D. J. (2012). Efficacy of pre-ascent climbing route visual inspection in indoor sport climbing. *Scandinavian Journal of Medicine and Science in Sports, 22*(1), 67–72.

Seifert, L., Boulanger, J., Orth, D., & Davids, K. (2015). Environmental design shapes perceptual-motor exploration, learning, and transfer in climbing. *Frontiers in Psychology, 6*, 1819.s

Seifert, L., Orth, D., Boulanger, J., Dovgalecs, V., Hérault, R., & Davids, K. (2014). Climbing skill and complexity of climbing wall design: assessment of jerk as a novel indicator of performance fluency. *Journal of Applied Biomechanics, 30*(5), 619–625.

Seifert, L., Orth, D., Herault, R., & Davids, K. (2013). Affordances and grasping action variability during rock climbing. In T. J. Davis, P. Passos, M. Dicks, & J. A. Weast-Knapp (Eds), *Studies in perception and action: seventeenth international conference on perception and action* (pp. 114–118). New York: Psychology Press.

Seifert, L., Wattebled, L., Herault, R., Poizat, G., Adé, D., Gal-Petitfaux, N., & Davids, K. (2014). Neurobiological degeneracy and affordance perception support functional intra-individual variability of inter-limb coordination during ice climbing. *PloS one, 9*(2), e89865.

Vigouroux, L., & Quaine, F. (2006). Fingertip force and electromyography of finger flexor muscles during a prolonged intermittent exercise in elite climbers and sedentary individuals. *Journal of Sports Sciences, 24*(2), 181–186.

Wagman, J. B., & Morgan, L. L. (2010). Nested prospectivity in perception: perceived maximum reaching height reflects anticipated changes in reaching ability. *Psychonomic Bulletin & Review, 17*(6), 905–909.

White, D. J., & Olsen, P. D. (2010). A time motion analysis of bouldering style competitive rock climbing. *The Journal of Strength and Conditioning Research, 24*(5), 1356–1360.

13 Visual-motor skill in climbing

*Chris Button, Dominic Orth, Keith Davids
and Ludovic Seifert*

Visual-motor skill is the capacity to detect relevant optical information from the environment and to coordinate movements in order to achieve an outcome. This chapter presents an overview of visual-motor behaviours used by climbers and how they can develop this important aspect of their climbing. Recent advances in eye movement tracking equipment have afforded new opportunities to study how climbers detect visual information to plan their routes and also to regulate their ongoing actions. An important phase for visual search behaviour occurs during pre-ascent inspections of a route in which numerous strategies have been identified in skilled climbers. For example, a common strategy for more difficult routes involves observing groups of holds in sequence in which more time is spent looking at holds in potentially difficult regions (cruxes). Whilst limited research has examined visual-motor skill during climbing, it has been shown that climbers develop more economic visual search patterns with practice, in which the overall number of exploratory fixations decreases, whilst performatory fixations remain relatively stable. In this chapter, we also consider how influential factors such as anxiety and fatigue affect visual-motor behaviour. Finally, some implications of this emerging field of study for climbing training and performance will be discussed.

The importance of visual-motor skill in climbing

One of the key challenges of climbing that is common to many other mountaineering activities (*e.g.* hiking, skiing, paragliding, etc.) is coordinating one's movements effectively within physically demanding and sometimes extreme environments. Undoubtedly, climbers use a variety of information sources to 'read' the environment and support their actions. Such information sources include visual, auditory, tactile, proprioceptive and prior experience. The primary concern for this chapter is how visual information is detected via eye movements before and during a climb.

The control of human movement has traditionally been conceived as consisting of three distinct phases: perception, decision making and action. In reality, each of these phases are so tightly connected and interrelated it is perhaps unwise to think of (and study) them as independent processes (Bootsma, 1989). As such, although this chapter focusses upon the perceptual characteristics of climbers, we will also discuss how perception influences planning, decision-making and movement behaviour in general. Clearly, skilled movement behaviour requires effective perception of one's local and global environment to allow climbers to regulate posture and limb movements effectively. Three kinds of task demands typically need to be satisfied for successful coordination of movements with environmental events. Performers need to:

- Ensure that they contact an object or surface in the environment at an appropriate moment in time.
- Ensure contact with appropriate velocity and force.
- Ensure contact at an intended spatial orientation (Savelsbergh & Bootsma, 1994).

In order to satisfy these task constraints, climbers need access to high quality perceptual information.

Climbers use vision to explore and detect important environmental characteristics that inform current and subsequent behaviour (e.g. surface texture and inclination, optimal anchorage points, potential routes or places to avoid, etc.). However, given environmental variables such as light quality and the weather, the appearance of many outdoor climbing environments can change from day to day and from moment to moment. Consequently, environmental features are sometimes easy to detect, they are clearly contrasted and reliable, whereas at other times, the same features may be more ambiguous and less obvious. The quality and intensity of light available partly determines the ease with which visual information can be detected. Contrast the relative perceptual challenges of climbing in natural daylight with that of climbing at night with just a head torch and the moonlight to guide one's path. However, equally influential for visual perception are the contours, textures and reflections of light that are presented by the climbing surface.

Visual information or optical flow generated as a climber explores his/her environment can be both invariant and variant. Some elements of the optical array change as the performer moves relative to the climbing surface and surrounding objects, and these features are therefore considered as variant. However, there is also an underlying essential structure that consists of what is invariant despite other superficial changes. Movement-induced changes in the informational array result in invariants becoming more apparent against the background of variants (Figure 13.1). That is, patterns within the optic structure can be detected by a climber's visual system through exploration and invariant structure can be revealed for supporting current and future actions. The process of detecting and using information to support movement is circular and reciprocal. In motor control terms, this important characteristic is called 'perception-action coupling' (Davids, Kingsbury, Bennett, & Handford, 2001) and it is apparent in the following climbing quote: 'observe an expert climber, he is always in motion, continuously moves on his feet, movements are small, but they help him to see, to analyze the environment in which he is moving' (Ivo Buda, 2013, http://www.climbingfree. net/en/blog-en/20-vision-eyesight-exercises).

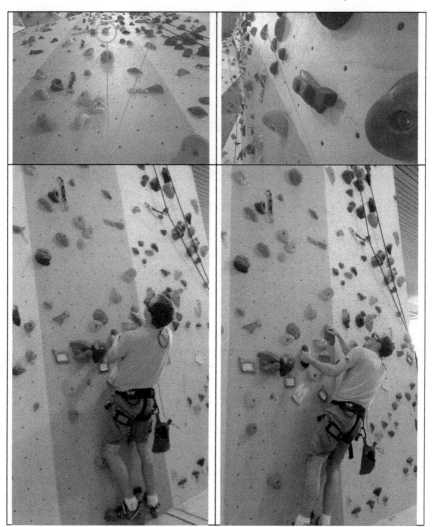

Figure 13.1 The optical flow presented to a climber as he examines holds on an indoor climbing route. There are variant and invariant optical characteristics in the visual array as the climber moves and changes his viewing perspective (left panels: looking straight up the wall; right panels: looking up the wall whilst leaning to the right)

The American psychologist Gibson (1979) proposed that humans perceive invariant information sources in terms of affordances for action, that is, what they offer, invite or demand of an organism in relation to action (see also Withagen, de Poel, Araújo, & Pepping, 2012). However, the *same* changes in local flow can afford different actions depending on the individual's current state (i.e. physical, mental, emotional) and experience. For example, skilled climbers can detect functional features different from unskilled climbers due partly to their superior knowledge but also because of their altered capacity to interact with those features.

For example, the features of a potential handhold may be 'seen' by an unskilled climber in simple physical terms (i.e. position, size, reachability) whereas a skilled climber can extract more sophisticated functional characteristics from the same information (i.e. usefulness within a sequence of moves, opportunity to rest). As described in Chapter 11 of this book, one important element of skill acquisition is the process of becoming better attuned to the affordances of invariant information perceived in specific movement contexts (see also Savelsbergh, van der Kamp, Oudejans, & Scott, 2004). Once attuned, the performer then needs to scale or calibrate their actions appropriately and thereby create an effective perception-action coupling (Jacobs & Michaels, 2007).

In the sports expertise literature there have been many attempts to examine the perceptual-motor skills of athletes in different performance contexts (for reviews, see: Mann, Williams, Ward, & Janelle, 2007; Vickers, 2007). It is now well established that athletes do not possess better visual anatomy than non-athletes but instead *how* they use their eyes differs considerably. Williams and Davids (1998) showed that expert athletes in some sports have more efficient (less random) visual search strategies than less able athletes. For example, elite athletes tend to have fewer and longer fixations when performing precise, accurate movements such as a basketball free throw or a golf putt. It is likely that such efficiencies in fixations are coupled with quicker and larger saccades between relevant information sources (Morgan & Patterson, 2009). However, a limitation of much of the existing gaze behaviour studies is that eye movement registration technology has constrained researchers to studies in which restricted participant movement was mandated.[1]

Measuring and analysing eye movements

Advances in mobile eye movement registration systems over the last 20 years have afforded new opportunities to study the visual-motor skills of climbers. The equipment now used to record eye movements is lighter and more portable than previous models and can be worn by climbers without impeding their perceptual or physical behaviours (e.g. http://www.eyetracking-glasses.com). As such, there is a small emerging body of research studies in which mobile or portable eye movement registration systems have/are being used to analyse the gaze behaviours of climbers in naturalistic climbing environments. It is towards these studies that we shall direct our attention for the remainder of this chapter.

First it is necessary to provide a few technical details about how portable eye movement registration systems function. The equipment is typically composed of a pair of modified glasses with miniaturised cameras mounted around the frames and a recording device to store video footage (the climber in Figure 13.1 is wearing such a system). Such systems usually detect the location of foveal vision within a scene through integration of two eye features: the pupil and reflection from the cornea. The fovea is the small region on the retina which provides the highest level of visual acuity. Portable eye movement systems compare the vector (angle and distance) between the pupil and the cornea, from which the system's software computes point of gaze. An additional camera records the viewpoint of the participant and this perspective is interlaced with the eye motion video. The vector displacements are calibrated (usually prior to testing) by asking participants to fixate upon objects of set locations positioned within the scene of view. A positional cursor highlighting the point of visual gaze is then digitised and superimposed onto the scene camera by custom written software. The accuracy of mobile eye movement systems is typically reported to be within 1 degree of visual angle (e.g. www.asleyetracking. com). However, there are numerous steps in the process of generating data that potentially introduce systematic error including manual calibration, inconsistent identification of both pupil and corneal reflection, and identification of fixations and locations of interest; hence, the actual accuracy is likely to be lower than that reported in user manuals. Despite such limitations the improvements seen in eye tracking technology in recent years is very impressive and likely to continue.

Pre-climb visual inspection

Pre-climb visual inspection, otherwise known as route preview, is thought to enhance climbing performance as the climber has the opportunity to identify, group and memorise key affordances offered by the to-be climbed surface and also to mentally plan and rehearse potential climbing movement patterns (Boschker et al., 2002). Once a climber has committed to a route it can be difficult to return or alter their path, hence it can be critically important to visually inspect potential climbing routes. Route preview is also considered important in indoor climbing competitions where a standard format ('on-sight') permits the climbers a timed inspection of the route before attempting to ascend without prior physical practice. Route previews are typically undertaken at ground level or the bottom of an ascent meaning that the quality of optical information may not be uniform and invariants may be more difficult to detect as the climber observes later features of the ascent.[2]

Two research studies provide indirect support for the role of route preview in identifying affordances for climbing (Boschker, Bakker, & Michaels, 2002; Pezzulo, Barca, Bocconi, & Borghi, 2010). In both studies, climbers were required to reproduce after a preview certain features of the climbing route (such as position and orientation of holds). Expert climbers typically recalled more clustered, 'chunks' of information and apparently focussed on the functional characteristics of the wall while the novices did not recall such clustered information and mostly reported the structural features of the holds. In each study, the active effort to perceive behavioural opportunities in the routes during preview was associated with more effective recall performance (Boschker, et al., 2002; Pezzulo, et al., 2010). However, it should be noted in these studies that neither preview nor subsequent climbing behaviours were measured and examined directly.

Perhaps unsurprisingly, experienced climbers can extract more functional information from a preview than less experienced climbers. Sanchez et al. (2012) examined the influence of a route preview on the performance of a subsequent climb. In this study, 29 climbers were allocated to three groups of different skill levels (intermediate: 6a or 6a+, advanced: 6c, and expert: 7b or 7c). The climbers attempted different routes that corresponded to their respective skill levels either with or without a preceding route preview of three minutes. Whilst the presence of a preview did not typically influence whether the climbers were able to complete the climbs (output performance) it did have an effect on climbing form (process performance). For example, integrating the task of preview with climbing modified the performatory behaviour of the intermediate and expert climbers (see Chapter 11 for a detailed explanation of performatory behaviour). With a preview, the more skilled climbers paused less frequently and for shorter periods of time at rest regions (Sanchez, Lambert, Jones, & Llewellyn, 2012). These findings indicate that the use of preview is an adapted skill and that it can contribute to climbing fluidity. Furthermore, climbers of different skill levels can compensate for a lack of preview by using within-route visual and/or haptic inspection assuming the difficulty of the route does not exceed their capability. It also highlights that, with the advantage of a route preview, climbers do not need to stop that long or that often, once on the wall, for route visual inspection.

More direct measures of visual perception have since further illuminated the visual-motor skills used during preview. A recent study by Grushko & Leonov. (2014) measuring visual search strategies during route preview (at intermediate and advanced levels of route difficulty) showed that a number of different eye movement patterns can be used by skilled climbers. Four globally different eye movement patterns were categorised from 23 young rock climbers as they previewed two routes suited to their skill level in an indoor climbing gym. The four search strategies were described as follows:

- *Ascending strategy*: climber looks from below to upwards and finishes preview on the top hold.
- *Fragmentary strategy*: climber looks at parts of a route and ignores a lot of holds and quickdraws.
- *Zigzagging strategy*: moving gaze from side to side as the climber looks through the route.
- *Sequence of blocks*: gradually looking though the route in blocks of two to four handholds, with particular attention being focussed on crux points (parts of the route that are more difficult).

The latter block sequencing strategy was used by 52 per cent of the climbers for viewing an intermediate difficulty route (6a+6b) and by 87 per cent of the climbers for a more advanced route (7a+/7b). The range of different strategies found by Grushko & Leonov (2014) suggests that climbers can use route previews of varying complexity for multiple purposes. For example, 'simple' previews may initially be used to identify the location of potential holds (and footrests), whereas more 'sophisticated' previews are necessary to plan potential sequences of movements. The data also seem to provide additional evidence that skilled climbers use the route preview to mentally rehearse climbing movements and that they spend most time looking at potentially difficult parts of the route. To our knowledge, this study is the only published data directly examining eye movements during preview and further research on this important element of climbing perceptual-motor skill is required.

Visual-motor behaviour while climbing

Dupuy and Ripoll (1989) measured the eye movements of five highly skilled climbers attempting the same set route in three conditions: 1) on-sight (without prior knowledge of the route), 2) after repetition (i.e. on the fifth attempt), and 3) maximal speed (to assess the influence of time pressure). A semi-portable eye movement registration device (Eye Mark Recorder IV, Nac Image Technologies) was worn by participants whilst climbing.[3] For the purposes of analysis the visual data were categorised into three dependent variables. *Prospective vision* (PV) was composed of preparatory fixations of relevant features such as holds and foot supports. *Visual-motor guiding* (GV) were regulatory fixations that occurred whilst the climber was moving for and grasping with the hands or seeking foot support. These fixations typically occur within an area close (local) to the climber defined by their reachability; however, part of the visual search occurs outside this reachability area (which might correspond to route finding, for example). For that purpose, *decentred visual exploration* (EVE) was categorised when the point of gaze was outside the recordable corneal reflection, that is, non-local fixations.

Climbers spent most time overall fixating non-local information (EVE), followed by prospective identification of features (PV), and visual-motor guidance fixations (GV) absorbed the least time (Figure 13.2). Both EVE and PV were

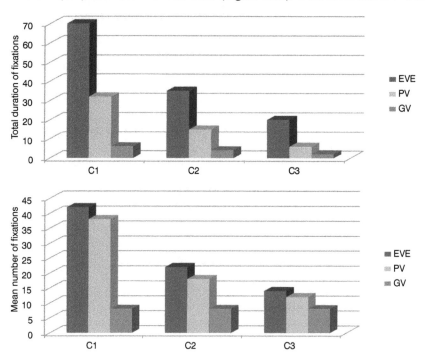

Figure 13.2 Mean visual search data of five skilled climbers. Black bars denote decentred visual exploration (EVE); the shaded bars denote prospective vision (PV); the white bars denote visual-motor guiding (GV). C1: on-sight, C2: fifth repetition of route, C3: maximum speed attempt

Source: Figure redrawn from Dupuy and Ripoll (1989).

economised under the conditions of repetition and temporal pressure; however, GV was unaffected under these constraints. Hence, during on-sight climbs, skilled climbers seemed to engage in a high proportion of visual search and planning particularly during initial attempts at a route. Dupuy and Ripoll (1989) suggest that prior experience of the route facilitates decision-making about which holds to use, and thus leads to a decrease in the amount of prospective visual and motor exploration required. Also when speed climbing, several motor actions are performed simultaneously which was associated with less overall prospective exploration. As visual-motor guidance was less affected by speed climbing and repetition, a tentative interpretation is that this process is optimised during initial attempts and remains relatively stable despite other changes in task constraints.

In contrast to Dupuy and Ripoll (1989) who examined skilled climbers, Nieuwenhuys et al. (2008) studied the visual search of unskilled climbers. Twelve inexperienced climbers wore a mobile eye tracking system while traversing two matched routes (a high route was 4.25 m) from the ground on average, whereas a low route was 0.44 m from ground level). Gaze position data was coded with greater sensitivity than in Dupuy and Ripoll's study, for example fixation locations were coded as corresponding to either 'handhold', 'wall', 'hand' or 'other'. Beyond the traditional gaze variables reported (number of fixations, average fixation duration in total and by location, and search rate[4]), Nieuwenhuys and colleagues also classified fixations as either performatory (the fixation occurred during a hip movement) or exploratory (the fixation occurred when the climber's hip was stationary).

Total fixation duration was longer in the high climb condition, although it should be noted that climb times were also much longer in this condition (Table 13.1). Interestingly, the climbers executed between two to three more exploratory fixations for every performatory fixation (which were longer) regardless of condition. Search rate was significantly lower in the high climb suggesting that participants were taking longer to extract information from fixations when more anxious.

Table 13.1 Summary of gaze behaviour from unskilled climbers contrasting between traverses associated with low (mean height 0.44 m) and high anxiety (mean height 4.25 m).

Variable	Low anxiety		High anxiety	
	M	SD	M	SD
Climbing time (s) **	29.4	4.79	45.5	12.84
Total fixation duration (s) **	7.8	2.16	12.4	4.82
Handholds (s) **	6.6	2.07	10.1	4.36
Wall (s) *	0.5	0.56	1.3	1.25
Other (s)	0.5	0.84	0.6	1.74
Number of fixations **	21.9	4.31	31.5	11.26
Average duration of fixations (ms) *	359	83	401	62
Average duration of performatory fixations (ms) *	603	194	719	165
Average duration of exploratory fixations (ms)	243	43	278	47

* p < .05, ** p < .01. Adapted from Nieuwenhuys et al. (2008) with permission of Copyright Clearance Centre

There are numerous differences between the study of Dupuy and Ripoll (1989) and that of Nieuwenhuys et al. (2008), including participant skill level, difficulty of route, outdoor versus indoor, sample size and so on; however, there are some general features that can be extracted. Visual search during climbing is predominantly focussed upon determining potential hand-holds in preparation for action. In comparison, much less time is spent looking at other features of the climbing surface or the climber's own body. Once the relevant hold has been identified the climber rapidly shifts their gaze (known as a 'saccade') to the next potential hand (or foot) hold. Presumably, the climber uses their awareness of reaching length to facilitate visual guidance of their limbs towards anchorage points, as performatory fixations are generally much shorter than exploratory fixations. Furthermore, climbers generally execute two to three times as many exploratory fixations as performatory fixations. Hence, the primary changes to visual search as a function of skill and experience appear to be in terms of improved economy of visual search with fewer, shorter fixations and a decreased search rate.

Partly inspired by these pioneering studies, Button and colleagues recently carried out a study of visual search behaviour during climbing (unpublished data). In particular they set out to determine whether repetition of a route led to improved economy of visual search behaviour. They recorded the eye movements of ten skilled climbers (6b–7a on the French rating scale) as they attempted six repetitions of two indoor climbing routes. The positions of the holds were the same for each route (both rated on the French scale as 6a–6a+). The nature of the holds used in the two routes was manipulated, that is: route 1) irregular holds: a range of different shapes of handholds were available; and route 2) regular holds: ten repetitions of only two types of handholds were available (to limit the ways in which the climbers could use the holds). The climbers conducted up to three minutes of preview prior to each attempt, and were instructed to climb with as much fluidity/efficiency as possible.

The preliminary data (Figure 13.3) indicate that skilled climbers utilise on average six to ten short fixations (approximately 130 milliseconds) per second whilst climbing a route of moderate difficulty. At first glance, the results appear to confirm Dupuy and Ripoll's (1989) findings in that the number of fixations decreased with experience of the route (Figure 13.3B). However, the simultaneous decrease in climb time (Figure 13.3A) indicates that this effect can be attributed to less overall time spent climbing. In fact, the duration of fixations (Figure 13.3C) does not appear to decrease as expected over trials; instead a subtle increase in duration occurred in both conditions. The search rate, which expresses the number of fixations made as a ratio of climb time, is a more direct indicator of economy and this variable shows a clear decreasing trend over practice (Figure 13.3D). Hence, as climbers became more familiar with the two routes they made longer fixations to fewer locations thereby confirming that experience alters the visual search behaviour of climbers.

Interestingly, climbing the *regular* hold route (squares) seems to require more frequent fixations than the *irregular* hold route (circles). Whilst the features of the holds in the *regular* hold route were more predictable, they elicited more visual search during the climb than the varied shapes of the *irregular* hold route.

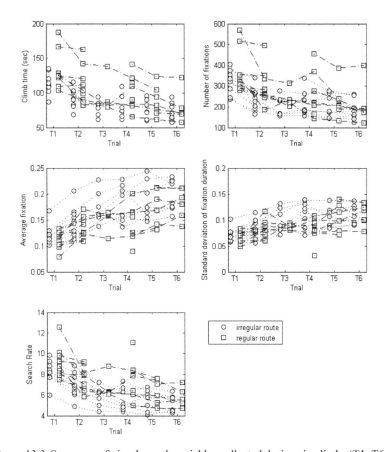

Figure 13.3 Summary of visual search variables collected during six climbs (T1–T6)

Anecdotally, after completing both routes, the climbers self-reported through a questionnaire that the *regular* hold route was physically more demanding as the lack of variety in holds restricted the number of grasp patterns they could use.

To summarise, although relatively few studies have directly examined visual-motor skills during climbing activities, some interesting data has emerged. As a function of skill and experience climbers may develop more economic visual search patterns in which the overall number of exploratory fixations decrease whilst performatory fixations remain relatively stable (Dupuy & Ripoll, 1989; Nieuwenhuys, et al., 2008). In the Button et al. pilot study, it was confirmed that fixation search rate decreases with practice, whilst average fixation duration increases.

Factors that influence visual-motor behaviour in climbing

Numerous factors are likely to influence the visual search characteristics that climbers use. For example, Pijpers and colleagues (2006) were interested in how visual attention is modified by anxiety. Climbers were asked to detect lights that were projected around them whilst they were climbing. Participants detected fewer lights when attempting a horizontal traverse on a high wall (high-anxiety condition) than on a low wall (low-anxiety condition). Hence, anxiety acts to narrow visual attention only towards local information sources. Furthermore, when participants were anxious, their perceived reach height was decreased indicating an influence on the likelihood of detecting affordances at the extremities of action boundaries.

In a follow-up study it was shown that physiological fatigue also influences the likelihood of affordance detection (Pijpers, Oudejans, & Bakker, 2007). In this study, a horizontal traverse was attempted numerous times by 16 novice climbers. Perceived and actual maximum reach height were measured at several times over a series of ten climbs. Figure 13.4 clearly shows that perceived maximal reach height is typically overestimated. After a few repetitions (trials 2–6) actual reach height remains fairly stable while perceived reach height decreases. Interestingly, the largest decreases in perceived reach height occurred after only a few trials when participants did not report any feelings of increased exertion. When perceived exertion was reported as 'high' (trials 6–10), neither perceived nor actual reach height decreased further. However, in a second experiment including trials to exhaustion where perceived exertion was reported as 'maximal', both actual and perceived reach height decreased to similar levels. Interestingly, the

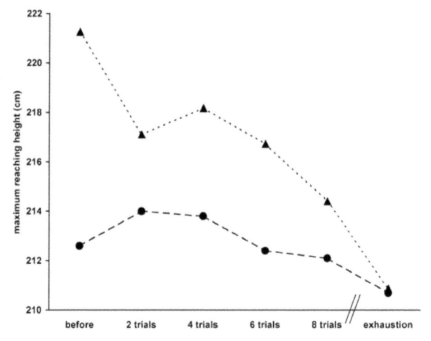

Figure 13.4 Perceived maximum reaching height (indicated by triangles) and actual maximum reaching height (indicated by circles) before climbing, after climbing 2, 4, 6 and 8 trials, and after climbing to exhaustion

most accurate perceptions of maximum reach occurred when participants were close to exhausted! Whether this phenomena arises as a subconscious protective mechanism to reduce the risk of falls from occurring remains to be established.

Practical applications

Several practical implications concerning visual-motor skill in climbing can be drawn from this chapter. Depending upon the situation and context (e.g. on-sight and lead climbs, unfamiliar routes, etc.) the visual search behaviours used during route preview can influence climbing form and, potentially, whether the climb is successfully completed. Hence, conducting a route preview is a good habit for climbers to practice. During preview, climbers should practice looking for groups of potential holds that correspond to their own action capabilities. They should also be encouraged to identify crux regions and plan (mentally rehearse) potential action strategies for these more difficult parts of a route (see Chapters 15 and 16). Whilst climbing, learners should be developing efficient visual search behaviours to explore and identify future holds. It is possible that emerging technologies such as apps that can provide three-dimensional reproductions of routes with potential routes highlighted may assist climbers to develop their search behaviours (Kajastila & Hämäläinen, 2014). With practice of a route, overall search rate should decrease, although for unfamiliar routes this characteristic is an important component of climbing regardless of skill level. Finally, learners should be aware of the factors that influence visual search behaviours (e.g. anxiety, fatigue, practice, etc.) and develop robust strategies to adapt to such factors. For example, practicing in conditions that induce mild anxiety helps to prevent attentional narrowing or more severe performance decrements (such as 'choking') from occurring when placed under high levels of anxiety (Oudejans & Pijpers, 2010).

Conclusion

Pre-climb visual inspection of a route can improve the fluency and efficiency of a subsequent climb. Skilled climbers typically extract clustered information during route preview and focus on the functional characteristics of the wall, while less experienced climbers mostly 'see' the structural features of the holds. Skilled route previewing behaviour consists of systematic visual search strategies in which groups of holds are attended to in sequence and linked to potential movement patterns. Importantly, it is not just the location of holds but the functionality of the holds that can help climbers to appreciate the 'climb-ability' of a potential route. More fixation time is devoted to harder parts of an ascent (i.e. crux points) where various potential movement configurations may exist. Whilst climbing, brief but frequent exploratory fixations are used to scan for holds and thereby facilitate planning of future behaviours. Longer and less frequent performatory fixations are used to guide hand and foot movements to intercept anchorage points. As a function of climbing practice, visual search rate decreases indicating improved economy of eye movements. Learners should be taught to look strategically for groups of holds that can be linked and mentally rehearsed with a series of movements.

Summary

- Skilled climbers use specific visual search behaviours to see more functional characteristics of the to-be climbed surface in contrast to less skilled climbers
- During route preview, climbers look for sequences of holds that support a series of actions and they spend most time viewing difficult sections of a route
- Effective route previews can enhance climbing efficiency
- Climbers use frequent exploratory fixations towards hand and foot holds to plan their potential actions, whilst less frequent performatory fixations are used to actually guide their movements
- Skilled climbers use more efficient visual search strategies than less skilled climbers (i.e. fewer, longer fixations on relevant sources of information, decreased search rate).
- Factors such as the location of difficult regions of a route (cruxes), anxiety and fatigue reduce the processing efficiency of climbers and can result in less efficient visual search behaviours.

Notes

1 For example, experimental tasks have often required participants to produce verbal judgments (e.g. Abernethy, 1990) or simulated movement (e.g. Savelsbergh, van der Kamp, Williams, & Ward, 2005) responses in preference over in situ measures in experimental conditions that are representative of typical performance environments (Dicks, Button, & Davids, 2009). Meta-analyses have revealed differences between laboratory studies and natural experimental settings for several variables related to perceptual expertise (Mann et al., 2007), hence there is a need for more in situ analysis of athletes' eye movements.
2 Although various aids to visual function now partly compensate for this (e.g. binoculars, belay specs, apps for viewing 3D topos (Kajastila & Hämäläinen, 2014)).
3 This early mobile system allowed the climber to move their head and body, but it was larger and heavier than contemporary systems and it had a wired connection to the recording device and a limited range of approximately 3–5 m.
4 The total number of fixations divided into the sum of the fixation durations.

References

Abernethy, B. (1990). Anticipation in squash: differences in advance cue utilization between expert and novice players. *Journal of Sport Sciences, 8,* 17–34.
Bootsma, R. J. (1989). Accuracy of perceptual processes subserving different perception-action systems. *The Quarterly Journal of Experimental Psychology, 41A*(3), 489–500.
Boschker, M. S., Bakker, F. C., & Michaels, C. F. (2002). Memory for the functional characteristics of climbing walls: perceiving affordances. *Journal of Motor Behavior, 34*(1), 25–36.
Button, C., Orth, D. & Seifert, L. (unpublished data). Comparing eye movements of skilled climbers when hold types are regular and irregular.
Davids, K., Kingsbury, D., Bennett, S. J., & Handford, C. (2001). Information-movement coupling: implications for the organisation of research and practice during acquisition of self-paced extrinsic timing skills. *Journal of Sports Sciences, 19,* 117–127.
Dicks, M., Button, C., & Davids, K. (2009). Representative task designs for the study of perception and action in sport. *International Journal of Sport Psychology, Special issue on Skill Acquisition and Sport Performance, 40*(4), 506–524.

Dupuy, C., & Ripoll, H. (1989). Analyse des stratégies visuo-motrices en escalade sportive. *Revue Siences et Motricité, 7*, 19–26.

Gibson, J. J. (1979). *The ecological approach to visual perception.* Hillsdale, NJ: Lawrence Erlbaum Associates.

Grushko, A. I., & Leonov, S. V. (2014). The usage of eye-tracking technologies in rock-climbing. *Procedia-Social and Behavioral Sciences, 146*, 169–174.

Jacobs, D. M., & Michaels, C. F. (2007). Direct learning. *Ecological Psychology, 19*(4), 321–349.

Kajastila, R., & Hämäläinen, P. (2014). Benefits of 3D topos for information sharing and planning in rock climbing. *Sports Technology*, 7(3–4), 128–140.

Mann, D. T. Y., Williams, A. M., Ward, P., & Janelle, C. M. (2007). Perceptual-cognitive expertise in sport: a meta-analysis. *Journal of Sport & Exercise Psychology, 29*(4), 457–478.

Morgan, S., & Patterson, J. (2009). Differences in oculomotor behaviour between elite athletes from visually and non-visually oriented sports. *International Journal of Sport Psychology, 40*, 489–505.

Nieuwenhuys, A., Pijpers, J. R., Oudejans, R. R., & Bakker, F. C. (2008). The influence of anxiety on visual attention in climbing. *Journal of Sport & Exercise Psychology, 30*(2), 171.

Oudejans, R. R. D., & Pijpers, J. R. (2010). Training with mild anxiety may prevent choking under higher levels of anxiety. *Psychology of Sport and Exercise, 11*(1), 44–50. doi: http://dx.doi.org/10.1016/j.psychsport.2009.05.002

Pezzulo, G., Barca, L., Bocconi, A. L., & Borghi, A. M. (2010). When affordances climb into your mind: advantages of motor simulation in a memory task performed by novice and expert rock climbers. *Brain and Cognition, 73*(1), 68–73.

Pijpers, J., Oudejans, R. R., Bakker, F. C., & Beek, P. J. (2006). The role of anxiety in perceiving and realizing affordances. *Ecological Psychology, 18*(3), 131–161.

Pijpers, J. R., Oudejans, R. R. D., & Bakker, F. C. (2007). Changes in the perception of action possibilities while climbing to fatigue on a climbing wall. *Journal of Sports Sciences, 25*(1), 97–110.

Sanchez, X., Lambert, P., Jones, G., & Llewellyn, D. J. (2012). Efficacy of pre-ascent climbing route visual inspection in indoor sport climbing. *Scandinavian Journal of Medicine and Science in Sports, 22*(1), 67–72.

Savelsbergh, G. J. P., & Bootsma, R. J. (1994). Perception-action coupling in hitting and catching. *International Journal of Sport Psychology, 25*, 331–343.

Savelsbergh, G. J. P., van der Kamp, J., Oudejans, R. R. D., & Scott, M. A. (2004). Perceptual learning is mastering perceptual degrees of freedom. In A. M. Williams & N. J. Hodges (Eds), *Skill acquisition in sport: research, theory and practice* (pp. 374–389). London: Routledge, Taylor & Francis.

Savelsbergh, G. J. P., van der Kamp, J., Williams, A. M., & Ward, P. (2005). Anticipation and visual search behaviour in expert soccer goalkeepers. *Ergonomics, 48*(11–14), 1686–1697.

Vickers, J. (2007). *Perception, cognition and decision training: the quiet eye in action.* Champaign, IL: Human Kinetics.

Williams, A. M., & Davids, K. (1998). Visual search strategy, selective attention, and expertise in soccer. *Research Quarterly for Exercise and Sport, 69*(2), 111–128.

Withagen, R., de Poel, H. J., Araújo, D., & Pepping, G.-J. (2012). Affordances can invite behavior: reconsidering the relationship between affordances and agency. *New Ideas in Psychology, 30*(2), 250–258. doi: 10.1016/j.newideapsych.2011.12.003

Part V
Psychology

14 Climbing grades

Systems and subjectivity

Nick Draper

Grading systems that assess the difficulty of the routes have been developed for all climbing disciplines. Typically, while graded initially by the person making the first ascent, those making repeat ascents and subsequent editions of climbing guidebooks serve to bring some further objectivity to this somewhat subjective process. A number of different grading systems have been established, not only for each climbing discipline, but also for different countries. In some countries, such as Turkey, the grading system used varies between crags even within the same discipline. This chapter presents an overview of the history of a number of the key grading systems used in rock climbing, highlights issues associated with making comparisons between grading systems, particularly in a research context, and discusses the appropriateness of using self-report climbing grades as a measure of performance ability when reporting climbing research. The chapter closes by recommending the 3:3:3 rule as a more robust method for reporting climbing ability and examining the potential, through the use of technology, to develop a more objective method through which to categorise the difficulty of a climbing route.

Introduction

The grade for a route informs climbers about the relative difficulty of a particular climb. For almost as long as climbing has existed as sport, certainly for more than 120 years, climbers have been giving grades to the routes they ascend, or in the case of indoor climbing the routes they build. Grading the difficulty of climbs is something common to all climbing disciplines whether that be mountaineering, rock climbing, deep water solo, bouldering or mixed climbing. Typically, the first to ascend the climb provides the initial grade for that route, although sometimes the original grade can be up or downgraded by consensus following repeat ascents. Although the grading of a climb is subjective in nature, the subsequent verifying process can bring some level of objectivity to the grade given for a climb.

The subjectivity in grading climbs perhaps presents some of the richest debate in the sport with climbers continuing to spend many an hour arguing the rights and wrongs of a grade for a particular climb, or the level of grades between one crag or another. The inherent subjectivity in grading climbs and the debate between climbers should always be kept in mind when researchers in the field use such scales for statistical analysis. While it might be attractive to attach a notion of ratio data to such scales, in reality the scales are perhaps ordinal at best and as such statistical analysis of data should be conducted with a degree of caution.

This chapter begins with a brief examination of the reasons climbs are graded and then takes an international perspective on the development of climbing grades. This is followed by a discussion of the issues regarding grade comparison tables, how climbing grades are reported in research, issues regarding the self-report nature of such reporting and finishes by examining who can claim to be a certain grade of climber and consequently the links between climbing grades and performance ability.

Why grade climbs?

The wide range of grading systems that have developed around the world highlight the importance placed by climbers on the need to grade climbs. Different grading systems, while generally capturing the difficulty of the climb, use a variety of components to contribute to the grade given for a climb. For instance, the UK traditional grade scale has two components, the adjectival grade and the technical grade. The adjectival component describes the overall difficulty of the climb taking into account the protection available, exposure and length of the route, rock quality and so on. The technical grade captures the (technical) difficulty of the hardest move, or sequence of moves, on a route. Regardless of differences between grading systems, climbers grade climbs to tell others about the difficulty of a route.

International approaches to grading climbs

As the sport has grown, a wide variety of locally and nationally developed systems of grading climbs have developed. A number of these systems can be seen in Table 14.1. The grading systems illustrated represent exemplars of those used in the Americas, Africa, Europe and Asia, and Australasia, but are only a fraction of the grading systems used by climbers around the world. Each grading system has its own unique history, development and usage such that it might be employed at a single crag only, in one specific region or nation or has become an internationally recognised and applied scale.

As early as the 1890s climbers had begun to use climbing grades to express the difficulty of routes in the Alps, the Benesch and the Welzenbach scales being examples. The Welzenbach scale, which consisted of Roman numerals from I (easiest) to V (hardest), was adopted in the 1960s by the International Climbing and Mountaineering Federation (UIAA) and renamed the UIAA scale (Table 14.1). The scale has been extended as can be seen in the table to accommodate more recent advances in climbing. One of the most widely used systems in Europe is the French grading system which begins at 1 for a very easy climb and is open-ended to accommodate advances in climbing. Within each number grade, as can be seen from Table 14.1, climbs can be graded with a letter (a, b or c) and be

Table 14.1 Climbing grades comparison table. IRCRA stands for the International Rock Climbing Research Association; YDS for Yosemite Decimal System; BRZ for Brazilian scale, UIAA for the Union Internationale des Associations d'Alpinisme and Font for Fontainebleau. Sources: Watts, Martin, and Durtschi (1993), Benge (1995), Draper et al. (2011a), Schöffl, Morrison, Hefti, Ullrich, and Küpper (2011), BMC (2007), Rockfax (n.d.), Club (2012)

Climbing Group	Vermin	Font	IRCRA Reporting Scale	YDS	French/sport	British Tech	Ewbank	BRZ	UIAA	Metric UIAA	Watts
			1	5.1	1		4	I sup	I	1.00	
			2	5.2	2	2	6	II	II	2.00	
			3	5.3	2+		8	II sup	III	3.00	
Lower Grade (Level 1) Male & Female			4	5.4	3-	3		III	III+	3.50	
			5	5.5	3		10	IV	IV	4.00	
			6	5.6	3+	4	12	IV	IV+	4.33	0.00
			7	5.7	4		14	V	V-	4.66	0.25
			8	5.8	4+		16	V	V	5.00	0.50
	VB	<2	9	5.9	5	5a		V sup	V+	5.33	0.75
									VI-	5.66	
			10	5.10a	5+		18		VI	6.00	1.00
Intermediate (Level 2)	V0-	3	11	5.10b	6a	5b	19		VI+	6.33	1.25
	V0	4	12	5.10c	6a+		20	VI sup	VII-	6.66	1.50
Intermediate (Level 2) Male	V0+	4+	13	5.10d	6b	5c	20		VII	7.00	1.75
	V1	5	14	5.11a	6b+		21	7a	VII+	7.33	2.00
		5+	15	5.11b	6c	6a					2.25
	V2	6A	16	5.11c	6c+		22	7b	VIII-	7.66	2.50
Advanced (Level 3) Female	V3	6A+ / 6B	17	5.11d	7a		23	7c	VIII	8.00	2.75
	V4	6B+	18	5.12a	7a+	6b	24	8a	VIII+	8.33	3.00
	V5	6C	19	5.12b	7b		25	8b			3.25
Advanced (Level 3) Male	V6	6C+ / 7A	20	5.12c	7b+		26	8c	IX-	8.66	3.50
	V7	7A+	21	5.12d	7c	6c	27	9a	IX	9.00	3.75
	V8	7B	22	5.13a	7c+		28	9b	IX+	9.33	4.00
Elite (Level 4) Female	V9	7B+	23	5.13b	8a		29	9c	X-	9.66	4.25
		7C	24	5.13c	8a+		30	10a			4.50
Elite (Level 4) Male	V10	7C+	25	5.13d	8b	7a	31	10b	X	10.00	4.75
	V11	8A	26	5.14a	8b+		32	10c	X+	10.33	5.00
	V12	8A+	27	5.14b	8c		33	11a	XI-	10.66	5.25
	V13	8B	28	5.14c	8c+		34	11b	XI	11.00	5.50
Higher Elite (Level 5) Female	V14	8B+	29	5.14d	9a	7b	35	11c			5.75
			30	5.15a	9a+		36	12a	XI+	11.33	6.00
Higher Elite (Level 5) Male	V15	8C	31	5.15b	9b		37	12b	XII-	11.66	6.25
	V16	8C+	32	5.15c	9b+		38	12c	XII	12.00	6.50

given a + to further highlight the difficulty of the route within a number and letter category. The Brazilian system begins with walking (grades I–II) and easy grades (III–V) with grade VI originally the hardest grade achievable. The 'sup' suffix as shown in Table 14.1 refers to 'superior' or harder routes within a number grade from I to VI. In the 1980s, as advances continued in the sport, Brazilian climbers adopted a French or sport style of grading, including a number and letter for climbs graded above 6 sup.

The Ewbank system, named after the developer, John Ewbank, was developed in the 1960s and is used in Australia, New Zealand and South Africa, although there are slight differences between the matching of the grades between the countries, for instance South African and Australian grades differ by 1 or 2 grades. As can be seen in Table 14.1, the scale begins at 4 for climbing, with grades 1–3 referring to walking or scrambling. As can be seen from the scale, Ewbank included only whole numbers in the scale and rejected the notion of having a technical and adjectival grade for each route. The grade for a route using the Ewbank scale reflects an overall feel of the climb, including the difficulty, length, exposure, protection and quality of rock.

The British system of grading for trad climbing, as was mentioned, as well as having a technical grade as shown in Table 14.1, also places an adjectival grade on the route. The technical grades scale originated at climbing areas such as the southern sandstone crags at Bowles and Harrison's rocks where soloing or top-roping was the norm and the key concern was with the technical difficulty of the route. The adjectival system originated at a time when British climbers were using nailed boots and hemp ropes, when the system was centred around the grade of 'difficult', which was the norm at the time, although with modern equipment such climbs are now viewed as easy routes. The scale developed over time to include the grades shown in Table 14.2, although some routes were additionally labelled as 'mild' or 'hard' such as Sail Buttress at Birchen Edge in the Peak District, which is graded as hard very difficult (HVDiff). In order to accommodate the improvements in technical difficulty, the adjectival system was extended such that it now includes divisions within the extremely severe grade from E1 to E11 grade. In traditional climbing (the leader placing their own protection en route), to which this system applies, the adjectival grade, as was mentioned above, should be seen in conjunction with the technical grade which describes the hardest move(s) on the route, such that routes could be classified at VS4b, VS4c or VS5a, which captures the degree of exposure on the route and the technical difficulty of the hardest move(s).

In North America, the most popular system (illustrated in Table 14.1) is the Yosemite Decimal System (YDS). The YDS was developed in 1953 by the Rock Climbing Section of the California Sierra Club to rate the difficulty of routes at Tahquitz Rock. In this classification system class 1 represents walking or hiking and class 5 the start of roped climbing. In this system the classification for the route was given to reflect the single most difficult move on the route, but more recently

Table 14.2 The British adjectival system

Easy (M)
Moderate (M)
Difficult (D)
Very Difficult (V Diff)
Severe (S)
Very Severe (VS)
Hard Very Severe (HVS)
Extremely Severe (E)

has evolved to reflect the overall feel of the route, so in this sense, in comparison to the British system, there has been somewhat of a move from a technical to an adjectival grading for routes. Similar to the extension to the adjectival system in the UK, the YDS developed to consist of ten divisions from 5.0 to 5.9, and has subsequently been extended to 5.15, with grades 5.10 and above being subdivided into a, b, c and d to accommodate the continued developments in the sport.

Table 14.1 illustrates the two most widely used bouldering grading systems, the 'V' or Vermin and the Font scales. The Vermin scale, named after John 'The Vermin' Sherman, represents the most widely used scale in North America, while the Font system was developed in Fontainebleau, France, and is the most widely used bouldering scale in Europe. Perhaps due to relative age of the sport or discipline, there are currently fewer systems for grading bouldering problems than for other forms of climbing; however, there are some interesting novel approaches, such as the 'Dan-Kyu' system which is widely used in Japan. Anyone familiar with the Japanese martial art of judo will know that Kyu means student or pupil and Dan means master, the Kyu grade belts being white (red) to brown, while a master (Dan grade) achieves the coveted black belt. Thus for bouldering, using this system, as a climber moves towards the Dan grade climbs, so the difficulty of the problems increase.

Issues with comparison tables in climbing

There are a number issues that arise when making comparisons between climbing grades. If climbers only took part in their sport at one crag and comparison between studies was not helpful in a research context there would perhaps be no need for climbing comparison tables. One of the great attractions for many climbers though is to visit different crags: to climb outdoors as well as indoors, to climb on limestone, granite, sandstone and gritstone, to climb in more sunny or mountainous areas than available at their local crags, to test themselves against classic climbs nationally and internationally or to find virgin rock to establish new routes. For climbers, medics and coaches, in a research context, the ability to draw comparison between studies improves our knowledge of climbing and potentially narrows the number of studies each research team might need to conduct for their area of focus. To obtain a full understanding of the relevance and implications of the findings of a particular study necessitates a translation of the ability rating of the participants and, as appropriate, the difficulty of climbs undertaken in the study. Comparison tables have grown as a result of the interest in travel shown by climbers and the increasing international research attention on the sport.

There are numerous examples of such comparison tables in research papers and climbing guides, such as Rockfax (n.d.), Peter and Peter (1990), Watts et al. (1993), Duff (2000), Padrenosso et al. (2008), Llewellyn and Sanchez (2008) and Draper et al. (2016). Even if we accept and recognise the subjective nature of climbing grades, issues arise, as can be seen from Table 14.1, as soon as one begins to construct such a comparison table. Firstly, there are differences between countries and systems regarding where 'climbing' actually starts, what constitutes rock climbing and what constitutes walking or scrambling. This creates issues with the initial alignment of grading scales. Then, as can be seen from the table, there are differences as to the number of steps and where these occur for each climbing scale. For instance, the YDS and sport scales have 32 grades, whereas the BRZ has 27, Ewbank 28 and UIAA 29, which makes in-scale alignment also problematic. It is for this reason that the IRCRA scale, which was developed by Draper et al. (2016) during the IRCRA 2014 Congress held in Pontresina, was developed with 32 divisions in order to match to the two scales with the largest number of grade divisions.

In a research context both the way a comparison table has been constructed and any statistical analysis coding system that is applied can affect the comparative potential of the findings. For instance, Llewellyn & Sanchez (2008) created a statistical code linked to the adjectival grades in the British scale (moderate to E9 grade) assigning a number to each division such that there were 16 grades in their analysis. Such an approach, which has been very common in climbing research to date, adds a further complexity to comparison between studies. It was for such reasons that the IRCRA created their scale in order to bring a more uniform approach to grading for future research publication and dissemination. Ultimately, it must be recognised that not only is the grading of a climb subjective, so also is the creation of a comparison table whether in a guidebook or a research paper. While both the grade of a climb and a comparison table, through experience and feedback, can be refined over time, there remains always an element of subjectivity to both climbing grades and comparison tables.

The relationship between climbing grades and performance ability

The exact nature of the relationship between climbing ability and climbing grade attained – as two distinct measures of performance – remains to be elucidated. In 2015 Draper and co-workers from the IRCRA published a position statement regarding ability groupings, comparison between scales and statistical analysis of data. The table published as the recommended way forward for researchers is shown in Table 14.1. Further analysis, as shown in Figure 14.1, between the established IRCRA scale and existing climbing grade scales shows that while the relationship between the scales is linear, the gradient and nature of the slope differs between scales.

To further elucidate the relationship between self-reported climbing grades and performance ability, a multi-centre study has been undertaken by members of IRCRA. This research, which will be presented at the 2016 International Rock Climbing Congress, will utilise a battery of tests to quantify climbing ability, objectively measure climbing performance on graded climbs and collect data on self-reported ability grade to further examine the relationship between these performance parameters.

Climbing grades and research: issues with self-report climbing grades

As can be seen from Table 14.3, the performance ability of climbers is most commonly described by participant grade self-report, with this increasingly representing the best

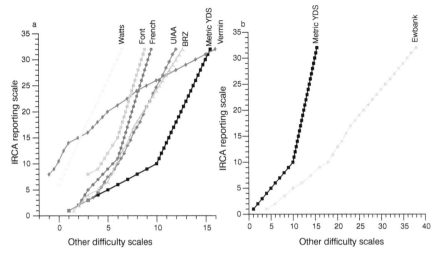

Figure 14.1 IRCRA Reporting Scale against existing difficulty scales. IRCRA stands for the International Rock Climbing Association; YDS for Yosemite Decimal System; BRZ for Brazilian scale, UIAA for the Union Internationale des Associations d'Alpinisme and Font for Fontainebleau

redpoint climb for the cohort in each study. The performance ability of climbers, as expressed through their highest climbing grade, has value for research purposes, firstly to enable categorisation of climbers within a study (for instance expert versus advanced or intermediate climbers) and secondly to facilitate comparison between studies. Until recently, however, the validity of self-report ability assessment had not been reported. Away from climbing there have been many studies which have examined the use of self-report in areas such as emotional intelligence, sports injuries and ability assessment (Mabe & West, 1982; O'Connor & Little, 2003; Piland, Motl, Ferrara, & Peterson, 2003; Valuri, Stevenson, Finch, Hamer, & Elliott, 2005).

Mabe & West (1982) completed a meta-analysis of 55 previous studies in the area of self-evaluation of ability and found a low mean validity co-efficient between self-evaluation and actual performance measurement (mean r = 0.29). However, they went on to suggest that when appropriate conditions of measurement are met then the validity co-efficient rose to mean r = 0.80. One of the key conditions of measurement highlighted was the rater's previous experience with self-evaluation. In the area of sports injuries, both Piland et al. (2003) and Valuri et al. (2005) found good levels of agreement between self-report and more objective/measured data. However, in the area of emotional intelligence, O'Connor & Little (2003) found a poor agreement between self-report and ability-based measures. This research suggests that there is a need to evaluate self-report as it relates to reporting climbing ability of climbers in any study. It was for this reason that Draper et al. (2011b) conducted a study of self-report ability in rock climbing.

Draper et al.'s (2011b) paper highlights the fact that the validity of self-report questionnaires is dependent on the respondent's previous experience and their

Table 14.3 Summary of self-report methods and reported grades in rock climbing studies post 2000

Authors and date	Participating climbers' experience	Climbing grades French/sport (YDS)
Janot, Steffen, Porcari, and Maher (2000)	Beginner and recreational	Not reported
Grant et al. (2001)	Recreational and elite	Traditional: Recreational, f4 to f5 (5.7 to 5.10a); Elite, >f5+ (>5.10a)
Noe, Quaine, and Martin (2001)	International competitors	Not reported
Boschker and Barker (2002)	Non-climbers	Non-climbers
Grant et al. (2003)	Intermediate	≥f6a (≥5.10b)
Watts, Joubert, Lish, Mast, and Wilkins (2003)	Experienced junior competitive climbers	Redpoint: f7a (5.11d), f5 to ~f8b+ (5.10a to ~5.14a)
Schoffl, Hochholzer, and Imhoff (2004)	German junior national team and recreational climbers	Redpoint: Team, f7c (5.12d); Recreation, f6b (5.10)
Schweizer, Bircher, Kaelin, and Ochsner (2005)	Experienced rock climbers	Not reported
de Geus, Villanueva O'Driscoll, and Meeusen (2006)	Competitive climbing experience	On-sight: f7b to f8a (5.12b to 5.13b)
Ferrand, Tetard, and Fontayne (2006)	Junior elite	f7b (5.12b)
Bertuzzi, Franchini, Kokubun, and Kiss (2007)	Elite and recreational	Recreational: f6a to f6c+ (5.10b to 5.11c); Elite: f7c to f8b+ (5.12d to 5.14a)
Hardy and Hutchinson (2007)	Experienced rock climbers	Traditional: f5 to f7b (5.9 to 5.12b)
MacLeod et al. (2007)	Intermediate	On-sight: f7a+ (5.12a), f6c to f7c (5.11b to 5.12d)
Schweizer and Furrer (2007)	Not specified (rock climbers)	On-sight: f7a+ (5.12a), f6b+ to f7c (5.11a to 5.12d); Redpoint: f7b+ (5.12c), f7a to f8b+ (5.11d to 5.14a)
Draper, Jones, Fryer, Hodgson, and Blackwell (2008)	Intermediate	~f3- to ~f4+ (~5.4 to ~5.8)
Llewellyn & Sanchez (2008)	Not specified (rock climbers)	~f6b (5.10d)
Watts et al. (2008)	Experienced climbers	f6c (5.11b)
Brent, Draper, Hodgson, and Blackwell (2009)	Novice, intermediate, advanced and elite	f6b+ (5.11a)

Authors and date	Participating climbers' experience	Climbing grades French/sport (YDS)
España-Romero et al. (2009)	High-level sport climbers	On-sight: Male, f8a (5.13b); Female, f7a (5.11d)
Sanchez, Boschker, and Llewellyn (2010)	Elite (Belgian climbing championship)	f7b+ to f8b (5.12c to 5.13d)
Draper, Jones, Fryer, Hodgson, and Blackwell (2010)	Intermediate	Traditional: f3- to f5+ (5.6 to 5.10a); Sport: f6a to f6c (5.10b to 5.11b)
Fuss and Niegl (2010)	Intermediate, advanced and elite	Intermediate: f6a to f6b (5.10b to 5.10d); Advanced: f6b+ to f7c (5.11a to 5.12d); Elite: f8a (5.13b)
Sherk, Sherk, Kim, Young, and Bemben (2011)	Intermediate and advanced	f5+ to f7c (5.10a to 5.12d)
Green and Helton (2011)	Intermediate	>f5 (>5.9)
Fryer et al. (2011)	Not specified (rock climbers)	Redpoint: f6b (5.10d)
Draper, Dickson, Fryer, and Blackwell (2011c)	Intermediate	On-sight: f5+ (5.10a); Redpoint: f6a+ (5.10c)
Schöffl, Schöffl, Dötsch, Dörr, and Jüngert (2011)	German Junior National Team	Female: f7b+ (5.12c), f7a to f7c+ (5.11d to 5.13a); Male: f8a (5.13b), f7c+ to f8c (5.13a to 5.14b)
Espana-Romero et al. (2012)	Experienced	f6c to f7b (5.11a to 5.12b)
Baláš, Pecha, Martin, and Cochrane (2012)	Beginners to national team members	f4 to f8c+ (5.7 to 5.14c)
Draper et al. (2012)	Intermediate	Redpoint: f5+ to f6b (5.10a to 5.10d); On-sight: f6a (5.10b)
Amca, Vigouroux, Aritan, and Berton (2012)	Experienced	f7b (5.12c)
Dickson, Fryer, Blackwell, Draper, and Stoner (2012)	Elite	Redpoint: f7c+ to f8a (5.13a to 5.13b); On-sight: f7b+ (5.12c)
Fryer et al. (2012)	Intermediate and advanced	On-sight: Intermediate: f5+ to f6a (5.10a to 5.10b); Advanced: f6a to f6c (5.10b to 5.11b)
Seifert et al. (2013)	Novices and intermediate	Novice: <f5 (<5.9); Intermediate: f6a (5.10b)
Fuss, Burr, Weizman, and Niegl (2013)	Experienced	Redpoint: f6c+ (5.11c); On-sight: f6b (5.10d)

continued ...

Table 14.3 continued

Authors and date	Participating climbers' experience	Climbing grades French/sport (YDS)
Green, Draper, and Helton (2014)	Intermediate and greater	<f6a (<5.10b)
Fanchini, Violette, Impellizzeri, and Maffiuletti (2013)	National and international competitors	f7b to f8c (5.12b to 5.14b)
Laffaye, Collin, Levernier, and Padulo (2014)	Novice, skilled and elite	Novice: <f6a (<5.10b); Skilled f6c to f7b (5.11b to 5.12b); Elite: ≥f8a (≥5.13b)
Seifert et al. (2014)	Not specified (rock climbers)	f6a (5.10b)
Balas et al. (2014)	Beginner to elite level	f3 to f8b (5.4-5.13d)

ability to accurately assess and evaluate this in the context of the questionnaire (Mikkelsson, Kaprio, Kautiainen, Kujala, & Nupponen, 2005). This is in agreement with the conditions of measurement highlighted by Mabe & West (1982). In the context of climbing, while for newer climbers this might be more difficult, for more experienced climbers this criterion would appear to be more easily met due to the nature of the sport. Climbers, from beginner level upwards, constantly have to recall previous experience and refer to local climbers (indoor guides etc.) and guidebooks to choose their next route. A climber's performance on each route informs them of their performance against (a) a particular level (grade) and (b) at a particular venue and consequently affects their choice for their next route. Given this aspect of the sport it would seem appropriate to hypothesise that climbers would be able to accurately self-assess and report their climbing ability via questionnaire. This fact, however, had not been verified in a climbing context until the work of Draper et al. (2011b).

In their study, involving 29 competitive climbers (17 male, 12 female), the participants completed a self-report questionnaire within which they recorded their highest on-sight ascent in the previous 12 months. To assess the validity of this data the climbers subsequently completed a sport lead, on an indoor climbing wall, of a route that increased in difficulty over the 19 m of ascent. The height achieved by the climber was associated with a particular climbing grade, the route having been set by the research team who had between 5 and 20 years' experience in competition route-setting. Results of the study indicated that there was good agreement between the self-reported and assessed climbing grades of the participants. Males slightly over-reported their climbing ability in comparison to their assessed ability (mean ability [± SD] being 23.9 [± 2.4] and 22.9 [± 2.7] Ewbank, respectively), while females conversely slightly under-reported their ability (20.1 [± 3.7] and 20.7 [± 3.1] Ewbank, respectively). There were, however, no significant differences between self-report and assessed grades for either males or females, which perhaps suggests that climbers do accurately recall their ability when completing questionnaires.

Although quite similar, Draper et al. (2011b) commented on the slight overestimation of ability for males and slight underestimation by females, suggesting that their results were similar to those in other areas of research. A number of previous studies had found respondents overestimated their abilities in order to cast themselves in a more complimentary light (Palta, Prineas, Berman, & Hannan, 1982; Niedhammer, Bugel, Bonenfant, Goldberg, & Leclerc, 2000; Spencer, Appleby, Davey, & Key, 2002; Jones, Knapik, Sharp, Darakjy, & Jones, 2007). Draper et al. (2011b) suggested that this was likely the case for the males in the study. Conversely, Sulheim, Ekeland, and Bahr (2007) noted a similar trend with the female skiers in their study, who also underestimated their ability, which the researchers attributed to a tendency towards a modest attitude. Draper et al. (2011b) suggested that this was also perhaps likely in their study.

Nevertheless, it would appear that using self-report grades to record the ability of a group may be justified in a climbing context because of the constant measuring of performance against the grade of each ascent, which is inherent within the sport. This constant calibration process is likely to mean that climbers can accurately gauge their ability when asked to record this for research purposes. As a result of the use of grades for routes or problems in all climbing disciplines, it would perhaps not be inappropriate to generalise these findings to other climbing disciplines. A note of caution perhaps should perhaps be heeded when working with children or novice climbers who might have insufficient experience to accurately estimate their ability. Future studies in this area might assess the reliability of self-report grades and conduct, with a larger group of climbers, a study in which the climbers ascend a number of routes of increasing difficulty to even more accurately assess their actual climbing ability.

When can you claim a grade?

The simple answer to this question might be once you have ascended a route at that grade. For instance, if you ascend one 6a (19 Ewbank, 5.10b YDS) sport route does this make you a 6a climber? The inherent subjectivity in grading, differences, perceived or actual, between the same grade climb at different crags, and nuances between different rock types and angles of climb (slab versus vertical or overhanging) perhaps suggest that to make a claim to be a 6a climber with one ascent would be inappropriate. Drum (2014) proposed an excellent solution for claiming a grade: the 3:3:3 rule. When wishing to claim a particular grade as their highest redpoint grade, the climber should have completed three successful ascents of that grade on three different routes within the previous three months.

A more objective method for grading climbs?

A further method through which to bring greater objectivity to grading climbs could be developed with the assistance of technology. With the aid of information and communications technology (ICT) it would be possible to place factors such as the following (in no particular order) into an algorithm to objectively quantify the difficulty of a route:

- Number, size, type and quality of the holds
- Quality of the rock
- Number of moves required
- Number of changes in position/stance required
- Rock type
- Angle of the rock face
- Availability of protection (for trad routes)
- Exposure of the route
- Location of the route, sea cliff, quarry, mountain route and so on
- Number of ascents
- The ratio of the crux move(s) relative to the difficulty of rest of the climb
- The height of the route (climb distance)

Once an initial grade was confirmed via the algorithm, the use of video and smartphone apps could then support an ongoing grade refinement process.

One might argue that such a process of bringing objectivity to grading climbs might undermine some of the post-climb discourse in the pub/bar/café/tavern. However, given the continued debate around goal line technology in football/soccer, often inconclusive evidence in rugby and cricket replays regarding tries and dropped catches, there would no doubt be room for discussion. Where humans and technology meet there is always room for error and subsequent discussion. As a consequence, the development of a more objective grading system using video and ICT as a comparison with existing grades is research I anticipate with excitement. I look forward to the ensuing discussion; see you for some après-climb debate in the pub!

Practical applications

The need for a chapter such as this was highlighted to me when I began to search for literature and previous research in the field. To say the least, there appears to be a dearth of research and literature relating to the grading of climbs, grading systems, their development and the establishment of grading scale comparison tables. Each evolved over time to attempt to quantify in a quasi-objective manner difficulty in climbing. It is not by accident perhaps that Watts entitled his review of climbing research 'the physiology of *difficult* rock climbing' (Watts, 2004).

The grade for any particular route is normally decided upon by the climber making the first ascent. Over time, the ascribed grade is given a further degree of objectivity through confirmation after repeat ascents. In the fullness of time the grade for a climb is normally widely accepted by the climbing community, although there are always exceptions where debate continues around the real difficulty of the climb, 'Long Tall Sally' at Burbage North on the Peak District gritstone being one such example. Some feel it is 'soft' in the grade, as an entry to the extreme category using the British adjectival system, while others defend its rating at E1. The (healthy) debate will no doubt continue into the future, as it will for those climbs which push the boundaries of the sport at grades such as E11, 5.15 and 9b, given the lack of climbers with the ability to repeat hard ascent and the politics of downgrading that can appear in such elite climbing circles.

Key practical aspects arising from the research and literature suggest that:

- Rock climbers appear to be relatively accurate when self-reporting their climbing ability so, consequently, in the absence of a more objective system this would seem to present a valid and reliable assessment of performance in a research context.
- The 3:3:3 rule could be used as a practical and consistent method to quantify a climber's current performance ability. Climbers wishing to claim a particular grade as their highest redpoint grade should have completed three successful ascents at that grade on three different routes within the previous three months.

Summary

- The initial grade given to a rock climb, assessed by the climber making the first ascent, is an inherently subjective process.
- Repeat ascents and verification, or modification, of the initial grade will serve, over time, to increase grade objectivity.
- Research indicates that self-report climbing grades are a valid measure of performance ability for males and females and can be used in research papers as part of the description of participants.
- The 3:3:3 rule might provide a more robust method through which to assess a climber's ability at any one grade level.
- Further research and new technologies may enable the development of a more objective method by which to quantify the degree of difficulty in a particular route.

Acknowledgements

I would like to thank Professor Phil Watts, Dr Arif Mithat and Dr Jiří Baláš who provided advice regarding grading scales in their countries, Professor Tino Fuss who developed Figure 14.1 and David Giles who developed Tables 14.1 and 14.3 for the chapter and completed the references.

References

Amca, A. M., Vigouroux, L., Aritan, S., & Berton, E. (2012). The Effect of Chalk on the Finger-Hold Friction Coefficient in Rock Climbing. *Sports Biomechanics / International Society of Biomechanics in Sports, 11*(4), 473–479.

Balas, J., Panackova, M., Strejcova, B., Martin, A. J., Cochrane, D. J., Kalab, M., Kodejska, J., & Draper, N. (2014). The Relationship between Climbing Ability and Physiological Responses to Rock Climbing. *Scientific World Journal, 2014*, 678387.

Baláš, J., Pecha, O., Martin, A. J., & Cochrane, D. (2012). Hand–Arm Strength and Endurance as Predictors of Climbing Performance. *European Journal of Sport Science, 12*(1), 16–25.

Benge, M. (1995). *Rock: Tools and Technique*. Carbondale, CO: Elk Mountain Press.

Bertuzzi, R. C. D. M., Franchini, E., Kokubun, E., & Kiss, M. A. P. D. M. (2007). Energy System Contributions in Indoor Rock Climbing. *European Journal of Applied Physiology, 101*(3), 293–300.

BMC. (2007). A Brief Explanation of UK Traditional Climbing Grades. Retrieved from https://www.thebmc.co.uk/Download.aspx?id=108

Boschker, M. S., & Barker, F. C. (2002). Inexperienced Sport Climbers Might Perceive and Utilize New Opportunities for Action by Merely Observing a Model. *Perceptual and Motor Skills, 95*(1), 3–9.

Brent, S., Draper, N., Hodgson, C., & Blackwell, G. (2009). Development of a Performance Assessment Tool for Rock Climbers. *European Journal of Sport Science, 9*(3), 159–167.

Club, T. A. A. (2012). *The American Alpine Journal*. Canada: The American Alpine Club.

de Geus, B., Villanueva O'Driscoll, S., & Meeusen, R. (2006). Influence of Climbing Style on Physiological Responses during Indoor Rock Climbing on Routes with the Same Difficulty. *European Journal of Applied Physiology, 98*(5), 489–496.

Dickson, T., Fryer, S., Blackwell, G., Draper, N., & Stoner, L. (2012). Effect of Style of Ascent on the Psychophysiological Demands of Rock Climbing in Elite Level Climbers. *Sports Technology, 5*(3–4), 111–119.

Draper, N., Canalejo, J. C., Fryer, S., Dickson, T., Winter, D., Ellis, G., Hamlin, M., Shearman, J., & North, C. (2011a). Reporting Climbing Grades and Grouping Categories for Rock Climbing. *Isokinetics and Exercise Science, 19*(4), 273–280.

Draper, N., Dickson, T., Blackwell, G., Fryer, S., Priestley, S., Winter, D., & Ellis, G. (2011b). Self-Reported Ability Assessment in Rock Climbing. *Journal of Sports Sciences, 29*(8), 851–858.

Draper, N., Dickson, T., Fryer, S., & Blackwell, G. (2011c). Performance Differences for Intermediate Rock Climbers Who Successfully and Unsuccessfully Attempted an Indoor Sport Climbing Route. *International Journal of Performance Analysis in Sport, 11*(3), 450–463.

Draper, N., Dickson, T., Fryer, S., Blackwell, G., Winter, D., Scarrott, C., & Ellis, G. (2012). Plasma Cortisol Concentrations and Perceived Anxiety in Response to on-Sight Rock Climbing. *International Journal of Sports Medicine, 33*(1), 13–17.

Draper, N., Giles, D., Schöffl, V., Fuss, F., Watts, P., Wolf, P., Baláš, J., España Romero, V., Gonzalez, G., Fryer, S., Fanchini, M., Vigouroux, L., Seifert, L., Donath, L., Spoerri, M., Bonetti, K., Phillips, K., Stöcker, U., Bourassa-Moreau, F., Garrido, I., Drum, S., Beekmeyer, S., Ziltener, J., Taylor, N., Beeretz, I., Mally, F., Amca, A., Linhat, C., & Abreu, E. (2016). Comparative Grading Scales, Statistical Analyses, Climber Descriptors and Ability Grouping: International Rock Climbing Research Association Position Statement. *Sport Technology*, 10.1080/19346182.2015.1107081.

Draper, N., Jones, G. A., Fryer, S., Hodgson, C., & Blackwell, G. (2008). Effect of an On-Sight Lead on the Physiological and Psychological Responses to Rock Climbing. *Journal of Sports Science and Medicine, 7*(4), 492–498.

Draper, N., Jones, G. A., Fryer, S., Hodgson, C. I., & Blackwell, G. (2010). Physiological and Psychological Responses to Lead and Top Rope Climbing for Intermediate Rock Climbers. *European Journal of Sport Science, 10*(1), 13–20.

Drum, S. (2014). Personal communication, 25 November.

Duff, A. C. (2000). *Yorkshire Gritstone Bouldering*. Sheffield, UK: Rockfax.

Espana-Romero, V., Jensen, R. L., Sanchez, X., Ostrowski, M. L., Szekely, J. E., & Watts, P. B. (2012). Physiological Responses in Rock Climbing with Repeated Ascents over a 10-Week Period. *European Journal of Applied Physiology, 112*(3), 821–828.

España-Romero, V., Porcel, F. B. O., Artero, E. G., Jiménez-Pavón, D., Sainz, A. G., Garzón, M. J. C., & Ruiz, J. R. (2009). Climbing Time to Exhaustion is a Determinant of Climbing Performance in High-Level Sport Climbers. *European Journal of Applied Physiology, 107*(5), 517–525.

Fanchini, M., Violette, F., Impellizzeri, F. M., & Maffiuletti, N. A. (2013). Differences in Climbing-Specific Strength between Boulder and Lead Rock Climbers. *The Journal of Strength & Conditioning Research, 27*(2), 310–314.

Ferrand, C., Tetard, S., & Fontayne, P. (2006). Self-Handicapping in Rock Climbing: A Qualitative Approach. *Journal of Applied Sport Psychology, 18*(3), 271–280.

Fryer, S., Dickson, T., Draper, N., Eltom, M., Stoner, L., & Blackwell, G. (2012). The Effect of Technique and Ability on the Vo2–Heart Rate Relationship in Rock Climbing. *Sports Technology, 5*(3–4), 143–150.

Fryer, S., Draper, N., Dickson, T., Blackwell, G., Winter, D., & Ellis, G. (2011). Comparison of Lactate Sampling Sites for Rock Climbing. *International Journal of Sports Medicine, 32*(6), 428–432.

Fuss, F. K., Burr, L., Weizman, Y., & Niegl, G. (2013). Measurement of the Coefficient of Friction and the Centre of Pressure of a Curved Surface of a Climbing Handhold. *Procedia Engineering, 60*, 491–495.

Fuss, F. K., & Niegl, G. (2010). Biomechanics of the Two-Handed Dyno Technique for Sport Climbing. *Sports Engineering, 13*(1), 19–30.

Grant, S., Hasler, T., Davies, C., Aitchison, T. C., Wilson, J., & Whittaker, A. (2001). A Comparison of the Anthropometric, Strength, Endurance and Flexibility Characteristics of Female Elite and Recreational Climbers and Non-Climbers. *Journal of Sports Sciences, 19*(7), 499–505.

Grant, S., Shields, C., Fitzpatrick, V., Loh, W. M., Whitaker, A., Watt, I., & Kay, J. W. (2003). Climbing-Specific Finger Endurance: A Comparative Study of Intermediate Rock Climbers, Rowers and Aerobically Trained Individuals. *Journal of Sports Sciences, 21*(8), 621–630.

Green, A. L., Draper, N., & Helton, W. S. (2014). The Impact of Fear Words in a Secondary Task on Complex Motor Performance: A Dual-Task Climbing Study. *Psychological Research, 78*(4), 557–565.

Green, A. L., & Helton, W. S. (2011). Dual-Task Performance during a Climbing Traverse. *Experimental brain Research, 215*(3–4), 307–313.

Hardy, L., & Hutchinson, A. (2007). Effects of Performance Anxiety on Effort and Performance in Rock Climbing: A Test of Processing Efficiency Theory. *Anxiety Stress Coping, 20*(2), 147–161.

Janot, J. M., Steffen, J. P., Porcari, J. P., & Maher, M. A. (2000). Heart Rate Responses and Perceived Exertion for Beginner and Recreational Sport Climbers during Indoor Climbing. *Journal of Exercise Physiology Online, 3*(1).

Jones, S. B., Knapik, J. J., Sharp, M. A., Darakjy, S., & Jones, B. H. (2007). The Validity of Self-Reported Physical Fitness Test Scores. *Military Medicine, 172*(2), 115–120.

Laffaye, G., Collin, J. M., Levernier, G., & Padulo, J. (2014). Upper-Limb Power Test in Rock-Climbing. *International Journal of Sports Medicine, 35*(8), 670–675.

Llewellyn, D. J., & Sanchez, X. (2008). Individual Differences and Risk Taking in Rock Climbing. *Psychology of Sport and Exercise, 9*(4), 413–426.

Mabe, P. A., & West, S. G. (1982). Validity of Self-Evaluation of Ability: A Review and Meta-Analysis. *Journal of Applied Psychology, 67*(3), 280.

MacLeod, D., Sutherland, D. L., Buntin, L., Whitaker, A., Aitchison, T., Watt, I., Bradley, J., & Grant, S. (2007). Physiological Determinants of Climbing-Specific Finger

Endurance and Sport Rock Climbing Performance. *Journal of Sports Sciences, 25*(12), 1433–1443.

Mikkelsson, L., Kaprio, J., Kautiainen, H., Kujala, U. M., & Nupponen, H. (2005). Associations between Self-Estimated and Measured Physical Fitness among 40-Year-Old Men and Women. *Scandinavian Journal of Medicine & Science in Sports, 15*(5), 329–335.

Niedhammer, I., Bugel, I., Bonenfant, S., Goldberg, M., & Leclerc, A. (2000). Validity of Self-Reported Weight and Height in the French Gazel Cohort. *International Journal of Obesity and Related Metabolic Disorders: Journal of the International Association for the Study of Obesity, 24*(9), 1111–1118.

Noe, F., Quaine, F., & Martin, L. (2001). Influence of Steep Gradient Supporting Walls in Rock Climbing: Biomechanical Analysis. *Gait Posture, 13*(2), 86–94.

O'Connor, R. M., & Little, I. S. (2003). Revisiting the Predictive Validity of Emotional Intelligence: Self-Report Versus Ability-Based Measures. *Personality and Individual Differences, 35*(8), 1893–1902.

Padrenosso, A., de Godoy, E. S., César, E., Barreto, A., Reis, V., Silva, A., & Dantas, E. (2008). Somatic and Functional Profile of Sport Rock Climbers. *Physical Education and Sport, 52*(1), 73–76.

Palta, M., Prineas, R. J., Berman, R., & Hannan, P. (1982). Comparison of Self-Reported and Measured Height and Weight. *American Journal of Epidemiology, 115*(2), 223–230.

Peter, A., & Peter, I. (1990). *The Handbook of Climbing*. London: Pelham Books.

Piland, S. G., Motl, R. W., Ferrara, M. S., & Peterson, C. L. (2003). Evidence for the Factorial and Construct Validity of a Self-Report Concussion Symptoms Scale. *Journal of Athletic Training, 38*(2), 104.

Rockfax. (n.d.). Grade Conversions. Retrieved from http://www.rockfax.com/publications/grades/

Sanchez, X., Boschker, M. S., & Llewellyn, D. J. (2010). Pre-Performance Psychological States and Performance in an Elite Climbing Competition. *Scandinavian Journal of Medicine & Science In Sports, 20*(2), 356–363.

Schöffl, I., Schöffl, V., Dötsch, J., Dörr, H., & Jüngert, J. (2011). Correlations between High Level Sport-Climbing and the Development of Adolescents. *Pediatric Exercise Science, 23*(4), 477.

Schoffl, V., Hochholzer, T., & Imhoff, A. (2004). Radiographic Changes in the Hands and Fingers of Young, High-Level Climbers. *The American Journal of Sports Medicine, 32*(7), 1688–1694.

Schöffl, V., Morrison, A., Hefti, U., Ullrich, S., & Küpper, T. (2011). The UIAA Medical Commission Injury Classification for Mountaineering and Climbing Sports. *Wilderness & Environmental Medicine, 22*(1), 46–51.

Schweizer, A., Bircher, H., Kaelin, X., & Ochsner, P. (2005). Functional Ankle Control of Rock Climbers. *British Journal of Sports Medicine, 39*(7), 429–431.

Schweizer, A., & Furrer, M. (2007). Correlation of Forearm Strength and Sport Climbing Performance. *Isokinetics and Exercise Science, 15*(3), 211–216.

Seifert, L., Orth, D., Boulanger, J., Dovgalecs, V., Hérault, R., & Davids, K. (2014). Climbing Skill and Complexity of Climbing Wall Design: Assessment of Jerk as a Novel Indicator of Performance Fluency. *Journal of Applied Biomechanics, 30*(5), 619–625.

Seifert, L., Wattebled, L., L'Hermette, M., Bideault, G., Herault, R., & Davids, K. (2013). Skill Transfer, Affordances and Dexterity in Different Climbing Environments. *Human Movement Science, 32*(6), 1339–1352.

Sherk, V. D., Sherk, K. A., Kim, S., Young, K. C., & Bemben, D. A. (2011). Hormone Responses to a Continuous Bout of Rock Climbing in Men. *European Journal of Applied Physiology, 111*(4), 687–693.

Spencer, E. A., Appleby, P. N., Davey, G. K., & Key, T. J. (2002). Validity of Self-Reported Height and Weight in 4808 Epic–Oxford Participants. *Public Health Nutrition, 5*(4), 561–565.

Sulheim, S., Ekeland, A., & Bahr, R. (2007). Self-Estimation of Ability among Skiers and Snowboarders in Alpine Skiing Resorts. *Knee Surgery, Sports Traumatology, Arthroscopy, 15*(5), 665–670.

Valuri, G., Stevenson, M., Finch, C., Hamer, P., & Elliott, B. (2005). The Validity of a Four Week Self-Recall of Sports Injuries. *Injury Prevention, 11*(3), 135–137.

Watts, P. B. (2004). Physiology of Difficult Rock Climbing. *European Journal of Applied Physiology, 91*(4), 361–372.

Watts, P. B., Jensen, R. L., Gannon, E., Kobeinia, R., Maynard, J., & Sansom, J. (2008). Forearm EMG During Rock Climbing Differs from EMG During Handgrip Dynamometry. *International Journal of Exercise Science, 1*(1), 2.

Watts, P. B., Joubert, L. M., Lish, A. K., Mast, J. D., & Wilkins, B. (2003). Anthropometry of Young Competitive Sport Rock Climbers. *British Journal of Sports Medicine, 37*(5), 420–424.

Watts, P. B., Martin, D. T., & Durtschi, S. (1993). Anthropometric Profiles of Elite Male and Female Competitive Sport Rock Climbers. *Journal of Sports Sciences, 11*(2), 113–117.

15 Psychological processes in the sport of climbing

Gareth Jones and Xavier Sanchez

This chapter provides an overview of the psychological processes that play a role in the sport of climbing in the form of schematic representations and an in-depth discussion on route previewing and self-efficacy. To date, climbing research has essentially focused on physiological aspects, anthropometric characteristics, biomechanical properties and injury epidemiology although psychology-based variables have also been suggested to play a significant role in predicting performance. Visual inspection in the form of route previewing and processing of climbing-related information is perceived by climbers as crucial. Both qualitative and quantitative research findings support such statements. Self-efficacy, a form of situational self-confidence, has been shown to positively influence both performance and motivation in the climbing populations studied. Relevant literature in these areas is addressed.

Introduction

The influence of psychological factors in sport performance has, in general, been extensively demonstrated. However, the study of the role of the psychological aspects in the performance of climbing has not yet been systematically dealt with by sport psychology. Though being considered unique from both scientific and sporting perspectives climbing has not attracted significant scientific interest from the field of sport psychology when compared to other disciplines such as physiology, biomechanics or even motor control. In the present chapter, after a short introduction to provide a rationale for the study of the sport of climbing within a psychological perspective, we provide the reader with a schematic overview of the psychological processes that play a role in the sport of climbing and discuss key findings with regards to route previewing as a critical performance-related psychological variable. The second part of this chapter focuses specifically on the role of self-efficacy and anxiety as key determinants of climbing motivation and, subsequently, performance.

The sport of climbing is considered unique in the fields of physiology 'in requiring sustained and intermittent isometric forearm muscle contractions for upward propulsion' (Sheel, 2004, p. 355), biomechanics as 'the role of the upper limbs and the predominantly vertical motion distinguish it from all other land-based movements' (Quaine & Martin, 1999, p. 233), and psychology given that individuals face 'challenging new courses and environment changes on a daily basis, prompting a more extreme psychological mindset' (Feher, Meyers, & Skelly, 1998, p. 173). From a sporting perspective (e.g. Goddard & Neumann, 1993; Stiehl & Ramsey, 2005), climbing is also unique because of: (a) the practice environment (outdoors or indoors, natural rock formations or artificial surfaces) and the practice modality (on sight, pre-practice, *flash*); (b) the different ways to assess route difficulty (e.g. English, Australian, French; see Draper, Giles, Schöffl, Fuss, et al., 2016, for the IRCRA reporting scale); and (c) the characteristics of the competition (i.e. leading, bouldering, speed and para-climbing).

To date, the study of climbing has essentially focused on (a) physiological aspects such as cardiovascular responses, muscular strength and flexibility, or anthropometric characteristics in particular (e.g. Sheel, 2004; Watts, 2004, for reviews on physiology and sport climbing; see also Chapters 2 and 3 in this book); (b) biomechanical measures such as postures, balance and muscle strength (e.g. Noé, Quaine, & Martin, 2001; Schweizer, 2001; see also Chapters 7 to 9 in this book); (c) injuries (e.g. Jones, Asghar, & Llewellyn, 2008; Jones, Llewellyn, & Johnson, 2015; Schöffl, Popp, Küpper, & Schöffl, 2015; see also Chapter 4 in this book); and (d) other climbing-specific matters such as the design and mechanics of mountaineering equipment (Fuss & Niegl, 2014). In comparison, 'little research has explored the psychological or neurogenic requirement of rock climbing at any age, though the former is a key element in accomplished climbers' (Morrison & Schöffl, 2007, p. 852).

Yet psychology-based climbing variables such as problem-solving ability, movement sequence recall, route finding skills, self-efficacy and emotions have been suggested as more comprehensive predictors of performance and performance outcome than physiological or biomechanical variables (e.g. Giles, Rhodes, & Taunton, 2006; Jones et al., 2015; Llewellyn et al., 2008; MacLeod et al., 2007; Sanchez et al., 2010, 2012).

Psychological aspects in climbing

The role psychological processes play in climbing performance has been examined. In a qualitative study, Sanchez and Torregrosa (2005) interviewed high-level climbers who had experience as climbing coaches, too. That is, in order to ensure that participants were accomplished climbers but also that they were able to explain, discuss and address the underlying processes and mechanisms that are involved in the actual activity of climbing, a threefold sample selection criterion was used: participants (1) had a degree in physical education and/or were a climbing coach/trainer; (2) had a minimum climbing level of '7a on sight' (according to the French rating system of difficulty); and (3) had climbed for a minimum of five years. An outline of a semi-structured interview was developed including areas from both general psychology and climbing. The predetermined psychological categories were grouped around the basic processes of capturing and processing of information (anticipation, attention–(re)concentration, memorising and imagery), the motivational aspects (self-efficacy, self-confidence and motivation) and the emotional mechanisms (stress, arousal and risk management).

A schematic overview of the aspects considered most noteworthy by the interviewees when identifying the role of psychological processes in climbing is shown in Figures 15.1, 15.2 and 15.3 (Sanchez & Torregrosa, 2005).

Sanchez and Torregrosa, (2005) found that visual inspection and processing of that information were perceived by the climbers as crucial skills to possess. That is, the capacity of memorising and mentally rehearsing the route were perceived by climbers as essential in order to improve (optimise) actual climbing performance. Indeed, the visual examination of the climbing route before undertaking the ascent, known as route finding before climbing or 'route previewing', had been suggested as one of the variables of a psychological nature that are determinant to successful climbing performance (e.g. MacLeod et al., 2007); route finding mistakes prior to climbing would be 'a major reason for falling during climbing' (Boschker, Bakker,

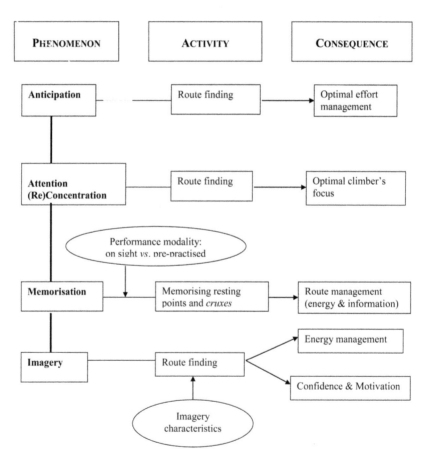

Figure 15.1 Basic processes of capturing and processing information in sport climbing.

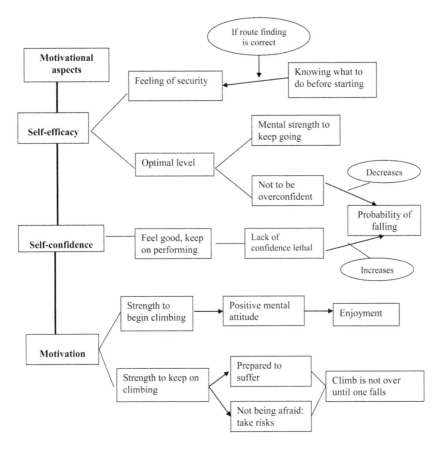

Figure 15.2 Motivational aspects in sport climbing

& Michaels, 2002, p. 25). In a more recent qualitative study (Sanchez, Torregrosa, Jones, Woodman, & Llewellyn, 2016), participants interviewed described route previewing as crucial when preparing for ascents, both cognitively (optimising decision making in relation to climbing progression) and physically (enhancing strategic management of physical effort and exertion). Route previewing may allow the climber to conserve the necessary energy for successful completion of 'crux' sections and ultimately the route. These factors, in turn, may reduce the risk of non-completion due to a fall.

The role of route finding in climbing performance has been examined experimentally (Dupuy & Ripoll, 1989; Sanchez et al., 2012). Sanchez and colleagues (2012) showed that climbers using visual inspection before climbing were not more likely to finish the ascent than those without the option of using visual inspection. Nevertheless, route preview did actually influence form performance in that climbers made fewer and shorter stops during their ascent following a preview of the route. Form performance differences remained when

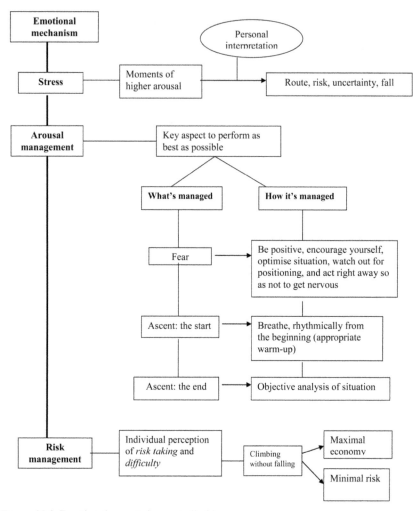

Figure 15.3 Emotional aspects in sport climbing

baseline ability levels were taken into account, although for shorter duration of stops only – the higher the level of expertise of the climbers the more they benefit from route previewing. The authors suggested that this may prove vital to the climber in reducing the effects of fatigue in lengthy climbs or repeated bouts of performance (Sanchez et al., 2012).

Such form performance differences between climbing with or without route preview found by Sanchez and colleagues (2012) in expert climbers were consistent with those observed by Dupuy and Ripoll (1989), who compared climbers' visual and motor behaviours while climbing two route sections with different handhold configurations. Dupuy and Ripoll (1989) found that their expert climbers were able to select the optimal climbing options to negotiate the route from their first attempt.

That is, reductions in resting points, during which the route can also be inspected (i.e. route finding *during* climbing), would indicate that experts, contrary to non-experts, were able to benefit from route preview (route finding *prior* to climbing). Hence, experts did not need to stop that long or that often, once on the wall, for route visual inspection. Overall, findings from these few studies having examined route previewing suggest that the ability to visually inspect a climb before its ascent may represent an essential component of performance optimisation in climbing (Dupuy & Ripoll, 1989; Sanchez et al., 2012; see also Chapter 13 in this book).

Another psychological aspect that was identified as critical to achieve an optimal climbing performance was self-efficacy (Sanchez & Torregrosa, 2005). The second part of this chapter addresses in particular this given psychological construct.

Self-efficacy

The relationship between personality characteristics, physiological arousal and performance in high risk sports such as climbing and mountaineering is complex. To date research has considered these issues using a range of motivational theories with sensation seeking a central premise. Although empirical evidence in risk related activities has found sensation seeking to be predictive of behaviour, research in high risk sports including climbing has produced mixed results (Llewellyn & Sanchez, 2008; Slanger & Rudestam, 1997). Kerr and Mackenzie (2012) acknowledge that sensation seeking in the form of adventure seeking may be a contributory factor but not a primary source of motivation. They suggest a range of meta-motivational states that influence participation are likely to exist, including goal achievement, social motivation, environmental connection and risk taking. In addition, both task mastery and self-efficacy have been proposed as motivational factors that influence participation and engagement in high risk sports (Ewert, 1994; Llewellyn, Sanchez, Asghar, & Jones, 2008; Slanger & Rudestam, 1997). The aim of this section is to discuss key aspects of self-efficacy theory, related research and its role in climbing specific populations.

Bandura's (1997) social cognitive theory proposed that the interaction of cognitive, behavioural, physiological and environmental factors determine motivation. Within the theoretical framework, self-efficacy is a central construct that denotes a 'belief in one's capabilities to organize and execute the courses of action required to produce given attainments' (Bandura, 1997, p. 3). Self-efficacy in essence is a form of situational self-confidence relating to a specific behavioural goal or related behavioural goals. Early research considered self-efficacy to have a vital role in the conceptualisation of behaviours in high risk sports (Ewert, 1994; Kontos, 2004; Slanger & Rudestam, 1997). Bandura (1997) proposed that individuals with high levels of self-efficacy are more likely to set demanding goals, apply more effort in the pursuit of these goals and persevere in spite of periodic set-backs (Bandura, 1997).

The 'Big Five' personality traits of openness to experience; agreeableness; neuroticism; extroversion; and conscientiousness (McCrae & Costa, 1997) have been examined in high risk sports (Diehm & Armatas, 2004; Tok, 2011).

Sensation seeking and impulsiveness have been found to load on the same factor as conscientiousness (Aluja, Garcia & Garcia, 2004; Zuckerman, 2005). Sensation seeking is defined as the desire and tendency to engage in risk related activities (Zuckerman, 1994) and impulsivity as 'the tendency to enter into situations, or rapidly respond to cues for potential reward, without much planning or deliberation and without consideration of potential punishment or loss of reward' (Zuckerman & Kuhlman, 2000, p. 1000). Both Llewellyn and Sanchez (2008) and Slanger and Rudestam (1997) stated that sensation seeking theory does not adequately explain how high risk sports participants manage their state anxiety when engaged in such activities. Tok (2011) investigated the 'Big Five' personality traits and found that high risk sports participants had high levels of openness to experience and extraversion but lower levels of conscientiousness and neuroticism. The author suggested sensation seeking and extraversion to be positively related and that extraversion may be a key factor in participation in high risk sports. Additionally Tok (2011) stated a facet of neuroticism is self-confidence and in finding that high risk sports participants had lower levels of neuroticism supports the premise that people take risks when they have higher levels of self-efficacy.

Self-efficacy beliefs are largely formulated through successful personal engagement experience, termed mastery experience, and is believed to exert the strongest effect on self-efficacy (Bandura, 1997). Mastery experience refers to an individual's ability to control their course of action and emotions and provides a highly influential source of information. Mastery experiences may be considered in the context of task completion and in the completion of task elements. In relation to climbing this would mean a successful overall ascent and successful completion of individual pitches within the ascent. Although common performance aspects exist in the sport of climbing and a degree of transferability exists between individual types and styles of climbing, it is important to consider task mastery as domain specific. In addition, mastery experiences are an important disinhibitory factor. Disinhibition refers to a lack of restraint that allows individuals to perform activities that are considered to be dangerous and/or of increased personal risk. Task mastery has been suggested as a significant motivational influence in high risk sporting pursuits (Ewert, 1994; Slanger & Rudestam, 1997). Self-efficacy and climbing performance may be considered to be reciprocally determinate, in that individuals high in self-efficacy are more likely to attempt more difficult climbs. Successful performance of more difficult ascents further facilitates the development of a resilient sense of efficacy and the likelihood of more challenging goals being set in the future. In climbing it is important that both self-efficacy belief and the actual level of skill of the individual are consistent. A sound judgment of one's belief and actual ability is necessary to develop a strong and robust form of self-efficacy, for example when on-sighting climbers should consider attempting routes that only slightly exceeds their current level of performance. Early research supports the influential role that enactive mastery experiences play in high risk sporting populations (e.g. Bandura, 1997; Brody, Hatfield, & Spalding, 1988; Norris & Weinman, 1996). Other factors that influence self-efficacy to a lesser degree are verbal persuasion, vicarious experiences and physiological states (Bandura, 1997).

A qualitative study by Jones and colleagues (Jones, Milligan, Llewellyn, Gledhill, & Johnson, 2015) provided a unique insight into the experiences of elite winter climbers in terms of their motivational orientation and risk taking behaviour. Data analysis revealed elements of self-efficacy theory in that mastery and engendered disinhibition emerged as key behavioural and psychological determinants that influenced individuals to attempt more difficult and riskier forms of winter climbing. Mastery was principally developed through the ascent of challenging new climbs whilst engendered disinhibition was comprised of social cognitive appraisal and self-perception (see Jones et al., 2015b for details). The authors suggest the attainments of other leading climbers provided a vicarious experience through which the participants within the study socially modelled their own chance of future success. This provided an additional motivating factor and played a disinhibiting role when preparing themselves for future difficult ascents. Self-efficacy theory supports the role played by interpersonal experiences and findings from this study indicated climbing partners provided another key source of social persuasion. Climbing partners offered encouragement and guidance which further influenced the participants' belief in their ability and a bond of trust was developed. However, if the interpersonal experience is disparaging this could threaten the perceived competence of the individual climber, resulting in reduced performance or failure. In regard to performance anxiety the elite winter climbers interviewed within the study interpreted increased levels of somatic anxiety as normal given the physically demanding nature of the routes undertaken and the repeated exposure to them.

Somatic anxiety and cognitive anxiety are considered key components of performance anxiety. The relationship between physiological response to a stressful situation and the interpretation of this response may, in part, be mediated by previous accomplishments. Pijpers, Oudejans, Holsheimer and Bakker (2003) investigated anxiety and performance relationships in climbing. Participants were novice climbers and the authors manipulated anxiety by using a climbing wall with routes set at varying heights. Data collected included self-reported anxiety levels and physiological measures such as heart rate and blood lactate. Results indicated anxiety was exhibited at three levels (subjective, physiological, behavioural) and that increased anxiety resulted in a greater uncertainty in regard to movement sequence and hold selection. A later study by Pijpers, Oudejans, Bakker and Beek (2006) investigated anxiety in perceiving and realising affordance. The authors concluded that anxiety affected both the detection of environmental information in relation to climbing movement and cognitively inhibited the participants from considering possible solutions to these. Increased anxiety that is not controlled narrows the individual's attention field; anecdotal responses from climbers to their climbing partners support this finding: 'I didn't see that hold.' Fluid characteristics of moment are a key component to success on physically demanding and difficult routes. The ability to control anxiety may be key to this and the role of self-efficacy a vital mediating factor. Repeated exposure to difficult and demanding movement sequences may allow the individual to view these as the norm. Higher levels of anxiety have been found to be associated with higher levels of effort and overall performance (Hardy & Hutchinson, 2007). Hardy and Hutchinson (2007) suggest other variables may be a key determinant that allow individuals to profit from anxiety induced effort which we propose may be self-efficacy.

In 2008, Llewellyn and Sanchez examined the potential role of self-efficacy on risk taking behaviour in rock climbers in part and hypothesised that the greatest risk takers would be those with the strongest beliefs in their capacity to manage the situation and the risks involved. The authors conducted a quantitative cross-sectional study and utilised Slanger and Rudestam's (1997) Physical Self-Efficacy (PSE) Scale. Findings indicated self-efficacy significantly predicted all forms of risk taking and those climbers high in self-efficacy and male were likely to take the greatest risks. Of note when experience and ability were introduced to the soloing and leading grade regression models, self-efficacy did not remain a significant predictor of risk taking, leading the authors to suggest that this association was mediated by self-efficacy. The authors concluded that experienced climbers operating at a higher performance level and belief in their ability to manage the level of risk effectively are likely to have the highest levels of self-efficacy. In addition reciprocal determination acts to motivate some to attempt more difficult climbs and riskier forms of climbing behaviour such as soloing.

The measure utilised by Llewellyn and Sanchez (2008) to assess self-efficacy was the PSE Scale, which consists of 18 items rating confidence on a scale from 0 to 100 in ten-point increments; higher scores reflect greater confidence (i.e. greater self-efficacy). The items of the PSE are based around six themes relating to what allows high risk sports participants to take risks: confidence in (a) performing; (b) managing fear; (c) avoiding making a mistake; (d) handling whatever anyone else with their experience can handle; (e) dealing with unexpected events; and (f) accomplishing what they set out to do. For each of these themes respondents are asked to rate their confidence for three categories of error: those in which a mistake would be potentially trivial, harmful or fatal. The internal consistency of the PSE in the present study was found to be excellent (α = .94), although the authors acknowledged a limitation of the study was that the PSE as a measure of self-efficacy was not developed specifically for climbing populations.

Llewellyn and colleagues (2008) conducted a quantitative cross-sectional study to investigate the relationship between self-efficacy and a wide range of rock climbing behaviours in active rock climbers recruited at both indoor and outdoor venues. Linear regression results indicated climbers high in self-efficacy engaged in risker forms of rock climbing both more frequently and at a higher level of difficulty. Associations were attenuated slightly with adjustment for covariates, but self-efficacy remained a significant predictor of all forms of climbing behaviour. A major strength of this study was the development and application of a validated measure of self-efficacy (Climbing Self-Efficacy Scale; CSES), specific to the domain of climbing (Llewellyn et al., 2008; Figure 15.4).

The CSES was designed as a psychometric measure of self-efficacy in relation to the sub-skills required for accomplished performance in climbing following Bandura's (1997) recommendations. Semi-structured interviews were conducted with rock climbers, climbing instructors and academic specialists in the areas of social cognitive theory, risk taking and sport psychology to inductively identify

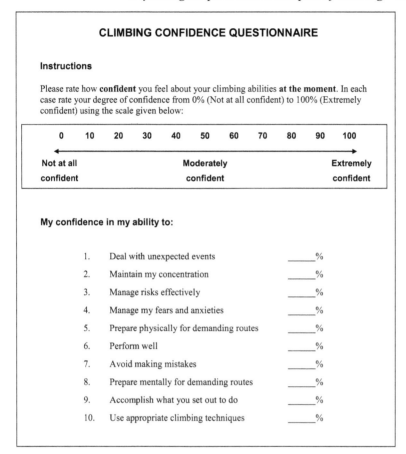

Figure 15.4 The Climbing Self-Efficacy Scale (CSES)

key variables in the domain of climbing. The items contained within the CSES were non-hierarchical and based around ten themes relating to how confident respondents felt about their current climbing abilities (Figure 15.4). In each case the degree of confidence was rated from 0 per cent (Not at all confident) to 100 per cent (Extremely confident). The total score (ranging from 0 to 1000) gives a measure of an individual's expectations or beliefs about their performance ability in climbing. Higher scores reflect greater confidence, that is, greater self-efficacy. The reliability of the CSES was examined using Cronbach's coefficient alpha, and results of $\alpha = .92$ in the pilot study, and $\alpha = .88$ in the main study both suggest excellent internal consistency (Kline, 2000). In the study the scale was completed by climbers prior to engagement in a variety of climbing behaviours such as sport leading, traditional leading bouldering and included on-sight and redpointing practices. Future studies may wish to consider its use.

Conclusion

Research examining the role of psychological factors in climbing is developing, although the psychological techniques that climbers utilise to optimise performance are borrowed from mainstream sport literature. Thus, psychological strategies will require specific modification to make them fit for purpose (Feher et al., 1998). This will benefit both general climbing populations and competitive performers alike.

The psychological aspects to be integrated into the general training programmes of all climbers should incorporate skills, techniques and strategies that promote the capacity for memorising and mentally rehearsing the route such as imagery and video modelling (Sanchez & Dauby, 2009). It is also necessary to consider the role of motivational aspects like self-efficacy. Bandura (1997) suggests that, once formed, strong efficacy beliefs allow individuals to cope with periodic difficulties and in doing so develop substantial mental resilience. Building a robust form of self-efficacy belief can protect the climber against the debilitating effects of anxiety and ultimately optimise performance and stimulate motivation (Jones et al., 2015; Llewellyn et al., 2008).

Summary

- Ability to visually inspect the route and correctly interpret the movement sequence required is critical to climbing performance.
- Self-efficacy is domain specific.
- A more experienced and able climber has higher levels of self-efficacy.
- Climbers higher in self-efficacy are likely to take greater risks.

References

Aluja, A., Garcia, O., and Garcia, L. F. (2004). Replicability of the three, four and five Zuckerman's personality superfactors: exploratory and confirmatory factor analysis of the EPQ-RS, ZKPQ and NEO-PI-R. *Personality and Individual Differences*, 36, 1093–1108.

Bandura, A. (1997). *Self-efficacy: the exercise of control*. New York: Freeman.

Boschker, M. S. J., Bakker, F. C., & Michaels, C. F. (2002). Memory for the functional characteristics of climbing walls: perceiving affordances. *Journal of Motor Behavior*, 34, 25–36.

Brody, E. B., Hatfield, B. D., & Spalding, T. W. (1988). Generalization of self-efficacy to a continuum of stressors upon mastery of a high-risk sport skill. *Journal of Sport and Exercise Psychology*, 10(1), 32–44.

Diehm, R., & Armatas, C. (2004). Surfing: an avenue for socially acceptable risk-taking, satisfying needs for sensation seeking and experience seeking. *Personality and Individual Differences*, 36(3), 663–667.

Draper, N., Giles, D., Schöffl, V. R., Fuss, F. K., Watts, P., Wolf, P., et al. (2016). Comparative grading scales, statistical analyses, climber descriptors and ability grouping: International Rock Climbing Research Association position statement. *Sports Technology*. doi: 10.1080/19346182.2015.1107081.

Dupuy, C. & Ripoll, H. (1989). Analysis of visual-motor strategies in climbing. *Science & Motricite*, 7, 18–24.

Ewert, A. W. (1994). Playing the edge: motivation and risk taking in a high-altitude wilderness like environment. *Environment and Behavior*, 26(1), 3–24.

Feher, P., Meyers, M. C., & Skelly, W. A. (1998). Psychological profile of rock climbers: state and trait attributes. *Journal of Sport Behavior*, 21, 167–180.

Fuss, F., & Niegl, G. (2014) Design and mechanics of mountaineering equipment. In Fuss, F., Subic, A., Strangwood, M., & Mehta, R. (eds.) *Routledge handbook of sports technology and engineering* (pp. 277–292). New York: Routledge.

Giles, L. V., Rhodes, E. C., & Taunton, J. E. (2006). The physiology of rock climbing. *Sports Medicine*, 36, 529–545.

Goddard, D. & Neumann, U. (1993). *Performance rock climbing*. Mechanicsburg, PA: Stackpole Books.

Hardy, L., & Hutchinson, A. (2007). Effects of performance anxiety on effort and performance in rock climbing: a test of processing efficiency theory. *Anxiety, Stress and Coping*, 20, 147–161.

Jones, G., Asghar, A., Llewellyn, D. J. (2008). The epidemiology of rock-climbing injuries. *British Journal of Sports Medicine*, 42(9), 773–778.

Jones, G., Llewellyn, D. J., & Johnson, M. I. (2015a). Previous injury as a risk factor for reinjury in rock climbing: a secondary analysis of data from a retrospective cross-sectional cohort survey of active rock climbers. *BMJ Open Sport & Exercise Medicine*, 1(1). doi: 10.1136/bmjsem-2015-000031.

Jones, G., Milligan, J., Llewellyn, D. J., Gledhill, A., & Johnson, M. I. (2015b). Motivational orientation and risk taking in elite winter climbers. *International Journal of Sport and Exercise Psychology*. doi: 10.1080/1612197X.2015.1069876,

Kerr, J. H., & Mackenzie, S. H. (2012). Multiple motives for participating in adventure sports. *Psychology of Sports and Exercise*, 13(5), 649–657.

Kline, P. (2000) *Handbook of psychological testing* (2nd ed.). London: Routledge.

Kontos, A. P. (2004). Perceived risk, risk taking, estimation of ability and injury among adolescent sport participants. *Journal of Pediatric Psychology*, 29(6), 447–455.

Llewellyn, D. J., & Sanchez, X. (2008). Individual differences and risk taking in rock climbing. *Psychology of Sport and Exercise*, 9, 413–426.

Llewellyn, D. J., Sanchez, X., Ashghar, A., & Jones, G. (2008). Self-efficacy, risk taking and performance in rock climbing. *Personality and Individual Differences*, 45, 75–81.

MacLeod, D., Sutherland, D. L., Buntin, L., Whitaker, A., Aitchison, T., Watt, I., Bradley, J., & Grant, S. (2007). Physiological determinants of climbing-specific finger endurance and sport rock climbing performance. *Journal of Sports Sciences*, 25, 1433–1443.

McCrae, R. R., & Costa, Jr. P. T. (1997) Personality trait structure as a human universal. *American Psychologist*, 52(5), 509–516.

Morrison, A. B., & Schöffl, V. R. (2007). Review of the physiological responses to rock climbing in young climbers. *British Journal of Sports Medicine*, 41, 852–861.

Noé, F., Quaine, F., & Martin, L. (2001). Influence of steep gradient supporting walls in rock climbing: biomechanical analysis. *Gait and Posture*, 13, 86–94.

Norris, R. M., & Weinman, J. A. (1996). Psychological change following a long sail training voyage. *Personality and Individual Differences*, 21(2), 189–194.

Pijpers, J. R., Oudejans, R. R. D., Bakker, F. C., & Beek, P. J. (2006). The role of anxiety in perceiving and realizing affordances. *Ecological Psychology*, 18(3), 131–161.

Pijpers, J. R., Oudejans, R. R. D., Holsheimer, F., & Bakker, F. C. (2003). Anxiety-performance relationships in climbing: a process-orientated approach. *Psychology of Sport & Exercise*, 4, 283–304.

Quaine, F., & Martin, L. (1999). A biomechanical study of equilibrium in sport rock climbing. *Gait and Posture*, 10, 233–239.

Sanchez, X., & Dauby, N. (2009). Imagery and video-modelling in sport climbing. *Canadian Journal of Behavioural Science*, 41, 93–101.

Sanchez, X., Boschker, M. S. J., & Llewellyn, D. J. (2010). Pre-performance psychological states and performance in an elite climbing competition. *Scandinavian Journal of Medicine and Science in Sports*, 20, 356–363.

Sanchez, X., Lambert, P., Jones, G., & Llewellyn, D. J. (2012). Efficacy of pre-ascent climbing route visual inspection in indoor sport climbing. *Scandinavian Journal of Medicine and Science in Sports*, 22, 67–72.

Sanchez, X., & Torregrosa, M. (2005). El papel de los factores psicológicos en la escalada deportiva: Un análisis cualitativo. *Revista de Psicología del Deporte*, 14, 177–194.

Sanchez, X., Torregrosa, M., Jones, G., Woodman, T., & Llewellyn, D. J. (2016). Identification of performance predictors in sport climbing. Submitted.

Schöffl, V., Popp D., Küpper T., & Schöffl, I. (2015). Injury trends in rock climbers: evaluation of a case series of 911 injuries between 2009 and 2012. *Wilderness & Environmental Medicine*, 26(1), 62–67.

Schweizer, A. (2001). Biomechanical properties of the crimp grip position in rock climbers. *Journal of Biomechanics*, 34, 217–223.

Sheel, A. W. (2004). Physiology of sport rock climbing. *British Journal of Sports Medicine*, 38, 355–359.

Slanger, E., & Rudestam, K. E. (1997). Motivation and disinhibition in high risk sports: sensation seeking and self-efficacy. *Journal of Research in Personality*, 31(3), 355–374.

Stiehl, J., & Ramsey, T. (2005). *Climbing walls: a complete guide*. Champaign, IL: Human Kinetics.

Tok, S. (2011). The big five personality traits and risky sport participation. *Social Behavior and Personality*, 39(8), 1105–1112.

Watts, P. B. (2004). Physiology of difficult rock climbing. *European Journal of Applied Physiology*, 91, 361–372.

Zuckerman, M. (1994). *Behavioral expressions and biosocial bases of sensation seeking*. Cambridge: Cambridge University Press.

Zuckerman, M. (2005). *Psychobiology of personality* (2nd ed.). New York: Cambridge University Press.

Zuckerman, M., & Kuhlman, D. M. (2000). Personality and risk taking: common biosocial factors. *Journal of Personality*, 68, 999–1029.

16 Exposure and engagement in mountaineering

Eric Brymer and Erik Monasterio

At its most extreme, mountaineering is traditionally associated with a search for varying degrees of risk and risk-taking. However, more recent research shows that mountaineering involves a considerable range of experiences that includes a search for mastery in challenging and unstable environments, unique camaraderie found in situations of mutual reliance in isolated, stressful and dangerous situations and the search for freedom and transcendence (Monasterio & Brymer, 2015). This chapter critiques the traditional risk focused approach that has dominated mountaineering literature and presents an alternative perspective. Based on this alternative perspective the chapter provides practical advice for mental preparation and coaching.

Introduction

In 1957 the Northwest Face of a large granite rock in the middle of Yosemite, known as the Half Dome, was climbed for the first time by a team of three climbers. The Northwest Face is sheer and approximately 650 metres high. While others had climbed easier routes with the aid of drills and bolts before, the Northwest Face had proved extremely challenging and there had been a few failed attempts in the early 1950s. This first ascent took the climbers five days. Over the years the time taken to climb this route has been reduced and the typical time to climb the Northwest Face of the Half Dome is now only two days. However, climbers still need ropes, protection and other equipment required for a two-day self-sufficient trip.

In 2008 a young man named Alex Honnold achieved what had previously been considered impossible. Honnold climbed the Northwest face of the Half Dome in a matter of hours without ropes or other protection. In 2012 Honnold climbed the Half Dome in less than two hours. In his first ascent Honnold described a moment a few hundred metres from the top where he needed to recompose himself, after losing focus, before completing the ascent. While Honnold's achievement maybe a well-known accomplishment with considerable media attention, mountaineers and climbers around the world have accomplished similar seemingly impossible acts for decades. Other well-known examples of mountaineering feats might include Reinhold Messner's solo ascent of Everest without oxygen in 1980 and Tom Hornbein and Willi Unsoeld's traverse of Everest in 1963 and Ueli Steck's various accomplishments in Europe and the Himalayas. Such amazing examples are not limited to the well-known or famous characters. However, it is also true that not all mountaineers or climbers will be able to perform at this level. So what is it that enables a climber like Alex Honnold, Ueli Steck or Reinhold Messner to accomplish such exploits when many skilled climbers would not be able to? While technical abilities are of course important, technical skills alone are not what makes the difference. The difference is often not how hard the climbing move is but how exposed the climber is when making the move (Brymer & Schweitzer, 2012; Brymer & Schweitzer, 2014). The difference that makes the difference is psychological. In the words of one extreme mountaineer interviewed for a phenomenological study on mountaineering;

> If you have to move up on that wall there (points to a low lying boulder), you might have two hundred people who can do it, you put it two hundred feet up and then only maybe fifty people can do it. If you put it two hundred feet up with no rope, then only two can do it. So really the move is exactly the same, it's just the problem is in your head

> (Ernie, free solo climber, late 60s)

The aim of this chapter is to critically assess the typical 'risk-taker' oriented notions of what it takes to climb at extreme levels with high exposure and present new information that indicates a more nuanced understanding that might better guide participants, coaches and those interested in facilitating mental preparation. Where appropriate first hand experiences from participants have been used to exemplify relevant points.

On risk and risk-taking

While the idea of risk-taking came from perceptions about gambling and included financial, emotional and psychological risk, risk in mountaineering is most often associated with physical risk and the chances of physical danger (Rossi & Cereatti, 1993). The traditional notion is that as exposure increases the level of risk also increases. A participant who climbs free solo or ascends Everest solo and without oxygen is traditionally assumed to be participating with high outcome uncertainty, high probability that something will go wrong and a high chance of death as an outcome (Slanger & Rudestam, 1997). Typically, mountaineers who participate at high levels of exposure are considered risk-takers or people who participate because they enjoy or perhaps need to take risks. Motives for participation in high-level mountaineering are most often attributed to a need for adrenaline or because participants like to test themselves through taking unnecessary pathological and socially unacceptable risks (Le Breton, 2000; Monasterio, 2007). Participants are most usually considered young males 'fascinated with the individuality, risk and danger of the sports' (Bennett, Henson, & Zhang, 2003, p. 98).

These assumptions are mirrored in science with the traditional theoretical perspective focusing on the risk-taking explanation. There are two main psychological theories that claim to explain mountaineering at extreme levels: sensation seeking and edgeworks. Sensation seeking (e.g. Zarevski, Marusic, Zolotic, Bunjevac, & Vukosav, 1998; Zuckerman, 2007) explains mountaineering as a psychological trait which drives a person to search out activities with physical risks (Rossi & Cereatti, 1993). Mountaineering is about the continual search for new thrills and excitement in an attempt to alleviate boredom. Edgeworks (Laurendeau, 2008) argues for a social explanation that encourages a participant to voluntarily go beyond the edge of control. The risk-taking perspective presents mountaineering as a means for living out a desire for physical risk. From these theoretical, risk-taking perspectives mountaineering participation is: 1) a need or search for uncertainty and uncontrollability; 2) a pathological and unhealthy activity that results in self-deception; and 3) a focus on undertaking an activity where death is probable for thrills and excitement.

A number of studies have considered broader personality variables, such as neuroticism, extraversion, harm-avoidance, conscientiousness, self-directedness and self-transcendence to provide a more nuanced account of mountaineering motivation. Freixanet (1991) found that extraversion was positively correlated, while neuroticism was negatively correlated to high-risk climbing, and that alpine and mountain climbers generally presented with a personality profile characterized by: extraversion, emotional stability, conformity to social norms, and seeking thrill and experience by socialized means. Monasterio et al. (2012) and Monasterio, Alamri, and Mei-Dan (2014) found that extreme athletes including elite mountaineers (Monasterio, 2005) exhibited a combination of high novelty-seeking and self-directedness, and low harm-avoidance and self-transcendence when compared to normative and those classed as low-risk sports participants. However, the large variation in the standard deviations across all measures was not indicative of a tightly defined mountaineering personality profile. This suggested that there are multiple motivators and coping strategies for mountaineers and other extreme athletes, even in situations that might lead to death.

While for some the attraction of risk and thrills might be part of an initial motive to participate, there is evidence that suggests that risk-taking is not the motivation behind mountaineering (Brymer, 2010) and that mountaineering at any level is not about maximizing risks (Slanger & Rudestam, 1997). Overconfidence while making a small lottery bet, where little is risked on the outcome, is not the same as mountaineering with serious and potentially fatal outcomes. Pain and Pain (2005) observed that contrary to the everyday assumption mountaineers are careful, well trained, well prepared and self-aware:

> Despite the public's perception, mountaineering demands perpetual care, high degrees of training and preparation, and, above all, discipline and control. Most of those involved are well aware of their strengths and limitations in the face of clear dangers. Findings of extensive research in climbers suggest that the individuals do not want to put their lives in danger by going beyond personal capabilities.
>
> (Pain & Pain, 2005, p. S34)

From this perspective mountaineers tend to be careful and self-aware with a high desire to remain in control. Pain and Pain (2005) observed that athletes expend considerable time and effort to develop high-level skills and a deep understanding of their particular activity and also undertake extensive planning. They deliberately become very familiar with all the variables including the environment, their equipment and even themselves.

The focus of the risk-taking perspective is that mountaineering is undertaken as a need or desire to search out risky activities. These perspectives, often the presuppositions of non-participants, are at best inconclusive (Brymer, 2005, 2010). While the problems with this approach from a research perspective have been examined elsewhere (Brymer, 2008, 2010, 2012) there are important ramifications from a coaching perspective that need to be recognized. The risk-taking approach makes certain assumptions that negatively constrain the development of expertise and puts up barriers to participating in mountaineering. First, the risk-taking approach has had an almost exclusive focus on mountaineering as a male pastime, which essentially ignores the many talented and experienced women who also participate in high-level mountaineering. Second, the risk-taking approach assumes that only those with a certain trait or personality will be interested in high-level mountaineering. Third, the risk-taking approach assumes that participation is a risk continuum and only those with the right personality or trait will be successful high-level mountaineers. The potential ramifications of points two and three above are that coaching only focuses on technique as it is assumed that the psychological aspects cannot be taught. A fourth issue with the risk-taking approach is that there is little recognition for the effort, commitment and skill required to participate. In addition, these approaches do not reflect the lived experience of participants (Celsi et al., 1993; Brymer, 2005, 2010). For example, Jim, an Everest mountaineer explained that he felt less risk while mountaineering than while in an everyday situation:

> Some of the biggest risks I face are on the roads because the most dangerous thing I encounter are people. They are the most unpredictable animal there is on the planet. So risk is a part of our daily lives and, although I acknowledge the risk when I go on an adventure I don't feel like I'm putting my life in any greater danger climbing Mt. Everest, but I do when I get out on the road. So we face risks in our lives every day and I don't really draw a big distinction. I do feel safer when I'm in the Himalaya than I do out in the home environment when I'm driving around.
>
> (Jim, extreme mountaineer, early 40s)

Nevertheless, the assumption that activities such as mountaineering, under conditions of high exposure, must be about risk, are seductive and hard to shake. For example, Brymer and Oades (2009) were careful not to focus on risks when reporting on their study. Allman, Mittelstaedt, Martin and Goldenberg (2009) interpreted their findings such that 'participants purposefully take risks' (Allman et al., 2009, p. 230). Brymer (2010) argued that sports such as high-level mountaineering should not be considered in terms of risk-taking alone. While there may be an element of difference between the most successful mountaineers and the everyday person, you do not need to be male to be successful and the psychological skills required to participate in high exposure mountaineering can be learned and coached. In addition, the finding that personality characteristics of climbers are different from those of the average person does not answer the question of why climbers climb or how they become successful in high exposed conditions. We must not confuse biology with cause and meaning. To play professional basketball you must be unusually tall, but very few tall people get to be professional basketballers. Biology is likely to contribute to what we do, but does not fully determine or explain why we do it. No two mountaineers are the same and the reasons that determine a person's choice to climb are as complex as human nature. It is important not too over generalize and take the findings of research too far. Whilst it does court danger, adventurousness is an attractive and admirable aspect of human nature and no doubt of great creative and evolutionary value. Interestingly, many participants make unprompted positive comments about the benefits of climbing and are keen to point out that they chose to climb despite (not because of) the perceived risks of the sport.

Revisiting the psychology of mountaineering

So if we accept the proposition that risk-taking is a) not the dominant aspect of mountaineering, b) no longer the focus that explains mountaineering motivations, c) not a good predicator for who might like mountaineering, and d) not a good predictor of those who may be successful at high-level mountaineering, what are the psychological aspects required to be successful? In this section we present another side to mountaineering that provides more information for the participant and coach. We will argue that there are three determinants to the psychology of successful mountaineering. The first is about emotional self-knowledge. This describes the ability to function in high stress situations while being comfortable feeling fear and even using fear as vital information. This also describes the ability to be comfortable being alone and the ramifications of this for decision-making. The second is about the commitment, planning and work required to develop high-level technical skills. The skills required do not just happen overnight as if by osmosis, it takes hard work. Further, a study by Monasterio, Alamri, and Mei-Dan (2014) which found that mountaineers scored high in self-directedness supports the notion that mountaineers are disciplined and methodical, and therefore likely to progressively acquire the complex skills required for mountaineering. The third is about the commitment required to know and be comfortable in the physical environment, no matter what the conditions. This third element also includes the appreciation that the natural world is more powerful than the individual and so working with nature rather than competing against nature is vital. Mountaineers do not conquer or compete with mountains.

Know the environment

A successful mountaineer has built up a deep relationship and understanding of the environment that they are moving in which comes with experience and a deliberate process of learning. As Brenda, an extreme mountaineer described:

> You tend to be very in tune with your environment and that means that you are going to react very intuitively I suppose to what's around you, once again if you have the experience to deal with whatever is going to be thrown at you.
> (Brenda, female mountaineer, mid 30s)

In the first instance, climbers must develop an understanding of the objective danger factors of the terrain where they are climbing. Climbing in glaciated regions requires an understanding of snow and ice conditions, avalanche proneness, rock quality and the effects of the weather conditions on these physical environments. Furthermore, an understanding of weather patterns (and the likelihood of being caught out in adverse weather) in the region where you choose to climb is imperative. While courses to develop skills in assessing these objective risk factors are freely available through alpine clubs and other agencies it is imperative that the climber is psychologically disciplined to the extent that they train hard not only on how to recognize important clues but also in managing reactions and decisions.

Commitment and skills

Mountaineering requires the progressive development of a complex set of skills and a focused intent on skill acquisition. Climbers need to be physically and psychologically well prepared, and have sufficient experience to cope with their chosen objectives. Often the outcome of an accident or a high stress situation is determined by the person's ability to focus, shift attention, moderate arousal and perform well under pressure. It is not sufficient to develop high-level skills to perform when the conditions are favourable. It is also vital to develop the capacity to maintain and optimize performance in stressful situations. Stressful and unpredictable situations present themselves frequently in the mountains and can include adverse weather conditions, unstable rock and ice conditions, falling into crevasses, injury, loss of orientation and altitude sickness. Insufficient attention to specific and focused mental training to deal with these stressful situations can significantly impair climbing performance and contribute to accidents. The skills and understanding acquired as part of mental training are transferable and applicable to other situation that demand maximal performance under stress such as may occur at work, during exams or in competitive sports.

Know thy self

The above are very explicitly tempered with this last idea that a climber needs to be highly self-aware to be successful at extreme levels. Assessment of danger requires an understanding of psychological and emotional dimensions. There is often a counter-intuitive inverse relationship between the perception of danger and the 'actual danger' in the mountains. Rock climbers can experience significant anxiety climbing over very steep terrain with good security points, when a potential fall is safe. The dangers in these settings are generally relatively small and the emotional distress excessive; the perception of danger is significantly greater compared to the actual or 'real' danger. The reason for this is the feeling of exposure created by vertical or near vertical climbing and the instinctive dread of falling into space. Many rock climbers fail to transcend this fear and their climbing development, mastery of technique, enjoyment and sense of achievement is significantly impaired. On the other hand mountaineers frequently and unwittingly expose themselves to extremely dangerous situations; they often wander down gentle angled snow slopes, late in the day blissfully unaware of avalanche potential. These gentle angled snow slopes (30–40 degrees) seem to be safe, as they don't have the sense of exposure that a vertical wall of rock has. At other times, climbers travel beneath unseen unstable seracs or rocks equally unaware of the dangers. The effects of dehydration, tiredness and altitude can be such that climbers became easily distracted, lose their focus of attention and fail to consider or underestimate the potential dangers in mountain environments. In the mountain environment therefore the perceptions of danger is frequently deceptively less than the actual or 'real' danger. This deceptive inverse relationship between 'actual danger' and perceived danger often leads to a false sense of security, contributes to inattention and complacency, and is a significant contributor to mountaineering accidents.

Successful extreme mountaineers often see fear as information that needs to be attended to for survival. For example, Jim articulated:

> I think fear is probably the most important single facet in survival. Yeah I think it's a good healthy emotion, fear. People are afraid of fear I think, generally and I get the feeling that most people see fear as a negative thing almost; you know I was really afraid and that means it's terrible. I don't know, fear is what keeps you alive, you know, it's your fear that stops you from standing right on the very edge; you know fear is the most important thing in survival; the most important thing.
>
> (Jim, extreme mountaineer, late 40s)

Extreme mountaineering, while often undertaken as part of a team, also means that the participant is often required to make decisions based on their own capacities and abilities, and as if on a solo expedition. Making these decisions with little awareness of personal capacities, emotional capabilities and an understanding of psychological readiness can lead to dangerous decisions. A successful mountaineer needs to be comfortable feeling vulnerable and still maintain the capacity to think and decide. Psychological and emotional dimensions can distort perceptions of danger, distract the climber's attention and can significantly impair performance. An understanding of the impact of these factors and training methods to overcome them should be an important part of a climber's preparation programme. This can lead to dramatic improvements in performance and may decrease the rate of accidents through better assessments and management of danger.

Practical advice for mental preparation and coaching

Preparation for extreme mountaineering requires three basic elements: a deep understanding of the mountaineering environment, a thorough understanding of the task involved in ascending and descending safely, and a thorough understanding of their psychological and physical capacities. Effective preparation for extreme mountaineering involves both the acquisition of knowledge of the specific performance environment and deliberate training in environments that effectively represent the intended performance environment. At first the training might be representative of small characteristics of the performance environment but gradually the different characteristics will need to be combined.

Mental preparation requires a capacity to focus in high stress/high danger situations, and the ability to tolerate the distress and discomfort that accompanies the intended climbing goal. It is too late to find out that you are not ready psychologically when things are going wrong above the death zone on K2, or a few hundred metres from the top of the Half Dome. It is imperative that these skills are honed in preparation. This will entail proper preparation, experiences that represent the performance environment, but perhaps guided in the first instance, and the use of techniques such as imagery, breathing retraining and stress management. Focus and appropriate relaxation allows you to do at 2000 feet what you do at 2 feet.

The third element, knowing the task, encourages climbers to think about skill acquisition. First, it is important to identify the skills specific to the climb very precisely and then develop the skills to deal with these. The central them here is to 'repeat' the skills in as many different combinations of environments as possible to develop the flexibility and adaptability to perform in a wide variety of contexts while still enhancing the capacity to problem solve and make appropriate decisions in the performance environment.

Summary

- Recent research suggests that extreme mountaineering may not just be about hedonism or risk-taking.
- There is considerable variability in the personality profiles of mountaineers, suggesting that there are multiple pathways to participation in mountaineering.
- Successful climbing requires a good knowledge of the environment, climbing and oneself.
- Coaching should focus on enhancing adaptability and the ability to problem solve.

References

Allman, T. L., Mittelstaedt, R. D., Martin, B., & Goldenberg, B. (2009). Exploring the motivations of BASE jumpers: extreme sport enthusiasts. *Journal of Sport and Tourism, 14*(4), 229–247.

Bennett, G., Henson, R. K., & Zhang, J. (2003). Generation Y's perceptions of the action sports industry segment. *Journal of Sport Management, 17*(2), 95–115.

Brymer, E. (2005). *Extreme dude: a phenomenological exploration into the extreme sport experience.* Doctoral dissertation, University of Wollongong, Wollongong. Retrieved from http://ro.uow.edu.au/theses/379

Brymer, E. (2008). *Extreme sports as ecotourism.* Paper presented at the Green Travel, Climate Change and Ecotourism, Adelaide. http://www.ecotourism.org.au/conference/pdfs/conf08/papers/Eric%20Brymer%20-%20Extreme%20sports%20as%20ecotourism.pdf

Brymer, E. (2010). Risk and extreme sports: a phenomenological perspective. *Annals of Leisure Research, 13*(1&2), 218–239.

Brymer, E. (2012). Transforming adventures: why extreme sports should be included in adventure programming. In B. Martin & M. Wagstaff (Eds), *Controversial issues in adventure programming* (pp. 165–174). Champaign, IL: Human Kinetics.

Brymer, E., & Oades, L. G. (2009). Extreme sports: a positive transformation in courage and humility. *Journal of Humanistic Psychology, 49*(1), 114–126.

Brymer, E., & Schweitzer, R. (2012). Extreme sports are good for your health: A phenomenological understanding of fear and anxiety in extreme sport. *Journal of Health Psychology*, 18(4) 477–487. doi: 10.1177/1359105312446770

Brymer, E., & Schweitzer, R. (2014). The Search for Freedom in Extreme Sports: A Phenomenological Exploration. *Psychology of Sport & Exercise*. 16, 4, 865–873.

Celsi, R. L., Randall, L. R., & Leigh, T. W. (1993). An exploration of high-risk leisure consumption through skydiving. *Journal of Consumer Research*, 20(1), 1–23.

Freixanet, M. G. (1991). Personality profile of subjects engaged in high physical risk sports. *Personality and Individual Differences, 12*, 1087–1093. doi: 10.1016/0191-8869(91)90038-D

Laurendeau, J. (2008). 'Gendered risk regimes': a theoretical consideration of edgework and gender. *Sociology of Sport Journal*, 25(3), 293–309.

Le Breton, D. (2000). Playing symbolically with death in extreme sports. *Body and Society*, 6(1), 1–11.

Monasterio, E. (2007). The risks of adventure sports/people. *The Alpinist*, 19 November. Retrieved from http://www.alpinist.com/doc/web07f/rb-erik-monasterio-mountaineering-medicine

Monasterio, E., & Brymer, E. (2015). Mountaineering personality and risk. In Musa, G., Higham, J., & Thompson-Carr, A. (eds.), *Mountaineering Tourism*. Abingdon: Routledge.

Monasterio, E., Alamri, Y. A., & Mei-Dan, O. (2014). Personality characteristics in a population of mountain climbers. *Wilderness & Environmental Medicine, 25*(2), 214–219.

Monasterio, E., Mulder, R., Frampton, C., & Mei-Dan, O. (2012). Personality characteristics of BASE jumpers. *Journal of Applied Sport Psychology, 24*(4), 391–400. doi: 10.1080/10413200.2012.666710

Monasterio, M. E. (2005). Accident and fatality characteristics in a population of mountain climbers in New Zealand. *New Zealand Medical Journal, 118*(1208): U1249.

Pain, M. T. G., & Pain, M. A. (2005). Essay: risk taking in sport, *The Lancet, 366*(1), S33–S34.

Rossi, B., & Cereatti, L. (1993). The sensation seeking in mountain athletes as assessed by Zuckerman's sensation seeking scale. *International Journal of Sport Psychology, 24*, 417–431.

Slanger, E., & Rudestam, K. E. (1997). Motivation and disinhibition in high risk sports: sensation seeking and self-efficacy. *Journal of Research in Personality, 31*, 355–374.

Zarevski, P., Marusic, I., Zolotic, S., Bunjevac, T., & Vukosav, Z. (1998). Contribution of Arnett's inventory of sensation seeking and Zuckerman's sensation seeking scale to the differentiation of athletes engaged in high and low risk sports. *Personality and Individual Differences, 25*, 763–768.

Zuckerman, M. (2007). *Sensation seeking and risky behavior* Washington, DC: American Psychological Association.

Part VI
Equipment, technology and safety devices in climbing

Part VI

17 The engineering of climbing equipment

Franz Konstantin Fuss and Peter Wolf

This chapter summarises the current means to measure contact forces between hand or foot and a hold. So far, most studies instrumented just one to four holds in a climb. However, interpretation of contact forces measured at one single hand hold is limited as other supports and the movement sequence itself must be taken into account. Therefore, affordable instrumentations have been presented recently. For practitioners, this chapter also summarises studies on the metrics extracted from contact force–time curves. For instance, it has been shown that finger injuries are less likely when in a double-handed dyno the target hold is grasped before the dead point, and that chalk on hand *or* hold provides the highest coefficient of friction. Finally, the advantages and disadvantages of various rope breaks and the functionality of rock protection devices are presented.

Introduction

The development of climbing equipment requires a sound understanding of various engineering disciplines, specifically, engineering design, mechanical engineering, ergonomics and design optimisation. With the advent of smart equipment, or instrumented equipment, an understanding of electrical and electronics engineering becomes increasingly important. This chapter gives an overview of engineering issues in climbing and mountaineering with a focus on practical applications and innovation. The chapter is divided in three sections: 1) contact force measurement and analysis, 2) grip enhancing agents, and 3) safety devices.

Contact force measurement and interpretation

This first section deals with contact forces between hand/foot and a hold on a climb. Contact forces in postural regulation, finger grip capacity in isolated, well-defined grip techniques, and tests of muscular strength in climbing specific body postures are addressed in Chapters 7, 8 and 9 respectively.

Instrumentations to measure contact forces on a climb

Prior to the interpretation of contact force–time curves on a climb, applied instrumentation for measuring these forces are presented briefly. The instrumentation of small bars or rails, for example by strain gauges as done by the research group of the University of Grenoble (see Chapter 7), facilitates the elaboration of the load distribution between upper and lower limbs during either simple climbing moves or dry tooling. To comprehensively analyse contact force–time curves in a more climbing specific setup, Fuss and Niegl (2006a,b) began to instrument typical handholds by one or two triaxial, piezoelectric force sensors, and mounted them on indoor climbing walls. Fuss and Niegl also demonstrated that an appropriate arrangement of two sensors on a handhold whose shape is represented by a single line enables visualisation of the centre of pressure progression on the surface of the hold (Fuss & Niegl, 2008a; Figure 17.1). When Fuss and Niegl started their work, sensors were directly fixed to a hold. Considering the manifold types of holds – with the exception of the standardised hold in speed climbing – this fixation hampered the extensive applicability of their manner of instrumentation. Thus, the instrumentation was redesigned by Fuss and Niegl such that one six axes force/torque sensor was combinable with interchangeable holds (Fuss & Niegl, 2008b). A similar instrumentation was also used to estimate slow moving, near static climbing poses from contact forces (Aladdin & Kry, 2012). To instrument any standard climbing wall such that the climber does not perceive the instrumentation, Simnacher and co-workers presented a custom-made device composed of three triaxial piezoelectric force sensors. The sensors were placed and preloaded between two steel plates being attached to the back side of the wall. The front plate was covered by a thin wooden disk in-plane with the wall and coatable with the same surface structure (Simnacher, Spoerri, Rauter, Riener, & Wolf, 2012).

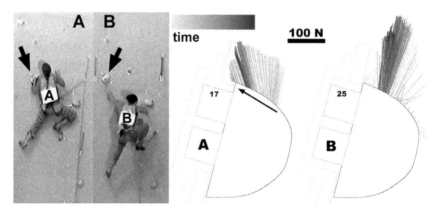

Figure 17.1 Instrumented hold mounted on wall (bold arrow; quarter final, Climbing World Cup 2002) and corresponding vector diagrams of climbers A and B (note that climber B slips off the instrumented hold); the vector diagram of climber A shows smaller force vectors (normalised to the body weight), moving consecutively over the hold's surface towards the wall and being inclined with respect to the surface (higher friction coefficient); the vector diagram of climber B shows higher force vectors, concentrated on the surface, and almost perpendicular to the surface

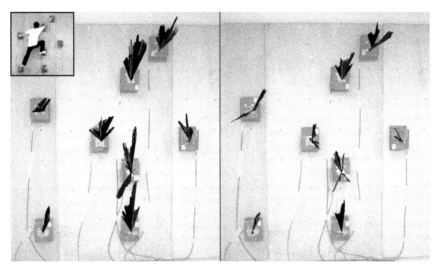

Figure 17.2 Fully instrumented climbing wall (with eight smart holds); left side: less experienced climber (higher forces, more chaotic force application); right side: more experienced climber (smaller forces, less chaotic force application); insert (upper left corner): climber on wall

The proposed instrumentations were all cost-intensive which is also reflected by the fact that only one to four instrumented holds have been used in studies with the exception of one study by Fuss and Niegl (2008b; eight holds, see Figure 17.2).

To affordably complement six degrees of freedom instrumentations, that is, devices measuring contact forces and moments in all spatial directions, Bauer and co-workers demonstrated that a one dimensional force sensor aligned to the main loading direction can contribute to a performance analysis in climbing. In order to avoid any alignment mechanism, they presented a two degrees of freedom instrumentation composed of two parallel arrangements of four low-priced weighing cells (Figure 17.3). This instrumentation showed an inferior linearity and hysteresis in comparison to the six degrees of freedom instrumentation developed by the same research group, for example horizontal linearity 10 per cent versus 0.18 per cent of the nominal force or horizontal hysteresis 2.5 per cent versus 0.05 per cent of the nominal force (Bauer, Simnacher, Stöcker, Riener, & Wolf, 2014). However, hardware costs were also reduced by factor 50, thus, a further development of the low-priced instrumentation has great potential to measure contact forces with a distinct loading direction within the plane of the wall which, for instance, can be expected at many footholds or at crimps.

If for whatever reason the instrumentation of climbing holds is not possible – for instance, in rock climbing – insole plantar pressure systems provide insights into vertical foot loads. These systems have been applied in gyms (e.g. Baláš et al., 2014; Zampagni, Brigadoi, Schena, Tosi, & Ivanenko, 2011); however, as loading direction and forces between hand and hold remain unknown, the interpretation of the results gained was limited. Another approach to elaborate contact forces without

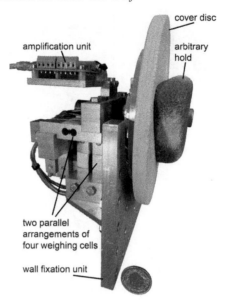

Figure 17.3 Two degrees of freedom instrumentation of an arbitrary hold

an instrumented hold is given by inverse dynamic modelling. First approaches have been presented (e.g. by Russell, Zirker, & Blemker, 2012); however, better models of human morphology and contact models incorporating different types of grasping are required to get sophisticated estimates of contact force–time curves.

In general, it has to be noted that the measurement of contact forces is still in its infancy. It seems that the community is still searching for practical instrumentations so that contact force–time curves can be reported for whatever reason. Quite often, the specifications of the applied instrumentation, for example in terms of crosstalk or hysteresis, have not been described which hampers the interpretation of the results gained.

Performance analysis based on contact force–time curves

Metrics of contact force–time curves complement performance analyses and expertise assessments in climbing. Thereby, the common assumption that mean force, maximal force and impulse at a handhold decrease as the climbing skills increase could be confirmed (Fuss & Niegl, 2006b; Baláš et al., 2014). In other words, the more skilled the climber is, the more the footholds are loaded. The contact time at handholds has also been observed to shorten, the more experienced the climber (Fuss & Niegl, 2006b).

However, as Fuss and Niegl (2008b) observed in their study on five individuals with a climbing level of 6a to 7b, French scale, it is not possible to use force variables, contact time, and impulse to rank individuals of a similar climbing level. In the same study, another extracted metric, the Hausdorff dimension, representing the entropy, that is, the irregularity or smoothness, of the contact force–time signal, was calculated based on a procedure described by Kulish, Sourin, and Sourina (2006). The Hausdorff dimension, normalised to the mean resultant force of either each single hold or all holds, was higher for the individuals of red point level 6a than for individuals of red point level 6b to 7a, French scale. Other smoothness related metrics may also support the assessment of expertise, such as the number of load changes and re-grips. A load change has been suggested to be present when the local minimum/maximum exceeded 20 N divided by the maximum force of the current force–time curve. A re-grip has been proposed to be present when a local minimum of the resultant force–time curve is smaller than two thirds of the neighbouring local maxima while the difference between the minimum and maximum is at least 50 N (Bauer et al., 2014).

The development of the contact force over time can also nicely be provided by four dimensional (4D) force vector diagrams as introduced by Fuss and Niegl (2006b, 2008a) for holds with a distinct shape (Figure 17.1) and by Wolf, Seiterle, and Riener (2012) for a broader range of holds and moves (Figure 17.4). Incorporating the information of the surface, that is, the position of the centre of pressure, also enables the ratio of the tangential to normal force components to be calculated (coefficient of friction, COF). Based on measurements of a sloper during the Climbing World Cup in Singapore in 2002, the COF of 23 female climbers were calculated. High COF values were observed for half of female climbers considered as the top group (world rank < 30) but only for 20 per cent of the climbers ranked worse (world rank > 60). A prediction of the world rank by the observed force ratio was not feasible as just one hold was instrumented while the ranking was based on the mean performance of several competitions. However, a highly positive correlation was found between a smoothness factor and the COF (Fuss & Niegl, 2006b, 2008a).

Contact time, mean force, maximal force, impulse and the Hausdorff dimension have also been observed to significantly decrease when a route was climbed a few times, that is, a training effect as expected was proven (Fuss & Niegl, 2006b,

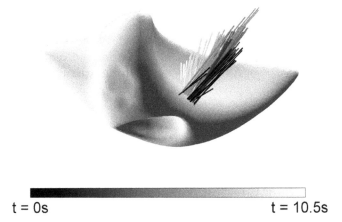

t = 0s   t = 10.5s

Figure 17.4 Development of the contact force over time

2008a). Such a training effect has also been reported in an investigation of the Swiss National Squad who climbed an unknown boulder several times: impulse and number of load changes at the instrumented holds (two crimps, one undercling, one sloper) were reduced from the very first attempts to the ninth/tenth attempt. In addition, absolute and relative between-trial reliability measures were improved, in particular for the more technically demanding moves in the second half of the boulder. Thus, the likelihood of detecting training effects depends on the level of familiarity with the route (Donath & Wolf, 2015). Remarkably, the study of Donath and Wolf (2015) was the first one reporting on reliability of metrics extracted from contact force–time curves in climbing. As only a few holds and a specific individual group (climbing experts) were investigated, further studies are needed to get a general idea of minimal detectable changes of contact forces. Thus, training effects in terms of metrics extracted from the contact force–time curves currently have to be interpreted with caution when no information on day-to-day variability is provided.

In addition, for top athletes, the definition of a training goal represented by a contact force metric might be tricky. Beginners and intermediate climbers can very likely improve in terms of load distribution or number of load changes. However, the pattern of the contact force–time curve is very likely highly individual for top athletes. Thus, coaches have to figure out what represents the best contact force pattern for the individual athlete. In order to identify better contact force patterns, knowledge of the relationship between contact force metrics and physiological variables might be helpful. Thereby, it has to be considered that physiological variables may change on a different timescale from contact force metrics. Up to now, the literature lacks contributing studies.

Instrumented climbing holds have also been used to investigate double-handed dynos (Fuss & Niegl, 2010). In contrast to textbooks commonly recommending gripping the target hold at the dead point, that is, at the highest position of the body centre of mass, climbers were more successful when they jumped higher than required. At the same time, peak contact forces were reduced. Thus, to likely be successful and to reduce finger injuries, the authors of that study recommend jumping at least 10 cm higher than required and grip the target hold before the dead point (Fuss & Niegl, 2010).

In speed climbing (Fuss & Niegl, 2006a), the force increases and the contact time decreases with the climbing speed. Holds that are more difficult to grip (e.g. slopers as compared to jugs) slow down the climber. The hand/finger force signal in speed climbing shows a pronounced shock spike immediately after contact, the magnitude of which increases with speed too.

Grip enhancing agents

Coefficient of friction

The COF is a ratio of forces (e.g. friction between hand and hold), changes of velocity (oblique impact of a ball) or distances (rolling friction of a ball), and is therefore unitless (dimensionless).

The type of friction, relevant to climbing, is the sliding friction; its effect, namely slipping of the hold, has to be avoided. The COF is calculated from the ratio of friction force FF to normal force FN.

$$COF = FF / NF \qquad\qquad\qquad (Eq.\ 17.1)$$

The term COF in Equation 17.1 is just a ratio and does not tell us whether the hand is gripping or even sliding on the surface of the hold. If FF equals zero, then the COF also equals zero. When increasing FF, the COF also increases, and the hand still grips until we reach the point of impending slippage. At this point, the COF equals the static coefficient of friction μ_s. After the point of impending slippage, when further increasing FF, the hand will slide off the hold and the COF equals the kinetic coefficient of friction μ_k. μ_s can be greater than 1, and can even reach values of up to 10, for example between glass and rubber, or tyre and concrete (drag racing cars can therefore accelerate at values greater than g, the gravitational acceleration). μ_k can be smaller or greater than μ_s; both μ_k and μ_s are dependent on normal force and area, and μ_s on speed. Between hand and artificial holds (made of resin), μ_k is greater than μ_s, and increases with the sliding speed (Fuss, Niegl, & Tan, 2004).

Equation 17.1 explains the principle of how to avoid slippage, that is, of how to increase FF: as FF = COF × NF, the options we have is to increase NF (put more weight on the hold) or increase the COF (and thereby μ_s, by using grip enhancing agents).

Free-body diagram analysis of a climber

In a climber, resting statically on a wall (Figure 17.5), the gravitational force produces a moment that tends to rotate the climber off the wall (Fuss & Niegl, 2012). The counter moments are produced by friction forces at hands and feet.

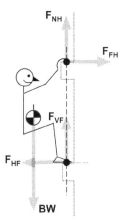

Figure 17.5 Climber in static position on a wall. Note: BW = body weight (gravitational force); F_{NH} = normal force component at hand; F_{FH} = friction force component at hand; F_{VF} = vertical force component at foot; F_{HF} = horizontal force component at foot

These friction forces generate a force couple that tends to rotate the climber towards the wall, that is, with a forward friction force at the hands, and a backward friction force at the feet (or toe force perpendicular to the wall). The gravitational force is balanced by the normal forces at hands and feet. The ratio of these normal forces depends on the performance level, and the NF is usually smaller at the hands in better climbers. However, according to Equation 17.1, reducing the load on the hands (NF) increases the COF and results in approaching the point of impending slippage. This is one of the reasons why better climbers exhibit a greater COF, closer to, but still before, the point of impending slippage (Fuss & Niegl, 2008a).

Chalk

Grip-enhancing agents belong to the standard equipment of a climber. The agents used are chalk (magnesium carbonate) and colophonium (rosin, sap of the pine tree); the latter is specifically used in sandstone. Chalk is available in solid form, powder and liquid form (alcohol suspension).

A study by Li, Margetts, and Fowler (2001) claims that chalk reduces the friction, as the data obtained between hand and rock plates suggest a μ_s of 2.5 with chalk, and of 3 without chalk. Even if μ_s can be greater than 1, the data seem excessively high and would correspond to inclination angles θ of 68 and 71 degrees, respectively, as

$$\theta = \tan^{-1} (COF) \hspace{4cm} \text{(Eq. 17.2)}$$

Hanging on a rock face inclined at these angles from the horizontal is impossible, and the COF data of Li et al. (2001) seem to be affected by a methodological error. The maximum inclination angle of an artificial climbing hold at the point of impending slippage measured by Fuss and Niegl (2008c) was 47.5°, corresponding to a COF of 1.09. Amca, Vigouroux, Aritan, and Berton (2012) reported a maximum COF of 1.14 on rock surfaces (inclination angle = 48.7°).

Fuss et al. (2004) investigated the COF between hand and an artificial climbing hold, under dry, wet and chalk conditions (powder chalk and liquid chalk). Powder chalk on hand *or* hold produces a significantly higher COF than liquid chalk, dry or wet hand, and powder chalk on *both* hand *and* hold. This means that holds polluted by chalk during the course of a competition exhibit a smaller COF if the climbers powder-chalk their hands. The COF was determined with a mini force plate, by plotting the COF against the centre of pressure (COP). The μ_s was identified from the faster COP movement after the point of impending slippage.

Amca et al. (2012) investigated the effect of chalk on the COF between hand and rock surfaces (sandstone and limestone) by increasing the inclination of the holds and recording the inclination angle at slippage (cf. Equation 17.2). In general, sandstone had a higher COF than limestone, and chalk improved the COF.

Safety devices

The protection of the climber is paramount in mountaineering, although, in spite of sophisticated safety devices, several fatal climbing accidents occur every year.

Only free climbers manage without safety devices. The standard climbing gear is comprised of ropes, carabiners, rope brakes, rock protection devices, helmets, shoes, ice axes and so on. Subsequently, two of these devices are explained: rope brakes and rock protection devices.

Rope brakes

The essence of rope brakes is the absorption of the energy of the falling climber. The two main techniques of belaying are dynamic and static belaying. In the former, the rope slips through the brake, thereby dissipating the kinetic energy of the falling climber through friction and heat. At the same time, the rope force between climber and brake decreases through friction, so that the belayer, holding the tail of the rope, is able to dampen the fall with a relatively small hand force. In the latter devices, the brake blocks the rope slip, and the energy is absorbed by the moving mass of the belayer.

Fuss and Niegl (2010) classified the rope brakes based on their design and function. Standard dynamic brakes are H-carabiners for the Italian hitch (HMS, noeud de demicabestan, nodo mezzo barcaiolo), figure-8, brake-bar carabiners and rappel racks, and belay rings (which evolved into the Sticht plate and the tubular brakes). Static brakes encompass tubular brakes with Magic plate function (for belaying of the second climber), as well as semi-automatic brakes that are a combination of brake-bar carabiners and tubular brakes. Hybrid brakes serve for both static and dynamic belaying, by manually switching between these two operational modes.

The basic function of rope brakes hinges on belt friction, that is, on the deflection of the rope about a component of the brake (or around itself as seen in the Italian hitch). In contrast to sliding friction (which requires a normal force; cf. Equation 17.1) with the linear equation of

$$T_1 = T_2 + \text{FF} = T_2 + \mu\,\text{NF} \tag{Eq. 17.3}$$

(where T_1 is the force produced by the falling climber, T_2 is produced by the belayer's hand and FF is the friction force), the belt friction is characterised by an exponential equation

$$T_1 / T_2 = e^{\mu\theta} = \beta = fmf \tag{Eq. 17.4}$$

where μ is the static belt friction coefficient, θ is the angle of contact (in radians), β is the brake factor, and fmf is the force multiplication factor. The more a rope is deflected by the brake (angle θ, see Figure 17.6), the higher is the brake factor. The brake factor and the force multiplication factor indicate the force amplification from T_2 to T_1.

According to Manin, Richard, Brabant, and Bissuel (2006), the ATC (air traffic controller, tubular brake) XP version is superior to the common ATC in terms of the brake factor, and the latter is slightly better than the Reverso, Figure-8, Pirana and the Italian hitch (HMS). According to Thomann and Semmel (2007), the Italian hitch (HMS) has a higher brake factor than the ATC (air traffic controller, tubular brake) and the Figure-8 brake. According to Stronge and Thomas (2014),

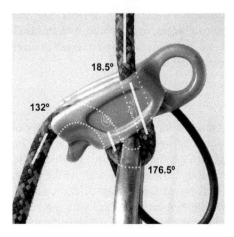

Figure 17.6 ATC Guide (with Magic plate function); the action lines of the rope are indicated as white lines; the total deflection angle θ is 327°; if the belt friction coefficient is 0.3 (Fuss and Niegl, 2010), then the brake factor is 5.54 (cf. Eq. 7.3)

tubular brakes with 'V-shaped' exit grooves (Verso, Reverso) have a higher brake factor than the ATC and the Figure-8.

Rock protection devices

Rock protection equipment connects the climber's gear (ropes, carabiners, harnesses) to the rock face and serves as an anchor for securing the rope. This equipment comprises of nails, pegs, pins, screws, rock anchors, pitons, chocks and frictional anchors. The latter two items are usually referred to as camming devices, fitting into cracks that jam when loaded. Frictional anchors are also known by the names of cams, friends and Camalots, and adapt to a wide range of crack widths. Their design follows a logarithmic spiral profile (Figure 17.7), which is characterised by a constant pressure angle and the following equation of

$$r = r_0 \, e^{b\varphi} \tag{Eq. 17.5}$$

where r and φ are polar coordinates, r_0 is the radius at $\varphi = 0$ and b is the tangent of the pitch angle θ (Figure 17.7), that is, the COF,s the ratio of friction to normal force

$$b = \tan \theta = \text{COF} = \text{FF/NF} \tag{Eq. 17.6}$$

The fact that the COF is a part of the logarithmic spiral equation connects to the term of frictional anchors. The load on the anchor, for example in the event of a fall, forces the opposing cam lobes apart, and thereby exerts a normal force on the wall of the crack. The (downward) load on the anchor is balanced by the upward friction force FF, which is proportional to the normal force NF. It has to be borne in mind that the COF is always smaller than the static friction coefficient μ_s, as approaching the latter would result in the cam sliding down the crack wall and ultimate failure.

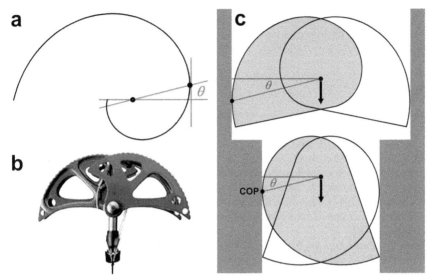

Figure 17.7 (a) Logarithmic spiral (b) and camming device; (c) camming device inserted in a crack with two different widths; θ = pitch angle; COP = centre of pressure; the downward arrow in (c) indicates the load direction

Source: From Fuss, F. K. and Niegl, G. (2014), © Routledge, 2014, reproduced with kind permission.

The design pitch angle θ, or camming angle, is smaller than the angle of an inclined rock plane at which a block of metal (aluminium) would start to slide. If the rock plane is made of granite, the angle is 18° (Foster, 2002) at a μ_s of 0.325 (tangent of 18°). In other rock materials the angle of impending slippage is around 15°, so that a safe pitch angle θ of 13.75° (COF = 0.245) prevents any slippage.

According to the standard EN 12276 (EN, 1998) the minimum strength requirement for all sizes and types of friction anchors is a downward load of 5 kN. If, for example, a manufacturer guarantees a minimum strength at a load of 6 kN, and the actual load is 4 kN, then the friction anchor would fail if the crack is flaring downward by more than merely 4.63° (Fuss & Niegl, 2014). Downward flaring cracks have to be treated with caution when using camming devices.

Summary

- Measurement and interpretation of contact forces are still in their infancy: not only the means to affordably instrument an entire root but also reliability studies to get an idea of minimal detectable changes of contact forces are lacking.
- The more experienced a climber is, the more footholds are loaded and mean force, maximal force and impulse at a handhold decrease.
- In double-handed dynos, jump higher than required and grip the target hold before the dead point.

- Powder chalk on hand *or* hold produces a significantly higher COF than liquid chalk, dry or wet hand, and powder chalk on *both* hand *and* hold.
- Downward flaring cracks have to be treated with caution when using camming devices.

References

Aladdin, R., & Kry, P. (2012). Static pose reconstruction with an instrumented bouldering wall. In *Proceedings of the 18th ACM symposium on Virtual reality software and technology* (pp. 177–184). New York: ACM.

Amca, A. M., Vigouroux, L., Aritan, S., & Berton, E. (2012). The effect of chalk on the finger-hold friction coefficient in rock climbing. *Sports Biomechanics*, 11(4), 473–479.

Baláš, J., Panáčková, M., Jandová, S., Martin, A. J., Strejcová, B., Vomáčko, L., ... & Draper, N. (2014). The effect of climbing ability and slope inclination on vertical foot loading using a novel force sensor instrumentation system. *Journal of Human Kinetics*, 44(1), 75–81.

Bauer, F., Simnacher, M., Stöcker, U., Riener, R., & Wolf, P. (2014). Interaction forces in climbing: cost-efficient complementation of a 6DoF instrumentation. *Sports Technology*, 7(3–4), 120–127.

Donath, L., & Wolf, P. (2015). Reliability of force application to instrumented climbing holds in elite climbers. *Journal of Applied Biomechanics*, 31(5), 377–382.

EN (1998). Mountaineering equipment – Friction anchors – Safety requirements and test methods, European Standard (EN 12276:1998; UIAA 125:2008). Brussels, Belgium: European Standards Commission, and Bern, Switzerland: Union Internationale des Associations d'Alpinisme.

Foster, S. (2002). *The Wild Country Cam Book*. Tideswell, England: Wild Country Ltd.

Fuss, F. K., & Niegl, G. (2006a). Dynamics of speed climbing. In E. Moritz, & S. Haake, (Eds), *The Engineering of Sport 6* (pp. 51–56). New York: Springer.

Fuss, F. K., & Niegl, G. (2006b). Instrumented climbing holds and dynamics of sport climbing. In E. Moritz, & S. Haake, (Eds), *The Engineering of Sport 6* (pp. 57–62). Munich, Germany: Springer.

Fuss, F. K., & Niegl, G. (2008a). Instrumented climbing holds and performance analysis in sport climbing. *Sports Technology*, 1(6), 301–313.

Fuss, F. K., & Niegl, G. (2008b). The fully instrumented climbing wall: performance analysis, route grading and vector diagrams-a preliminary study. In F. K. Fuss, A. Subic, & S. Ujihashi (Eds), *The Impact of Technology on Sport II* (pp. 677–682). London, England: Taylor and Francis Group.

Fuss, F. K., & Niegl, G. (2008c). Quantification of the grip difficulty of a climbing hold. In M. Estivalet, & B. Brisson (Eds), *The Engineering of Sport 7* (pp. 19–26). Paris, France: Springer.

Fuss, F. K., & Niegl, G. (2010). Design and mechanics of belay devices and rope brakes. *Sports Technology*, 3(2), 65–84.

Fuss, F. K., & Niegl, G. (2012). The importance of friction between hand and hold in rock climbing. *Sports Technology*, 5(3–4), 90–99.

Fuss, F. K., & Niegl, G. (2014). Design and mechanics of mountaineering equipment. In F. K. Fuss, A. Subic, M. Strangwood (Eds), *Routledge Handbook of Sports Technology and Engineering*. London, England: Routledge / Taylor & Francis.

Fuss, F. K., Niegl, G., & Tan, M. A. (2004). Friction between hand and different surfaces under different conditions and its implication for sport climbing. In M. Hubbard, R. D. Mehta, & J. M. Pallis (Eds), *The Engineering of Sport 5* (pp. 269–275). Sheffield, England: International Sports Engineering Association.

Kulish, V., Sourin, A., & Sourina, O. (2006) Human electroencephalograms seen as fractal time series: mathematical analysis and visualization. *Computers in Biology and Medicine*, 36, 291–302.

Li, F. X., Margetts, S., & Fowler, I. (2001). Use of 'chalk' in rock climbing: sine qua non or myth? *Journal of Sports Science*, 19, 427–432.

Manin, L., Richard, M., Brabant, J. D., & Bissuel, M. (2006). Rock climbing belay device analysis, experiments and modelling. In E. Moritz, & S. Haake, (Eds), *The Engineering of Sport 6* (pp. 69–74). Munich, Germany: Springer.

Russell, S. D., Zirker, C. A., & Blemker, S. S. (2012). Computer models offer new insights into the mechanics of rock climbing. *Sports Technology*, 5(3–4), 120–131.

Simnacher, M., Spoerri, R., Rauter, G., Riener, R., & Wolf, P. (2012). Development and application of a dynamometric system for sport climbing. 18th Congress of the European Society of Biomechanics, Lisbon, Portugal.

Stronge, W. J., & Thomas, M. (2014). Effectiveness of mountaineering manual belay/abseil devices. *Sports Engineering*, 17(3), 131–142.

Thomann, A., & Semmel, C. (2007). Die Bremskraftverstärker. *Bergundsteigen*, 2, 60–65.

Wolf, P., Seiterle, S., & Riener, R. (2012). Visualisierung der Kräfte zwischen Hand und Griff im Klettern. In *Proceedings (Extended Abstracts) of the 9. Symposium der Sektion Sportinformatik der Deutschen Vereinigung für Sportwissenschaft* (pp. 46–49). Konstanz, Germany: Konstanzer Online Publikations System.

Zampagni, M. L., Brigadoi, S., Schena, F., Tosi, P., & Ivanenko, Y. P. (2011). Idiosyncratic control of the center of mass in expert climbers. *Scandinavian Journal of Medicine & Science in Sports*, 21(5), 688–699.

18 Simul-climbing progression and falls analysis

Philippe Batoux

When mountain climbers are roped together, they sometimes move together or simultaneously, using the 'simul-climbing' technique on both glaciers and rock (with protection points between them). This mode of progression, which has the advantage of saving time, is considered safe. Yet, at least theoretically, the forces generated during a fall with a simul-climbing progression are very high and therefore dangerous for the other partners, and many accidents have been reported. This chapter presents an analysis of falls that have occurred during simul-climbing progression and recommendations for the alpinists deduced from these analyses. In high mountain ice field, we simulated different kinds of falls that could happen during simul-climbing progression. We analysed particularly (1) the fall of the second climber causing the leader's fall and (2) the leader's fall. In addition we measured the forces during a crevasse fall on horizontal glacial terrain, (1) with and without friction knots in the rope, and (2) as a function of the distance between the climbers. The results of our studies suggest new techniques and different ways to use equipment to minimize the consequences of falls. The simul-climbing progression is a safe way to climb if you follow the right instructions.

Introduction

French mountaineering is today a regulated sport practiced in specific environments (Decree No. 273713, 3 April 2006), but the risk of a serious accident is ever-present. The mode of progression depends on the nature of the terrain to be covered and the experience of the climbers. When the terrain is steep and difficult, climbers progress from pitch to pitch, with one climber climbing and the other acting as the belayer while solidly connected by anchors. When a climber falls in this type of progression we call it a standard fall. This technique is the safest but it means that the climbers progress one by one with protection points installed, so it is also slow. When the terrain is less difficult, the climbers progress simultaneously, keeping the rope taut between them. Most ascents cannot be made one climber at a time because of the time involved, and the climbers must choose between a fractioned progression, with the climbers switching between being leader and second, a technique which offers greater security, and simultaneous progression, which is much faster. Mountaineering clubs (e.g. Swiss

Alpine Club, Course No. 5660, Summer training, www.sac-cas.ch) specifically teach the technique of simultaneous progression. Paradoxically, most accidents occur on fairly easy terrains. Between 1993 and 2009, 492 climbers died in the Swiss Alps, with 139 deaths related to simul-climbing progression, or 28 per cent of the cases (Mosimann, 2009; Boutroy, et al. 2014). Experts also are at risk of this type of accident, as indicated by the statistics of the organization of professional French mountain guides (SNGM). Following numerous accidents during simul-climbing progression, the Safety Commission of the German Alpine Club conducted several studies (Schubert, 1986, 2012; Braun-Elwert, 2008) that showed that the lead climber could be pulled backward by the fall of the second climber when the tension on the rope exceeded 40 kg. These studies, however, only considered ascents without the placement of intermediate protection points, which was a particular case of the problem.

We present here the findings from a series of studies on simul-climbing progression including intermediate protection points. The dynamic behaviour of the various pieces of equipment during a climber's fall has already been investigated. Pavier (1998) developed a theoretical simulation of a climber fall based on a visco-elastic model of the rope. He performed experimental testing with different fall factors to establish the number of falls to failure. These data were used to derive a failure curve for the rope that may be combined with the theoretical simulation to predict the number of falls to failure.

Bedogni (2002) established a mathematical model in belaying techniques. The model describes the fall of a climber with a single anchor and different belaying techniques: harness connected brake and wall connected brake. In the model the rope is considered very simply as a spring having a constant characteristic based on the elasticity modulus and the length of the rope portion between two anchors. The brake is modelled as a force multiplier and assumed to be constant for a given rope and given braking device. Bedogni's model used the classical motion equations solved by Taylor forward finite differences. A comparison with the experimental data has been performed with a good correlation between experimental and simulated data. This mathematical model is efficient to compare different belaying techniques such as the difference of masses between belayer and leader, the fall height, different ropes stiffness and so on. Bedogni and Zanantoni (2005) have specified the Bedogni's model; they worked on the major role of the belayer and more particularly his hand/arm. They identified two phases in the hand/arm action: an inertial phase and a muscular phase. They added those considerations to the model and compared fix point belay, body belay and different braking devices. Again, the comparison with the experimental data gave a good correlation between experimental and simulated data. They established the advantages and disadvantages of different belay techniques.

However, an overall rope model (able to describe the behaviour to the yarn level) remains to be developed. The problem is very complex, considering that a rope is composed of 6,000 nylon yarns, with a kern mantel construction type consisting of a twisted nylon kern and a nylon mantel to protect the kern. It follows that all mathematical models need experimental measures to characterise each rope. The most detailed study to simulate rope behaviour during a climber fall was provided by Bedogni and Manes (2011). Their study proposes a model to describe the rope behaviour when stretched, representing the force as a function of strain and strain rate. Model parameters have been calibrated on experimental data measured from a specific mountaineering commercial rope. Jauffres et al. (2003) built a model slightly different from Bedogni's with a nonlinear model of the rope. The model includes several anchors creating friction. The model was validated with comparison with experimental data on the Petzl Company's drop tower. Jauffres et al. (2003) attempted to establish a standard (UIAA EN) for the braking capacities of braking devices, but despite their efforts the standard never happened. Dürrbeck et al. (2008) studied factor two falls on different belays with different braking devices. In an overhanging climbing wall, they dropped 80 kg tires to simulate a climber fall. They placed a dynamometer on each anchor of the belay and compared different constructions, including the failure of an anchor. Dürrbeck et al. (2008) highlighted the advantages and disadvantages of the different types of belays. Bedogni et al. (2011) studied load repartition on the anchors of different types of belays and different belaying techniques. A failure of one of the anchor points was analysed as well. The authors used a three dimensional (3D) dynamometer in order to avoid the inertia of the cells during the vertex swinging. Bedogni et al. (2011) compared the experimental data with the mathematical model (Bedogni, 2002) with a good correlation between experimental and simulated data. The authors concluded that a mobile connection generates lower loads on the anchor points but when an anchor fails and a belayer is hanging, the load on the remaining anchor point is higher with a mobile connection. Charlet and Meyer (2002) were interested in the effects of energy absorbers. Energy absorbers are used with dubious protection points when climbing ice or rock. The energy absorber reduces the impact force on protection in a fall: the absorber begins to deploy at 2.5 kN. Charlet and Meyer (2002) concluded that the absorber may work on small falls but require more stitches for big falls. The energy absorber increases the drop height and should be placed carefully if there is ledge below the anchor.

Based on field tests these studies described and built a numerical simulation of a standard fall but simul-climbing progression has never been studied. The previous mathematical models cannot be used in our case because the fall involves the two climbers at the same time. Before experimentation, we imagined that the leader, pulled by the second climber would crash on the anchor: it has never happened. Experimental studies must be performed. Our findings result in (1) recommendations for types of ascent based on the terrain and (2) a better definition of the conditions for choosing simul-climbing progression.

We studied several types of simul-climbing progression. We focused on simul-climbing progression on an ice field with intermediate anchor points placed between the climbers, which cause big problems for climber safety. Although the leader's fall has been already studied, it corresponds to a standard fall; the fall becomes more complicated when the second climber's fall causes the leader to fall. Several such cases have occurred during ice wall ascents: the ice screws, installed during the pitch by the climber, were ripped out, causing the climbers to become unclipped. Ropes and ice screws are considered personal protective equipment (PPE) and come under EN 892 and UIAA 101, and EN 568 and UIAA 151 standards, respectively, and should not pull out with conventional use. One hypothesis is that the leader, pulled backward by the second's fall, hits the screw and, without sufficient rope elasticity, the force of the impact generated on the screw is assumed to be extremely high. Other possibilities can be envisaged: the force is exerted on a rope under tension; in this case, its elasticity is reduced and the force exerted on the anchor is significantly increased. However, these explanations remain theoretical, as no experimental measure has ever been taken during this type of fall. Measures in real-life situations are very difficult to obtain. In order to simulate this type of fall, we need to let two masses of 80 kg fall simultaneously in the ice field. In order to have reproducible falls, we choose to replace human body by rigid masses. A body never falls in the same way, which makes it difficult to compare falls. We did the study in an ice field, where we found the best conditions for reproducible falls: the rigid masses slide on the ice and friction strengths are very low, which is very different from rock. We found a very good laboratory near the summit of Pointe Lachenal, (6°53'41"E 45°51'53"N) at an elevation of 3613 metres: a 45° ice field 120 metres high. A high-speed camera tracked the interactions between the rope, the carabiners and the anchor points, including the double circulation of the rope (i.e. circulation of the rope in the two directions), the whip-like response of the rope when the fall was stopped, and vibratory phenomena on the carabiners. The observation with the high-speed camera of simultaneous falls of two dummies was a key element that provided insight into the mechanisms that are operating and the potential causes for a failure in the safety chain. Climbing equipment is designed and standardized for a specific use. Climbing ropes are developed to absorb the energy from the worst fall of a climber – but only of one climber. When a climb becomes difficult, one climber progresses while another belays the first climber while being solidly attached to a belay point. The potential energy of a climber's fall is thus at most two times that of the climber's distance above the belay point. If he is the height of the climber above the belay point, he can fall at most 2*h; the energy of the fall is m*g*2*h and this fall is called a factor two. This is the worst climbing fall that can happen, and the ropes are designed so that the lead climber is not injured in a fall of this type (shock force less than 12 kN during the first fall, imposed by the EN 892 and UIAA 101 standard). For many reasons, climbers sometimes use their equipment in ways that no one had in mind when the equipment was designed. To save time, they can progress simultaneously and thus can fall at the same time if the second climber falls, pulling the lead climber backward. In this case, the energy released is: 2*m*g*h, with m as the mass (kg) and h as the height (m), which is the same as in the classic fall: a fall of 2*m from a height of h, whereas in the case of factor two, falls of 2*h (Figure 18.1).

To avoid the situation of the second climber's fall causing the leader to fall, mountaineers often use ascenders (Tibloc™ or Micro Traxion™ from Petzl, Ropeman™ from Wild Country). These ascenders were designed for ascending a rope and not for catching a fall. Is the fall of the second climber stopped by this type of product? Does the leader feel tension? Is the rope damaged?

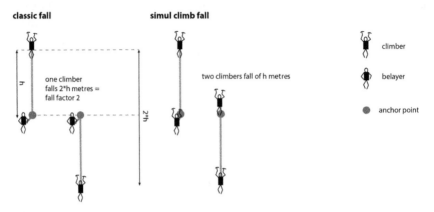

Figure 18.1 Fall factors during normal and simul-climbing falls

In the second part of the chapter, we also investigated crevasse falls. We focused on a second type of progression: the case of two climbers roped together and progressing simultaneously over a glacier. We measured the force transmitted by the rope on the climber arresting the fall as a function of the rope distance between the climbers and the presence or absence of friction knots in the rope.

For all our tests we use a chain of three synchronized one dimensional (1D) dynamometers (SRT©, Grenoble, France), with a sample frequency of 241.61 Hz. We registered 6.2 seconds, also known as 1498 points.

Falls with protection points

The standard fall

The objective was to measure the force on the ice anchor when the lead dummy fell and to compare the finding with those of simultaneously falling dummies. We thus made an 80 kg dummy fall on the same ice slope and under the same conditions as follows: the dummy was connected to a belay point by a 30 m dynamic rope (Figure 18.2). The belay point was equipped with a dynamometer and placed 25 m below. The anchor (a huge v-thread) was 5 m below the climbing protection point. An operator released the lead dummy.

In the prior configuration and without taking the rope length into account, the potential energy of the system was $2*m*g*25*\sin(45)$ (two masses falling from a $25*\sin(45)$ height in metres). In this configuration of a classic fall, the potential energy was the same because a single mass was falling but from a $2*25*\frac{\sqrt{2}}{2}$ height in metres. The forces measured on the anchor should thus have been comparable, but the force measured on the anchor point during the classic fall was 29 per cent less than that during the simultaneous fall. The juxtaposition of the arresting forces of the two masses thus created a dynamic that has yet to be explored. In the case

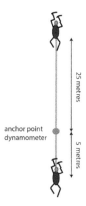

Figure 18.2 Configuration of the simul-climb tests

where the rope was attached to a belay and only the lead dummy fell, the rope's elasticity caused it to slide in the carabiner and part of the energy was absorbed by this rope/carabiner friction. In the case of the two dummies falling, the falls were arrested simultaneously, with no movement (or almost none) of the rope through the carabiner. This difference in friction partly explains the difference in force measured on the climbing protection point.

A fall causing the leader's fall

In a simulation of the simul-climbing progression of two climbers, we measured the force on the protection point when the fall of the second caused the fall of the leader. On an ice slope with an average angle of 45°, two 80 kg dummies were roped together with a 30 m climbing rope in a simul-climbing progression with a figure-eight knot. A dynamometer was embedded in the belay point 25 m below the lead dummy. The second dummy was released using a remote system and located 5 m below the belay (Figure 18.3). We have studied the worst fall that may happen: only one anchor point between the two climbers. If we placed more anchors the leader fall is smaller and the energy generated by the falls well below.

The lead dummy was held in position by a fusible cord that breaks under a tension of 850 N. The release of the second dummy caused the release of the lead dummy. Four rope models were used: the Beal Ice Line 8.1 mm (tested as a single rope), the Beal Joker 9.1 mm (tested as single), the Beal Diablo 9.8 mm (tested as single) and the Beal Ice Twin 7.7 mm (tested as a double rope). All knots were tightened to 800 N in the National School of Skiing and Mountaineering (ENSA) laboratory. To ensure the reproducibility of our tests and compare as objectively as possible the different types of rope, we used rigid 80 kg dummies. A human body of the same weight generates about 30 per cent less force because it becomes deformed during a fall and is connected to a harness (Gagneux 2010).

Figure 18.4 shows the forces measured on the anchor point (in Newtons) versus time (in seconds). We conducted a series of two tests. For each rope, Figure 18.4

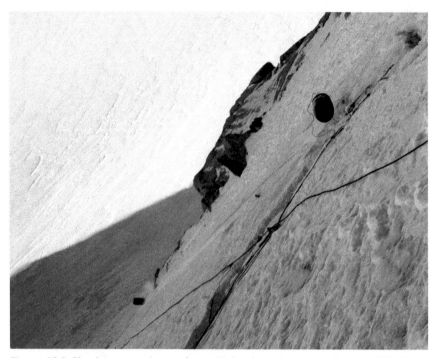

Figure 18.3 Simultaneous release of two 80 kg dummies to simulate the fall of two climbers on the north face of Pointe Lachenal

shows the highest strength obtained through all the trials. A part of the energy of falling is absorbed by the deformation of the rope on the anchor. During our tests, the rope that transmitted the lowest force on the anchor during the fall was the Ice Line (Table 18.1 and Figure 18.4).

The protection points were ice screws (we used screws with a length of 0.21 m and 0.17 m). None of the ice screws broke or was pulled out. Three screws became twisted during tests with the Joker and Diablo ropes for loads greater than 9000 N. The standard (EN 568) for a screw is 10000 N, but the ice screws on the market today are much more resistant (the ones we used were 15000 N). The ice screws were placed into smooth high-quality ice, which is not necessarily always

Table 18.1 Maximal force generated on the protection point by the simultaneous falls of the second and the leader, depending on the type of rope

Rope	Max force (Newton)
Ice Line	8600
Ice Twin (2 strands)	9720
Joker	9300
Diablo	10650

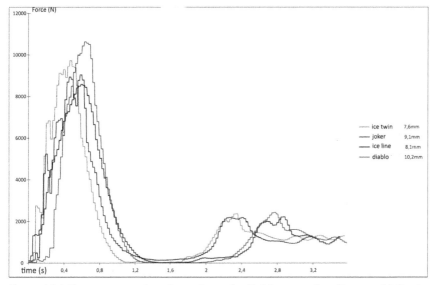

Figure 18.4 Forces measured on the anchor point (in N) versus time (in seconds) for the following types of rope – single, double and twin

possible to do. The risk was that they would be ripped out under the forces that we measured. Depending on the quality of the protection point, having a rope that generates the lowest force possible can be vital for the climber. These tests were filmed with a high-speed video camera (Vision Research Phantom Miro M120); the speed was 400 frames per second. The images show that the rope displayed complex movements (loops, spins, figure-eights) around the carabiner (Figure 18.5). The rope was slack for the duration of the fall. For the first tests, we chose to use a locking carabiner. During one of the tests, the rope loosened the security screw lock on the carabiner, and it seems possible that with such movements the rope could cause the gate to open and slip out (Figure 18.6).

We observed no 'crashes' of the lead dummy into the anchor (for guiding the rope). On the videos, it was clear that when the second dummy pulled on the lead, the second slowed down and the lead dummy greatly accelerated; for this reason, it always fell lower than the anchor point. Indeed, because the lead dummy's speed was greater than that of the second dummy and the slope was just about constant, the lead covered more distance in the same amount of time and thus came to a stop below the climbing protection point. The fall of the lead dummy was extremely violent. The percussions during rebounds on the ice slope or any obstacle (e.g. rock) can cause serious injury to the lead climber. To reduce the speed, the climber can lower the fall height by placing more protection points.

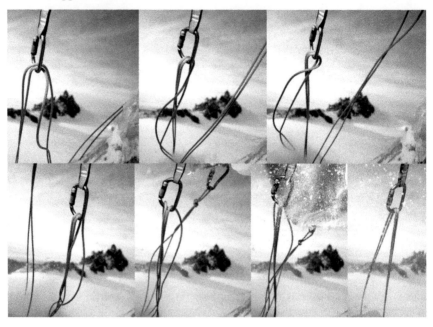

Figure 18.5 Screenshots from the high-speed film: movements of the Ice twin rope with both ropes running through the carabiner

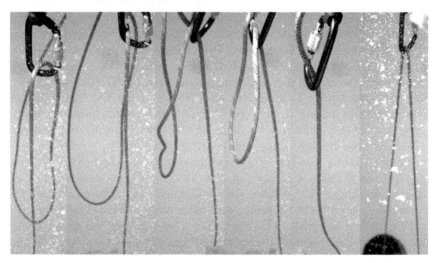

Figure 18.6 Screenshots from the high-speed film: movements of the Ice Line rope during a simul-climbing fall; the rope opened the screw

Second climber's fall during simul-climbing progression with mechanical ascender on the protection point

We measured the forces exerted on the climbing protection point and the lead climber when the second climber fell with an ascension mechanism on the anchor.

Table 18.2 Maximum force measured on the climbing protection during the fall of the second on the self-blocking pulley. We did three trials and the result is the average, the standard deviation was less than 5 per cent

Rope and ascender	Force (Newton)
Ice Line and Tibloc™	1850
Ice Line and Micro Traxion™	1860

Would the rope pull on the leader hard enough to cause a fall? Would the mechanical ascender damage the rope? The protocol was similar to that explained in the previous section; the second dummy was released using a remote system: (1) with the Tibloc™ ascender. The Tibloc™ was placed on the carabiner at the bottom of the quickdraw. The falls were made with 40 m of slack. (2) With the Micro Traxion™ for self-belay. The Micro Traxion™ was placed on the carabiner at the bottom of the quickdraw. The falls were made with 40 cm of slack. The forces on the anchor point at the ascender were low (Table 18.2). The rope sheath was not damaged and the ascender created no additional tension on the lead climber. If a second climber is likely to fall, positioning an ascender on the anchor is recommended.

Lead climber's fall during simul-climbing progression with a mechanical ascender on the belay point

In this study, our goal was to measure the force on the climbing protection point when the leader falls with an ascender system on the anchor point and to determine whether the rope was damaged. On ice with an average 45° slope, two 80 kg dummies were connected by a 30 m dynamic rope. A protection point fitted with a mechanical ascender (Tibloc™ or Micro Traxion™) was placed 15 m from the two dummies. A dynamometer was installed on the climbing protection point. The second dummy was placed on a small ledge and the lead dummy was released. The dummies were not in the same vertical axis.

Our results indicated that neither the Tibloc™ nor the Micro Traxion™ damaged the rope. In the test with the Micro Traxion™, the lead dummy came back higher and faster toward the belay than with the Tibloc™ due to the pulley system, which limited the friction. The impact force on the climbing protection point was relatively low because the second dummy rose back up once the lead dummy stopped falling.

Because small falls are better than long falls, the Tibloc™ was better than the Micro Traxion™ (with the latter's pulley system, the second dummy rose and hit the climbing protection point, and the pulley of the Micro Traxion™ increases the fall height; with the Tibloc™ the friction on the carabiner slows down and reduces the fall).

During the testing presented previously, configured with the Tibloc™ and the Ice Line rope, and with the two dummies in the same vertical axis, the lead dummy collided with the second dummy that was hanging on the Tibloc™ and the rope broke. This observation highlighted a scenario that we had not imagined

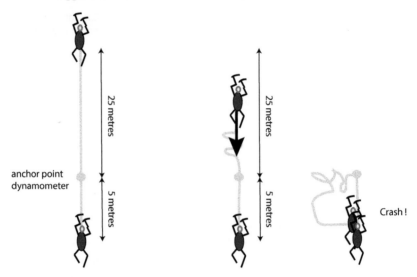

Figure 18.7 Leader fall with the second climber held by a Tibloc™

and that is dangerous for roped-in climbers: the lead climber's fall is arrested by the second, himself stuck on the Tibloc™. We placed a 1D dynamometer (with a sample frequency of 241.61 Hz; SRT©, Grenoble, France) on the anchor and we recorded a force of 4000 N on the anchor before the rope broke at the level of the Tibloc™ with a force far lower than the resistance of this type of rope.

If the leader has just crashed down into the second, the ascender stops this last fall. In this configuration, the fall factor may greatly exceed 2: in the case of Figure 18.7, the fall was 30 m with 5 m of rope – for a factor of 6! When the rope is stopped because it is crushed by the ascender teeth, obviously it breaks.

Given the findings of the tests reported previously, this system can be used for simul-climbing progression on snow/ice terrains with a slope of about 45/55°. Nevertheless, this type of ascent carries the risk of a collision between the leader and second, so we recommend arranging the protection points in a zigzag pattern to avoid the climbers colliding.

In general, given the forces generated on the anchor point and the violence of the leader's fall, simul-climbing progression cannot be recommended. It can be considered when the second's risk of falling is low, and if the risk of the leader and second colliding is limited. The forces generated on one anchor point are the lowest if double ropes are used to alternately carabinerize the two strands. If there is concern about the second falling, a mechanical ascender on the anchor should be considered, as long as there is no risk of collision between the two climbers. To avoid the risk of collision, we recommend placing an anchor before each difficult section and anchor with a mechanical ascender after each difficult section.

Crevasse falls

In glacier climbing, climbers progress with a simul-climbing progression of a distance of at least 12 m without carrying extra coils in order to limit the consequences of a crevasse fall. As it is always difficult to stop a crevasse fall, we asked the following questions:

- Do friction knots on the rope lower the force generated on the climber?
- Does the rope distance between the climbers affect the forces generated on the climber?

To answer these questions, we conducted many tests in a crevasse near the Gros Rognon at the Col du Midi. We made a rigid 80 kg dummy fall into a crevasse repeatedly while connected by different ropes to an anchor equipped with a 1D dynamometer (with a sample frequency of 241.61 Hz; SRT©, Grenoble, France) (Figure 18.8). We tested different dynamic ropes and then the tests were repeated with knots on the rope.

The ropes used for testing were as follows:

- Twin and double ropes: Beal Gully 7.3 mm
- Twin rope: Beal Ice Twin 7.7 mm
- Double rope: Beal Ice Line 8.1 mm
- Multi-standard rope (double, single and twin): Beal Joker 9.1 mm

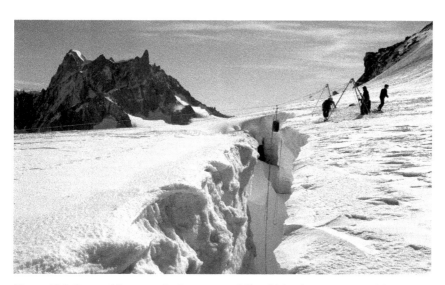

Figure 18.8 Repeatable protocol of a crevasse fall: a 80 kg dummy was positioned over the crevasse on a fixed rope resting on a tripod

What was the impact of the friction knots?

A crevasse fall is hard to catch, which we have observed in many real-life training sessions and have verified with measurements. Mountaineers tie auto-blocking knots in the rope to make it easier to stop a fall, and we measured the impact of these knots.

When a crevasse fall is being arrested, the arresting climber slides over the snow. To simulate this displacement, we devised a braking system that reproducibly slides at a force of 800 N. The system was a hoist that slides at a mean tension of 750 N (variations from 700 to 800 N). Our objective was to measure the force generated during a crevasse fall under two conditions: with friction knots in the rope and with no knots, and with different types of rope (attached or double rope).

We developed a knot with good characteristics: only a small drop in the rope resistance and high volume relative to its length. The knot design is described by Batoux (2014). On a snowy and gently sloping glacier, a dummy was suspended above the crevasse using a release system on a rope attached to a tripod. A braking system with a 1D dynamometer (with a sample frequency of 241.61 Hz; SRT©, Grenoble, France) was installed to ensure braking over a distance of 3.5 m and then a catch on the dead-man (Figure 18.9).

Each test was filmed in order to determine how far the knots penetrated into the snow. The knots were figure-eights pre-tied to 800 N in the laboratory. The first knot was placed 3 m from the dummy, then two other knots were placed every 2 m. We conducted three falls with a 12 m Ice Line rope, three falls with a 12 m

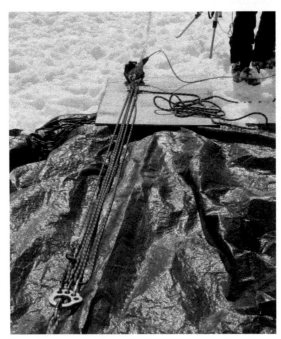

Figure 18.9 The braking system: the rope slides through the pulleys at a mean tension of 75 daN to simulate a climber holidng a crevasse fall

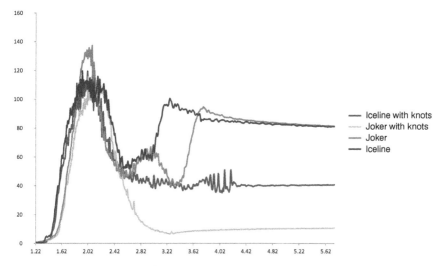

Figure 18.10 Comparison of the force transmitted to the rescuer during a crevasse fall with a double rope (Beal, Ice Line and Ice Twin) and a single rope (Beal Joker and Diablo) with and without friction knots

Ice Line rope with friction knots placed every 2 m, three falls with a 12 m Joker rope, and three falls with a 12 m Joker rope with friction knots placed every 2 m. We used new rope for each fall. The curves shown in Figure 18.10 are averages of the curves obtained at each test. The snowpack has many different layers of snow and ice crusts, and those layers are not regular. Although we made the tests in the same area, variations of the snowpack generated variations on the braking effect of the knots.

Our results indicated that with the single rope, the knots reduced the maximum force generated on the rescuer from 1380 to 1100 N, a 20 per cent reduction. At the end of the fall, the tension on the rope without knots was 800 N but it was only 100 N on the rope with knots, a reduction of 87.5 per cent. It became zero when the braking system was disengaged. This means that the rescuer had no tension when setting up the hauling mechanism. With the double rope, the knots had no impact on the maximum force generated on the rescuer. Conversely, the tension decreased significantly more rapidly with the knotted rope. At the end of the fall, the tension on the rope without knots was 800 N, whereas it was only 400 N on the rope with knots, a 50 per cent reduction. In this configuration, at the arrest of the fall in each test, the knot nearest the dummy came out of the snow. It therefore does not seem worthwhile making knots any closer to the climber who is falling. These results demonstrate the effectiveness of friction knots. As expected, the knots were far more effective on the thickest rope. It should be kept in mind that during tests in a cold and inconsistent snow (like powder) performed previously the knots had no impact. The current measurements were carried out in dense snow.

In conclusion, stopping a crevasse fall is difficult, and it is even more so when the climbers have no crampons or are progressing with snowshoes or touring skis. The difficulty is further compounded when the climber who has fallen is much heavier than the rescuer. In dense or/and wet snow, knots help considerably in stopping a crevasse fall. We recommend the use of friction knots, especially if the weight difference between climbers is significant. As soon as the friction knots are tied, it is important to rope in an N configuration (i.e. two thirds of the rope length stored in the backpacks) (Batoux, 2014) so that a strand of rope without knots can be thrown to the victim. Using a hauling system on a rope with knots will be ineffective.

Effect of the rope length

In this study, we assessed the impact of the rope distance between climbers when one falls into a crevasse. According to the theory of fall factors, the force on the belayer required to stop the fall should decrease with greater distances. But is this the case? Is there an optimal distance?

On a snow-covered glacier with a slight slope, a dummy was suspended above a crevasse by a trigger-release mechanism on a rope attached to a tripod (Figure 18.8). A 1D dynamometer (with a sample frequency of 241.61 Hz; SRT©, Grenoble, France) was installed on the dead-men. To increase reproducibility, figure-eight knots for attaching the dummy and the dynamometer were tied in at 800 N in the laboratory. We used a Beal double-strand Gully cord 7.3 mm. We did three falls (with new rope for each fall) with rope distances between dummies of 4, 7, 10, 13, 16, 19 and 21 m (Figure 18.11). The curve is the average of the maximum of each distance. We did three falls for each distance with new rope at each trial. The standard deviation was low for each length, less than 5 per cent.

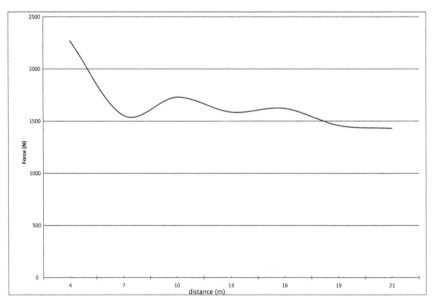

Figure 18.11 Force generated on the rope depending on the rope distance between the climbers

Given that the fall height was constant, we assumed that by increasing the rope length and thus lowering the fall factor, the force on the rescuer would drop as the distance became longer. The strength decreased between 4 and 7 m and then increased up to 10 m, decreased to 13 m and then increased again up to 16 m and finally decreased. The EN 892 and UIAA 101 standards for dynamic single ropes impose a 800 N length below 10 per cnet. To obtain the lowest possible impact force, the ropes are close to this limit. With a 16 m space between climbers, the fall height increased by 0.9 m from a tie-in at 7 m. Theoretically, the force on the rescuer should decrease in strict relation to a decrease in the fall factor. Yet we found that although the force decreased between 4 and 21 m, it increased between 7 and 10 m. This anomaly is difficult to understand. The fall was easier to arrest with a 7 m distance between climbers than 10 m or 16 m. It again became easier to arrest with a distance of 19 or 21 m.

We assume a kind of resonance in the rope/snow/victim system. We have tested only one rope, so are these characteristics unique to the Gully rope? These variations were not predicted by the theory by which the fall factor for a constant fall height suggests a strict decrease in the force on the rescuer when the roping distance increases. But this theory holds in 'laboratory conditions'; in our case, the rope goes through the snowpack, with many different layers of snow and ice crusts. When the rope is stretched, its diameter decreases, which will have an effect on its behaviour in the snowpack. A study with other types of ropes and more measures will be needed to better understand these phenomena. Without knowing the characteristics of each rope, the longest distance is the one recommended.

In conclusion, short rope distances (5 m or less) should be avoided for glacier travel because the forces generated make it impossible to stop a crevasse fall. With the Gully rope, the longest distance between climbers seems to be the best for arresting a fall.

Using rope with a mechanical ascender

Many climbers use a mechanical ascender to save time and adjust the rope distance more easily without having to untie their rope. We wanted to determine whether it would be safe to use a mechanical ascender like the Ropeman™ (Wild Country), Tibloc™ (Petzl), Micro Traxion™ (Petzl) or Duck (Cong) for glacier travel. Would the rope be damaged during a crevasse fall? On a snow-covered glacier on sloping terrain, a dummy was suspended above the crevice by a trigger-release system on a rope attached to a tripod. The tripod was connected to an 8.1 mm double rope and a 7.6 mm twin rope fixed by an ascender to a dead-man with a dynamometer. We used the high-speed video camera to film the rope in the ascender to see whether there was slippage. We provoked three falls with a Joker rope run through to a Ropeman™ at 12 m, using a new rope for each test, three falls with an Ice Twin rope run through a Tibloc™ at 12 m, three with an Ice Line rope run through a Micro Traxion™ at 12 m, and three falls with a Joker rope run through a Duck at 12 m. To film, we positioned the ascenders on the surface and not on the falling dummy.

We placed three synchronized 1D dynamometers (with a sample frequency of 241.61 Hz; SRT©, Grenoble, France) on each extremity of the rope between the falling dummy and the rescuer. The force generated on the falling dummy was 20 per cent greater than on the rescue dummy. If we had fixed the ascenders on the falling dummies, the findings would have been worse.

Our results indicated that using a mechanical ascender had no influence on the forces involved. The ropes did not slide in the cams during falls. Given the forces generated by crevasse falls, there is no risk of the rope breaking. In all cases, the ropes were crushed by the cams. Using a spiked ascender, the rope sheath was pierced by the spikes. In conclusion, given the damage to the ropes, we discourage the use of mechanical ascenders for tying in.

Roping on a cordelette and self-locking knots

We performed factor one falls in the ENSA laboratory with self-locking knots. We dropped an 80 kg guided rigid mass tied with different locking knots. We did the test in the configuration of the worst possible fall in a crevasse: in a factor one fall, the mass fell 3 m. The greater the difference in the diameter between the rope and the cordelette, the more effective the knots were in terms of low slipping on the rope.

Some of the knots slid systematically: Machard (Batoux, 2014). Some knots get stuck after a fall: Prussik (Batoux, 2014). Some slid in certain conditions, especially if the difference in diameter between the rope and the cordelette was small (less than 2 mm): the braided Machard. (Tying on with French knots and braided Machard knots did not damage the rope; the rope slippage in the knot was negligible, and the rope underwent no damage from being crushed or from friction burn.)

In conclusion, using auto-blocking knots like the braided Machard or the French knot is possible and is even recommended for the middle person of a team of three. It is important to tighten the knots and check them during the climb. If the difference in diameter between the rope and the cordelette is less than 2 mm, the French knot is recommended.

Summary and practical applications

Our field tests provided data that was at times at odds with the theoretical models. We were able to recommend the following practices. When progressing on a snowy and icy slope, we suggest the following if alternating progression is not suitable:

- simultaneous progression, placing protection points and ensuring that there are always at least two between the climbers.
- the use of ascenders on the belay points, making sure to place them in such a way as to avoid a collision between the leader and second in case the leader falls.

For glacier travel, we recommend:

- friction knots on the rope to facilitate crevasse fall arrest, especially if the weight difference between the two climbers is high, or snowshoes or cross-country skis are being used.
- putting the rope with the friction knots into an N configuration in case a hauling system needs to be installed.
- keeping the longest distance between climbers, as the N configuration remains possible with friction knots. Using auto-blocking knots like the braided Machard or the French knot is possible for tying and is even recommended for the middle person of a team of three.

Acknowledgments

These studies were conducted by ENSA with funding from the French Ministry of Sports and the National Institute of Sport, Expertise and Performance (INSEP), research and development convention No. 12-R-34. I thank our partners: the National Center of Ski and Mountaineering Instruction of the Gendarmerie (CNISAG) (Frédéric Amardeil, Vincent François, Cyril Gravier, Jean Nicolas Louis, Sébastien Lucéna, Sébastien Thomas and Blaise Agresti), the French Mountaineering and Climbing Federation (FFME) (Nicolas Bonnet and Gaël Bouquet des Chaux), the French Civil Security (Florent Dubar, Patrice Fauvel, Richard Peyre and Michel Pierre), the Air Transport Gendarmerie, the National Training Center for Ski and Mountaineering (CNEAS) (Yoann Haberey, Philippe Tamburini and Nicolas Thiebault), and the following mountain equipment manufacturers: Béal, Petzl and Simond. I also thank the National School of Skiing and Mountaineering (ENSA), especially, Valérie Aumage, Jean Franck Charlet, Gérard Descorps, Michel Fauquet, Paul Robach, Bruno Sourzac and Jean Sébastien Knoertzer. I also thank the National School of Skiing and Mountaineering (ENSA), especially, Valérie Aumage, Neil Brodie, Jean Franck Charlet, Gérard Descorps, Michel Fauquet, Paul Robach, Bruno Sourzac and Jean Sébastien Knoertzer.

References

Batoux, P. (2014). *Utilisation de la corde en alpinisme*. Internal publication of National School of Skiing and Mountaineering (ENSA), Chamonix, France.
Bedogni, V. (2002). *Computer mathematical model in belaying technique*. CAI-CMT, Turin, Italy.
Bedogni, V., Bressan, G., Melchiorri, C., & Zanantoni, C. (2011). *Stance load equalization*. CAI-CMT-UIAA. Safety Commission Meeting, Yverdon, Switzerland.
Bedogni, V., & Manes, A. (2011). A constitutive equation for the behaviour of a mountaineering rope under stretching during a climber's fall. *Procedia Engineering*, 10, 3353–3358.
Bedogni V., & Zanantoni, C. (2005). *Analysis of the belaying methods*. UIAA 3:7–11. CAI UIAA, Italy.

Boutroy, E., Corneloup, F., Lefèvre, B., Reynier, V., Roux, F., & Soulé, B. (2014). *Accidentologie des sports de montagne*. État *des lieux & diagnostic*. Fondation Petzl, Grenoble, France.

Braun-Elwert, G. (2008). *Verbunden bis in der tod*. Bergundsteigen, 2. Austrian Alpen Verein, Austria.

Charlet, J.-F., & Meyer, F. (2002). *Etude des absorbeurs d'énergie*. Report from ENSA-UIAA, Padou, France.

Dürrbeck, S., Hellberg, F., & Semmel, C. (2008). Untersuchungsbericht Standplatzuntersuchung. Deutcher Alpen Verein, Germany.

Gagneux, T. (2010). *Modélisation des chutes sur différents supports afin d'établir une corrélation entre les essais sur masses rigides et les chutes d'humains [Modelling of falls according to different supports, in order to determine a correlation between testing on rigid mass and human falls]*. Masters thesis, National School of Applied Sciences, Lyon, France.

Jauffres, D., Mahfoudh, J., Manin, L.O., & Richard, M. (2003). *Modélisation de la chute en escalade*. Masters thesis, INSA Lyon, France.

Mosimann, U. (2009). Les excursions de haute montagne sont-elles dangereuses? La problématique des accidents par entraînement. *Les Alpes*, 7, 16–19.

Pavier, M. (1998). Experimental and theoretical simulation of climbing fall. *Sports Engineering*, 1, 79–91.

Schubert, P. (1986). Ausrustung Sicherung – Sicherheit *DAV Alpin Lehrplan* 6.

Schubert, P. (2012). Sichereit und Risiko in Feld und Eis (Alpine Lehrschrift). Band 3. Ed. Deutcher Alpen Verein, 224.

Index

3:3:3 rule 227, 237, 239

Abernethy, B. 181, 193, 222
accident 74, 78, 87, 90, 238, 262–65,
   276–77, 299–300
acclimatization 76–8, 81, 95, 97–8, 100,
   102, 105
accuracy 123, 127, 164, 167, 169, 170,
   172–76, 181–2, 185–6, 192, 194, 200,
   214, 222
active recovery 19, 36, 43–5, 47, 56, 68,
   146, 205
acute mountain sickness (AMS) 76, 78–9,
   95, 97, 105–6
adaptability 181–2, 188, 190, 192, 194, 264
adaptation 19, 39, 41–2, 44, 47, 66, 70, 78,
   82, 90–1, 95, 98, 100–2, 105, 107, 119,
   129, 130, 140–1, 144–5, 148, 155, 158,
   166, 176, 181–2, 189, 192, 194, 197,
   202, 204–6, 209
Adé, D. 166, 176–7, 195, 209
adjectival system 228, 230–2, 238
aerobic 19–20, 24, 31–2, 44–7, 55, 77–8,
   91–3, 100, 102, 104, 107, 131, 136,
   143–4, 155–6, 161–2, 193, 241
affordance 177, 185, 191, 193–5, 197, 199,
   201–5, 207–9, 212–4, 220, 222–3, 242,
   251, 254–5
Allman, T.L. 260, 265
altitude hypoxia 76–81, 87, 90–5, 97,
   99–102, 104–7
Aluja, A. 250, 254
Amca, A.M. 131, 135, 143, 153
anaerobic 31–2
anthropologist 3
anthropometry 50–2, 56, 115, 243
anxiety 40, 45, 194–5, 202, 208–10, 217,
   220–223, 240–1, 244, 250–2, 254–5, 263
Armatas, C. 249, 254

arthritis 65–6, 72–3
attention 181, 194, 201–2, 220–1, 245,
   262–3
attunement 185–6
Aubel, O. 10, 15

Bakker, F.C. 184–5, 187, 193–5, 202,
   208–9, 214, 220, 222–3, 246, 251,
   254–5
Baláš, J. 20–2, 24–5, 27, 30, 40, 45, 115,
   118, 127, 148–9, 151–5, 159–61,
   235–6, 239, 271–2, 280
Bandura, A. 249–50, 252, 254
Batoux, P. 182, 193, 296, 298–9
Bayer, T. 64, 67, 72
Bedogni, V. 283–4, 299
Benesch scale 228
Bennett, G. 197, 199, 208, 211, 222, 258,
   265
bent–arm hang 147, 159–60
Bertuzzi, R.C. 19–20, 22, 25, 27, 30–2,
   34–5, 39, 41–2, 45–6, 49, 56, 234,
   240
Billat, V. 21–2, 28, 36, 45, 53, 55, 114,
   128, 132, 143, 151, 161, 184, 193
Biomechanics 56, 73–5, 109, 111, 119,
   124, 128, 144–6, 150, 163–4, 176–7,
   195, 209, 239, 241–2, 244, 256,
   280–1
blisters 83, 85
blood lactate 31–9, 42–4, 46–9, 132, 146,
   251
body: balance 111–2, 129, 136; equilibrium 112, 117, 119, 127–8, 166–7,
   191; weight 117–9
Bollen, S.R. 60, 65, 72, 129, 133–4,
   140–1, 143–4, 148, 155–6, 161
Booth, J. 20, 22, 24, 29, 31–2, 36, 45, 49,
   55, 132, 143

Borghi, A.M. 209, 214, 223
Boschker, M.S. 184–5, 187, 193, 195, 199–201, 203, 205, 208, 214, 222, 234–5, 240, 242, 246, 254, 256
Boulanger J. 56, 186, 188, 193, 195, 205, 208–9, 242
bouldering 2, 12, 33, 37, 47, 59–60, 73, 121, 123, 127, 150–1, 158–9, 163, 182–3, 191, 196, 209, 227, 231, 240, 245, 253, 280
Brandenburg, J. 19
Brazilian scale 229, 233
British scale 230–2, 238
Brody, E.B. 250, 254
Brymer, E. 196, 208, 257–60, 265
Button, C. 181, 188, 195–7, 199, 208, 210, 218–9, 222

calibration 120, 124, 185, 214, 237
California Sierra Club 7, 230
Callosity 70–1
Cauchy, E. 76, 83, 84, 86, 89–90
centre of mass 54, 111–3, 115, 117, 123–4, 165, 187–8, 205, 274
Cereatti, L. 258–9, 266
chalk 239, 269, 276, 280, 281
Chambre, D. 12, 15–16
Chartier, R. 3, 15
climber's grip capacities: biomechanical measurements 132–4, 140–141; crimp and slope grip techniques 130–1, 133–4, 138–9; forearm muscle fatigue 136–8; hold size 135–6; individual physiological profiles 138
climber's hand muscle adaptations: finger extensor muscles 141; finger flexor muscle 141; wrist muscles 141–2
climber's internal hand forces: biomechanical modeling 138; finger pulley forces 139–40; muscle forces 138–40
climbing: artificial climbing 2, 9, 112, 114, 276; clean climbing 10; free climbing 7, 9–11, 15, 193, 208; red-point and "jaunir" 10, 20–2, 25, 27–31, 33–9, 42, 44, 51, 120, 150–1, 199, 204, 233–5, 237, 239, 253, 273
climbing speed 12, 22, 24, 29–30, 34, 47, 49–50, 181–5, 217, 270, 274,
climbing self-efficacy scale 252–4, 266
club 5–8, 16, 229–30, 240, 283
coefficient of friction 67, 75, 196, 206, 239, 241, 269–70, 273–7, 291–9
cold effect 44, 76, 82–4, 87–90, 167, 295
cold water immersion 19, 43–4

competition 6–8, 10, 12, 20, 39, 42, 44, 46, 59, 103, 143, 151, 165–6, 195, 202, 236, 242, 245, 256, 276
constraint 3, 48, 52, 76, 111, 114, 119–20, 123, 127, 135, 167, 181–3, 188–97, 202–3, 207, 209, 211, 217
contact forces: analysis 272–4; instrumentation 269–72
coordination 112, 114, 128, 131, 139, 164–6, 170, 173, 175, 177, 188–90, 193, 195, 209, 211
Cordier, P. 52–5, 184, 187, 193, 196–9, 205, 208
core temperature regulation 76–7, 82–3, 86–9, 148, 158, 165
Costa, P.T. 249, 255
Courtemanche, S. 111, 120–1, 127
culture: ascetic 9; cultural history 1–4, 12, 14–5; fun 11, 13–4; hedonism 9, 13–4, 264; urban 3, 13

Davids, K. 56, 166, 177, 181, 186–90, 193–97, 199, 203, 206, 208–11, 213, 222–3, 242
decision–making 78, 211, 217, 261
degeneracy 177, 189–95, 209
dehydration 84, 263
determinant 46, 111–2, 162, 175, 241, 246, 251–2
Diehm, R. 249, 254
disinhibition 250–1, 256, 266
dislocation 64, 67
distortion 63
Donath, L. 158
Draper, N. 21, 24, 28, 31, 34–5, 37, 39–40, 43, 45–6, 49, 56, 152, 158–9, 161–2, 184, 194, 208, 227, 229, 231–7, 239–41, 245, 254, 280
Dupuy, C. 216–9, 223, 247–9, 254
dynamometer 134, 150, 155–7, 162, 284, 286–7, 291–4, 296–8
dyspnoea 79

economy 47–55, 100, 186–7, 218, 221
Edelman, G.M. 189–90, 194
efficiency 48–9, 53–6, 78, 100–2, 115, 173, 177, 186–7, 191–2, 198–9, 205, 207–8, 218, 221–2, 241, 255
electromyography 42, 128, 132, 145, 176, 177, 209
endurance 19–20, 41–2, 44, 46–7, 80–1, 91–2, 94, 98–101, 104, 106–7, 137, 144, 146–8, 154–5, 158–62, 202, 239, 241–2, 255

endurance: finger flexor 154–8; shoulder 159
energy 19, 31–2, 39, 45–6, 48–6, 120, 143–4, 147, 161, 177, 185–7, 193, 196, 240, 247, 277, 284–8
entropy 52–6, 187, 193, 197–9, 203–4, 208, 273
environment 12–14, 77, 81–4, 90, 100, 111–2, 120, 165–7, 181, 185, 190, 192, 196–9, 202, 206–7, 210–11, 245, 255, 260–4
Ericsson, K.A. 67, 73
España-Romero, V. 20, 23–4, 32, 36, 45, 49–51, 56, 148, 162, 235, 240–1
Ewbank, J. 229
Ewbank scale 229–30, 232–3, 236–7
Ewert, A.W. 249–50, 255
exhaustion 20, 22, 32, 44–5, 87, 101, 136, 147, 155, 168, 173, 220, 241
expenditure 46, 48–56, 144, 187, 196
experience 70, 81, 165–6, 174–5, 188, 191, 199–201, 204–5, 210, 212, 217–9, 232–7, 245, 249–54, 259–65, 282
expertise 52, 119, 133, 136, 164–6, 175–6, 181–4, 190–3, 204, 208, 213, 222–3, 248, 260, 272–3, 299
exploration 181, 192–5, 205–6, 209–11, 216–7, 265
exploratory 53, 182–8, 192–3, 204–7, 210, 217–22, 254
exposure 76–80, 82, 87–94, 98–102, 105–6, 182, 228, 230, 238, 251, 257–63
extreme 4, 7, 10, 13, 51, 68–9, 73–4, 77–8, 82, 150, 167, 196, 210, 238, 245, 257–65

Fajen, B.R. 185, 194
fall: crevasse 293–9; factor 286; simul climb 286–92; standard 286
Fanchini, M. 151, 162, 236, 240–1
fast twitch (FT) 101
fatigue 32, 41, 44, 54–5, 64, 66, 78–9, 91, 101–2, 113, 115, 129–33, 136–8, 143–5, 164–7, 169, 171–3, 175, 177, 184, 196, 209–10, 220–3, 248
fingertip 60, 129–33, 135–7, 141, 143–5, 209
flexibility 91, 151, 162, 188, 241, 245, 264
fluency 52–3, 56, 166, 185, 187–8, 191, 195, 209, 221, 242
force 40, 55, 59, 64–5, 70–2, 111–33, 136–46, 150–53, 161, 163, 189, 193, 269–82, 286–93, 297–8
fracture 59, 64, 66–7, 70–3

Frauscher, F. 63, 73
free-body diagram 275
friction 67, 75, 196, 206, 239, 241, 269–70, 273–99
friction: knots 293–6; carabiner 291
frostbite 76, 83–5, 87, 89–90
Fryer, S. 20–1, 24, 27–8, 30–5, 37, 39–42, 45–6, 49–50, 53, 56, 149, 155, 157, 161–2, 184, 194, 196, 205–6, 208, 234–5, 240–1
Fuss, F. 205–6, 208, 235, 239–41, 245, 254–5, 269–81

Gibson, J. 147, 162, 185, 194, 199, 202, 208, 212, 223
Girard, O. 91, 94, 98–9, 101, 104–6
Goldenberg, B. 260, 265
grading system 7, 23, 84, 227–32, 237–40, 254, 280
Grant, S. 150, 158–9
grasp 111, 130, 175, 185, 202, 208, 219
graspability 185, 201, 205–6
grip 19, 41–4, 60–1, 63–4, 66–7, 72, 74, 114, 129, 130–41, 143–8, 151–5, 157, 159–61, 163, 173, 193, 202, 208, 256, 269, 274–5, 279–80
Grushko, A.I. 215, 223
Guevel, A. 142, 145
guidance 216–18, 251

Haake, S. 169, 176, 280–1
hammering 167, 172, 177
handgrip 43, 46–7, 144, 146, 148–9, 151–2, 160–3, 173, 177, 243
hangboard 130
Hardy, L. 202, 208, 234, 241, 251, 255
harm avoidance 259
Havelange, V. 175–6
headache 78–80
heart rate 23, 25–6, 28–9, 38–40, 44–6, 56, 76–7, 87, 97, 132, 155, 194, 208, 241, 251
heat transfer and loss of heat 82, 87, 277
heel hooking 68, 189
hemoglobin mass (Hbmass) 95, 98–100, 102–3
Henson, R. 258, 265
Hérault, R. 56, 166, 177, 187–8, 193, 195, 205, 208–9, 242
Herry, J.P. 77, 79–80, 82, 90
high altitude: cerebral oedema (HACE) 78–9; pulmonary oedema (HAPE) 78–9, 81, 87
high-intensity intermittent training (HIIT) 101
hip trajectory 53, 68–9, 123, 184, 187–8, 192, 198, 207, 217

historical 1–3, 92, 94
Hochholzer, T. 60, 64, 66, 69, 73–4, 234, 242
Hoibian, O. 1, 3, 8–9, 13, 16
hold shape 111, 135, 186, 189, 196, 205, 209, 218, 270, 273
Hutchinson, A. 202, 208, 234, 241, 251, 255
hyperbaric bag 81–2, 85
hypobaric hypoxia (HH) 91–2, 95–8, 102
hypothermia 76, 83, 86–90

ice climbing 1, 13, 74, 164–70, 173, 175–7, 181–2, 184, 186, 189–91, 192–3, 195, 209
ice tool 164–9, 172–5, 177, 182, 186
iloprost 83
immobility 167, 184–5, 188, 192, 206
impulsive 250
indirect calorimetry 48–50
indoor(s) 1–2, 13, 21, 31, 37, 40, 43, 45–7, 56, 59–60, 70, 74, 120, 124, 144–5, 163, 181–3, 185, 190–2, 195, 208–9, 212–15, 218, 223, 227, 231, 236, 240–1, 245, 252, 256, 270
injury 45, 59–60, 63–75, 83–90, 131, 143, 161, 233, 243, 245, 255–6, 262, 269, 274, 289
instrumented climbing holds 269–74
intermittent: hypoxic exposure (IHE) 92–3, 100; hypoxic training (IHT) 92, 94–5, 100–1, 103–4
International Rock Climbing Research Association (IRCRA) 73, 229, 232–3, 240, 245, 254
inverse dynamics 119, 122–3, 127–8
Issurin, V. 191, 194, 202, 208
Itagushi, Y. 170, 176

jerk 53, 56, 187, 195, 209, 242
Jones, G. 21, 28, 31, 35, 45, 49, 56, 184, 195, 206, 209, 215, 223, 234–5, 237, 240–1, 244–5, 247, 249, 251, 254–6

Kerr, J.H. 249, 255
kinematic and electromyographic evalua-tion: cocking phase 164, 169–71, 173, 175–6; limb coordination 177, 189–90, 195, 209; stretching muscles 138, 140–1, 164, 167, 172, 175, 187, 189
Klauser, A. 60, 63, 72–3
Kontos, A.P. 249, 255
Kry, P.G. 111, 120, 127, 270, 280

Laffaye, G. 159, 162, 202, 208, 236, 241
Laurendeau, J. 259, 265
Laursen, B. 170, 176
lead climbing 30–1, 39, 151, 158, 160, 191
learning 78, 179, 188, 193–9, 202–9, 223, 262
Lenay, C. 175–6
live high: train high (LHTH) 92–5, 98–9, 102–4; train low (LHTL) 92–6, 98–100, 102–4; train low and high (LHTLH) 93–4, 103–4
Llewellyn, D.J. 184, 195, 206, 209, 215, 223, 231–2, 234–5, 241–2, 245, 247, 249–52, 254–6
Loret, A. 11, 16

Magiera, A. 51, 56
Martin, B. 45, 51, 56, 112, 114, 116, 128–30, 133, 136, 144–5, 148, 161, 163, 176–7, 186, 194, 229, 234–5, 239, 242–3, 245, 255–6, 260, 265, 280
mastery 12, 181, 193, 300
maximal oxygen uptake (VO2max) 48–9, 99–102, 106
McCrae, R.R. 249, 255
McIntosh, S.E. 83, 90
McKenzie, S.H. 20, 22, 26, 47, 70, 73, 132, 145, 249, 255
McLeod, D. 42, 46, 149, 155–6, 162, 234, 241, 245–6, 255
mechanical ascender 290–2, 297–8
Michaels, C.F. 185, 187, 193, 208, 213–14, 222–3, 247, 254
Michailov, M. 20–2, 46, 148, 151, 162
Millet, G. 91–5, 98, 100–2, 104–6
Mills, W. J. 82, 87, 90
mimicking 27, 112, 136, 150
Mittlestaedt, R. 260, 265
Mohr, W. J. 87, 90
Monasterio, E. 257–9, 261, 265
mood alterations 79
Moritomo, H. 173, 177
motion capture 123, 167, 169–70, 172, 187
motivation 244, 246, 249, 254, 255, 256, 259, 261, 265–6
motor behaviour and motor learning 55, 133, 139, 144, 147–8, 176, 179, 181, 189, 192–6, 202, 205, 208–9, 211, 217, 222–3, 240–1, 244, 248, 254
mountaineering 1–9, 11–5, 59, 74, 76, 91, 154, 165, 173, 177, 181–2, 190, 210, 227–8, 242, 245, 249, 255, 257–65, 269, 276, 280–2, 284, 287, 299
Müller, S. 191, 195

muscle(s) 9, 19–20, 30, 40–3, 68–9, 101, 129–31, 135, 137–43, 145, 147–8, 155, 159, 164, 169, 170–5, 209

nausea 79
necrosis 66, 86
neurological deficit 67, 79
neuromuscular 42, 91, 133, 151, 161
Newell, K.M. 135, 144, 191, 194, 196, 199, 209
Newton law 112, 148, 161, 287–8, 291
Nieuwenhuys, A. 184, 187, 194, 217–9, 223
nitric oxide (NO) 95, 97, 105
Noé, F. 114, 117–8, 128–30, 144, 207, 234, 242, 245, 255
normobaric hypoxia (NH) 91–3, 95–8, 102, 104–6
Norris, R.M. 250, 255
Nougier, V. 116, 127, 186, 194

Oades, L. 260, 265
optical flow 176, 210, 211–4
optimization 55, 112, 119–28, 138, 167, 208
Orth, D. 56, 181, 186–7, 195–6, 203–10, 222, 242
orthopaedic 72–4, 163
Ottogali, C. 5, 16
Oudejans, R.R. 184, 194–5, 202, 209, 213, 220–1, 223, 251, 255
outdoor(s) 11, 13–14, 21, 29, 40, 50, 60, 182, 187, 191, 193, 205, 208, 211, 218, 231, 245, 252
overuse syndrome 59, 67, 70, 72, 73
oxygen consumption and uptake 19–31, 41, 44, 48–9, 77–8, 91, 99, 102, 104, 106, 162, 257–8

Pailhous, J. 52, 55, 184, 187, 193, 197, 208
Pain, M. 63–4, 67–8, 70–2, 259–60, 265
para-climbing 245
Pasquier, M. 83, 86, 90
pathology(ies) 59, 67, 68, 71, 130, 138, 144
pedagogy 206, 209
perception 177, 181, 185–6, 191–5, 197, 199, 201–11, 215, 222–3, 259, 263
perception-action coupling 199, 211, 213, 222–3
perceptual-motor 195–7, 209, 213, 215
performatory 184–6, 192, 205–6, 210, 215–22
personality 242, 249–50, 254–56, 259–61,

264–6
persuasion 250–1
Pezzulo, G. 202, 209, 214, 223
phenomenology 176, 258, 265
Philippe, M. 42, 46, 132–3, 136, 141, 144, 149, 155–6, 162, 282, 299
physical 3, 8–9, 12–13, 45–8, 55, 72, 76–81, 88, 97, 101–2, 111, 120, 127, 143, 146, 161, 163, 165, 175, 193, 199, 209, 212–14, 241–2, 245–7, 252, 258–65
physical performance 77, 97, 102
physiology 17, 19, 45–7, 56, 104–7, 130, 143–5, 162–3, 176, 208, 238–45, 255–6
physiotherapy 68
Pijpers, J.R. 184–5, 194–5, 202, 205–6, 209, 219–23, 251, 255
pitons 6, 8–10, 278
pliometric 144
Poizat, G. 166, 176–7, 195, 209
post-climb(ing) 32–3, 35–9, 42, 49–50, 238
postural control 111–12, 114, 117, 119, 124, 127–8, 184, 187–8, 196, 206–7, 269
posture(s) 111–12, 114–5, 117–8, 120, 123, 127–8, 144–5, 167, 186, 189, 211, 242, 255–6
Pouponneau, C. 174–7
power(ful) 9, 12, 49–51, 55, 92–4, 100, 104, 143–51, 158–62, 174, 199, 202, 208, 241
practice 2, 6, 8, 10, 13–14, 55, 70, 89–90, 119, 129, 141, 163–5, 181, 187–91, 194–210, 214, 218–23, 245
preparatory 216
proprioceptive 210
protection 7, 9–10, 30–1, 59, 61–2, 72–3, 76, 82, 87, 89, 141, 228, 230, 238, 257, 269, 276–8, 282–92, 298
proximo-distal 164, 170, 175
psychology 176, 193–5, 208–9, 222–5, 241, 244–5, 252–5, 261, 265–6
pulley 59–63, 68, 71–5, 129, 131, 138–40, 144–6, 150, 153, 163, 291
pulling force 54

quadruped locomotion 164–6, 191
Quaine, F. 111–17, 128–39, 144–6, 152–3, 163, 173, 177, 196–7, 202, 209, 234, 242, 245, 255–6

Raspaud, M. 7, 16
reachability 185, 201, 205–6, 213, 216
recovery 19–20, 36, 43–7, 50, 56, 68, 97, 101, 144, 146, 155, 162, 205–6
redundancy 144

refreezing 76, 85, 89
rehydration 87
relaxation 42, 264
repeated sprint training in hypoxia (RSH) 93–4, 101–4
re-oxygenation 19, 42, 44, 79, 81–2, 136, 155
repetitions and fatigue, alteration of hanging, fatigue of wrist and hand muscles 50, 52–3, 55, 101, 158, 169, 197, 216–8, 220
representation 118, 140, 181, 208
reproducibility 188, 285, 287, 294, 296
resistance training in hypoxia (RTH) 93–4, 102–4
Reveret, L. 111
rewarming 76, 83–5, 87, 89
Richalet, J.P. 76, –7, 79, 80, 82, 89–90, 93, 100, 106–7
Ripoll, H. 216–9, 223, 247–9, 254
risk 4, 9, 14, 31, 54, 60, 72–3, 76–90, 129, 138, 150, 194, 221, 241, 246–52, 255–66, 282–3, 289, 292, 298
risk-taking 254, 257–61, 264
Robert, T. 119–22, 128, 164, 169–70, 177
rope 10, 23–4, 29–31, 38–9, 44–6, 56, 64, 182, 240, 258, 269, 277–99
Rosalie, S. 191, 195
Rossi, B. 131, 144, 258–9, 266
Rouard, A. 164, 177
Rougier, P. 114, 117, 127–8
route: finding 53, 184–7, 196, 204, 207, 216, 245–9; preview 201, 214–15, 218, 221–49; visual inspection 195, 209, 214–15, 221, 223, 244, 246–9, 256
Rudestam, K. 249–50, 256, 258–59, 266

safe(ty) 13–14, 59, 76, 84, 118–19, 167, 192, 263, 267, 269, 276–7, 279–85, 297, 299
safety devices: rock protection devices 278–9; rope brakes 277–8
Sanchez, X. 56, 184, 187, 195, 205–6, 209, 214–15, 223, 231–2, 234–5, 240–2, 244–56
scale 92, 153, 182, 197, 200, 213, 218, 228–33, 238, 242, 245, 252–3, 266, 272–3
Schaal, S. 119, 128
Schmidt, R.A. 99, 105–6, 181, 195
Schöffl, V. 42, 45, 56, 59–64, 66–8, 70, 72–4, 140, 145, 148, 152, 158, 161–3, 229, 235, 240, 242, 245, 254–6
Schweitzer, R. 258, 265

Schweizer, A. 59–60, 62–8, 72–5, 131, 133–34, 139, 145, 149–50, 152, 154, 163, 234, 242, 245, 256
Seifert, L. 53, 56, 164–7, 176–7, 181–2, 184, 186–9, 191, 193, 195–6, 201, 203–6, 208–10, 222, 235–6, 240, 242
self-efficacy 244–6, 249–56, 266
self-evaluation 233, 241
sensation 249–50, 254, 256, 259, 266
sensor(s) 82, 111, 114, 119–22, 127, 132, 134, 193–4, 208, 270, 271, 280
Sheel, A. 20, 22, 26, 30, 40, 47, 132, 145, 244, 245, 256
shivering 76, 82, 87, 89
Sibella, F. 52, 56, 184–5, 187, 195
simulation 111, 120, 123–4, 127, 209, 223, 283–4, 287, 300
skill 9, 52, 56, 130, 137, 176, 182–4, 188, 190–215, 218–23, 242, 250, 254, 260, 262, 264
skin 79, 82–3, 89
Slanger, E. 249–50, 252, 256, 258–9, 266
snowy 173, 182, 294, 298
social distinction and classes 3, 9, 11, 14
sociology 265
somatic 242, 251
soft tissue problems, deep friction 67
solo(ing) 13, 182–3, 227, 230, 252, 257–8, 263
Soo, Y. 173, 177
speed 12, 20, 22, 24, 29–30, 34, 47, 49–50, 55–6, 78, 87–8, 147–8, 151, 159, 165, 176, 181–5, 192–5, 216–7, 245, 270, 274–5, 280, 289
spinal 144
sprains 59, 67, 70
stability 68, 111–12, 114, 124, 158, 175, 188–9, 191, 195, 197, 202–3, 207, 259
static 49–50, 53, 55, 111, 113, 124, 127, 130, 136, 147, 151, 164, 166, 170, 184–5, 206, 270, 275–8, 280
stationary 53, 207, 217
stiffness 144, 173, 176, 283
strength 45, 47, 55, 63, 91, 101–5, 129, 139–64, 167, 173, 192–4, 201–2, 207–9, 239–2, 245, 252, 269, 279, 288, 297
striking 166–76
subjective(ity) 61, 165–6, 174–5, 227, 231–2, 239, 251
suffering 70–1
support 24, 30–1, 42, 49–53, 89, 95, 111–18, 124, 130, 158, 166, 176–7, 181–5, 189, 193–6, 201–11, 214–16, 222, 238, 244, 251, 273

surgical interventions 67–8, 70, 74, 193
Sylvester, A.D. 65, 75

technique(s) 3, 6–8, 15, 39, 46, 56, 62,
    68, 73, 111, 123, 130–40, 143, 146,
    151, 161, 163, 177, 193–4, 201, 206,
    208, 240–1, 253–4, 260–4, 269, 277,
    282–4, 299
technology 9, 45–6, 56, 127, 161, 176,
    194–5, 208–9, 213–14, 223, 227,
    237–8, 240–1, 254–5, 267, 280–1
therapy 68, 70, 83, 163
thermoregulatory 104
Theureau, J. 174, 177
three-holds 184–5
three-point-support 114–15
thrombolytics 83
Tok, S. 249–50, 256
tope rope climbing 30–1, 39, 182, 183,
    202, 230
torque(s) 60, 66, 112–13, 119–24, 127,
    135, 141, 145, 169, 170, 173, 187,
    270
Tosi, P. 22, 29, 32, 34, 47, 49, 50, 53, 56,
    187, 195, 271, 281
training 6, 7, 11, 15, 19, 41, 43–4, 50, 55,
    63, 80–1, 89, 91–6, 99–107, 129–30,
    136–39, 141–4, 147–8, 158, 160–3,
    175, 191–203, 207–10, 223, 242,
    254–5, 259, 262–4, 273–4, 283, 294,
    299
training adaptations: forearm vasculature
    41–2
training economy 50
transfer 82, 114, 117, 127, 190–7, 202–9,
    242
trauma 64, 67, 72, 75, 83, 87
traumatology 73, 243
tying-in with mechanical ascender 297–8
tying-in with self–locking knots 298

UIAA 12, 65, 70, 154, 160, 165, 228–9,
    232–3, 242, 280, 284–5, 297, 299
use–ability 185–6

variability 106, 151, 160, 177, 194, 195,
    209, 264, 274
vasoconstriction 76, 82, 87, 89
vasodilation 82, 84, 87, 155
velocity 36, 41, 116, 133, 143, 159, 164,
    169, 173–5, 187, 211, 274
vicarious 250–1
victim(s) 84–5, 89, 296–7
Vigarello, G. 4, 16
Vigouroux, L. 129–46, 152–3, 161, 163,
    177, 189, 193, 196–7, 202, 209, 235,
    239–40, 276, 280
vision 8, 11, 211, 213, 216, 289
visual 78, 186, 194–5, 208–23, 244,
    246–9, 256

Wagman, J. 201, 209
wall–collision 69–70
Wall, C.B. 150, 158, 163
Warme, W. J. 63, 75
Warren, W.H. 188, 195
Watts, P. 22, 24, 26, 29, 32, 34, 36, 38, 40,
    42–3, 47–51, 53–4, 56, 118, 128–30,
    132, 141, 146, 148, 150–2, 163, 229,
    231, 233–4, 238–40, 243, 245, 254, 256
Welzenbach scale 7, 228
Wilk, K.E. 177
wind 82, 87–8, 89
Wolf, P. 67, 75, 207, 240, 254, 269–74,
    280–1

Yan, X. 78, 90
Yosemite Decimal system (YDS) 8, 16, 51,
    229–37

Zafren, K. 83, 87, 90
Zampagni, M 187, 195, 271, 281
Zarevski, P. 259, 266
Zhang, J. 258, 265
Zuckerman, M. 250, 256, 259, 266

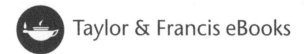

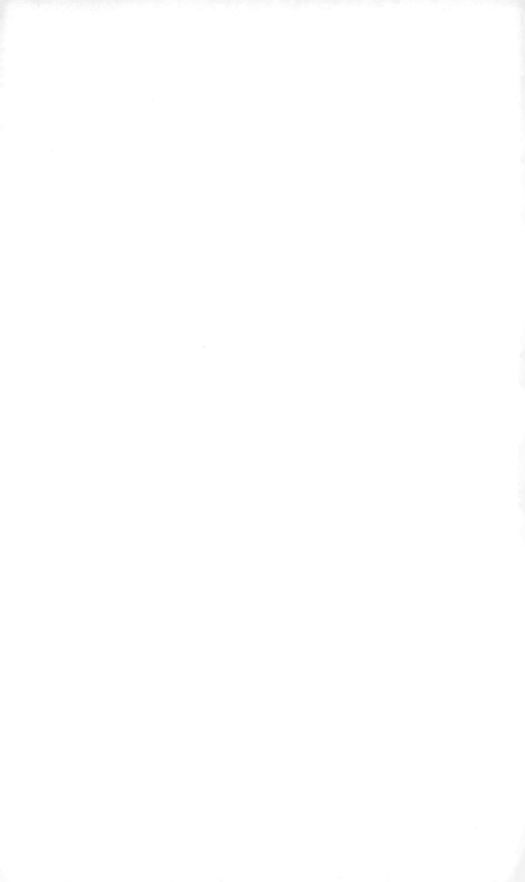

For Product Safety Concerns and Information please contact our EU
representative GPSR@taylorandfrancis.com
Taylor & Francis Verlag GmbH, Kaufingerstraße 24, 80331 München, Germany